D1482977

Head and Neck
Imaging
A Teaching File

SECOND EDITION

Anthony A. Mancuso, MD
Professor and Chairman, Department of Radiology
Professor of Otolaryngology
University of Florida, College of Medicine
Gainesville, Florida

Sharat Bidari, MD
Clinical Assistant Professor
University of Florida, College of Medicine
Gainesville, Florida

With contributions from:
Bruno Termote, MD
Department of Radiology
Jessa Ziekenhuis
Hasselt, Belgium

Berit M. Verbist, MD, PhD
Leiden University Medical Center
Leiden, The Netherlands

Reordan DeJesus, MD
Neuroradiology Fellow
Duke University Hospital
Durham, North Carolina

. Wolters Kluwer | Lippincott Williams & Wilkins
Health
Philadelphia · Baltimore · New York · London
Buenos Aires · Hong Kong · Sydney · Tokyo

Executive Editor: Charles W. Mitchell
Product Manager: Ryan Shaw
Vendor Manager: Alicia Jackson
Senior Manufacturing Manager: Benjamin Rivera
Senior Marketing Manager: Angela Panetta
Design Coordinator: Stephen Druding
Production Service: Aptara, Inc.

Printed in China

Library of Congress Cataloging-in-Publication Data

Mancuso, Anthony A.
  Head and neck imaging : a teaching file / Anthony A. Mancuso, Sharat Bidari ; with contributions from Bruno Termote ... [et al.]. – 2nd ed.
     p. ; cm.
  Rev. ed. of: Head and neck radiology / Anthony A. Mancuso. c2002.
  Includes bibliographical references and index.
  ISBN 978-1-60913-712-0 (alk. paper)
  1. Head–Imaging–Atlases. 2. Neck–Imaging–Atlases. 3. Head–Imaging–Case studies. 4. Neck–Imaging–Case studies. I. Bidari, Sharat. II. Termote, Bruno. III. Mancuso, Anthony A. Head and neck radiology. IV. Title.
  [DNLM: 1. Diagnostic Imaging–Atlases. 2. Diagnostic Imaging–Case Reports. 3. Head–Atlases. 4. Head–Case Reports. 5. Diagnosis, Differential–Atlases. 6. Diagnosis, Differential–Case Reports. 7. Head and Neck Neoplasms–diagnosis–Atlases. 8. Head and Neck Neoplasms–diagnosis–Case Reports. 9. Neck Injuries–diagnosis–Atlases. 10. Neck Injuries–diagnosis–Case Reports. 11. Stomatognathic Diseases–diagnosis–Atlases. 12. Stomatognathic Diseases–diagnosis–Case Reports. WE 17]
  RC936.M335 2012
  617.5′107572–dc23

                                                                            2011021911

Care has been taken to confirm the accuracy of the information presented and to describe generally accepted practices. However, the authors, editors, and publisher are not responsible for errors or omissions or for any consequences from application of the information in this book and make no warranty, expressed or implied, with respect to the currency, completeness, or accuracy of the contents of the publication. Application of the information in a particular situation remains the professional responsibility of the practitioner.

The authors, editors, and publisher have exerted every effort to ensure that drug selection and dosage set forth in this text are in accordance with current recommendations and practice at the time of publication. However, in view of ongoing research, changes in government regulations, and the constant flow of information relating to drug therapy and drug reactions, the reader is urged to check the package insert for each drug for any change in indications and dosage and for added warnings and precautions. This is particularly important when the recommended agent is a new or infrequently employed drug.

Some drugs and medical devices presented in the publication have Food and Drug Administration (FDA) clearance for limited use in restricted research settings. It is the responsibility of the health care provider to ascertain the FDA status of each drug or device planned for use in their clinical practice.

To purchase additional copies of this book, call our customer service department at (800) 638-3030 or fax orders to (301) 223-2320. International customers should call (301) 223-2300.

Visit Lippincott Williams & Wilkins on the Internet: at LWW.com. Lippincott Williams & Wilkins customer service representatives are available from 8:30 am to 6 pm, EST.

10 9 8 7 6 5 4 3 2 1

RRS1107

To Bill Hanafee, for all of his wisdom, leadership, and kindness, and Paul Ward . . . who together created a model of what can be accomplished for interdisciplinary patient care with a spirit of mutual respect and everlasting friendship.

AAM

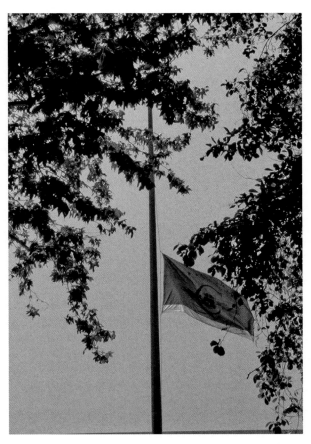

Bruin flag at UCLA Pauley Pavilion at half mast in honor of Bill's service—Summer 2010.

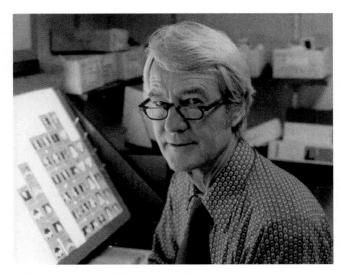

Bill in his office at UCLA, circa 1970s, preparing teaching material

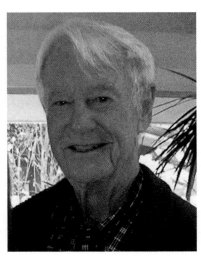

Bill in retirement in North San Diego County, likely getting ready to shoot a round of golf with his longtime friend and colleague Paul Ward

To our patients whose suffering is reflected in the images on these pages . . . may we all learn from them and, with the utmost compassion, improve daily our ability to find the best possible outcomes for those afflicted with often devastating diseases.

AAM
BMV

To my Dad Subhas and late mother Lalita for teaching me the values of hard work and perseverance, to my uncles Bhopal and Laxman for their mentorship throughout my medical school, to my loving wife Divya for her constant support and my dear son Dhruv who makes everything worthwhile.

SB

To my wife, thank you for your love and support. To my parents, thank you for everything you did and still do for us. To Anthony Mancuso, thank you for your excellent teaching and the opportunity to participate in this project.

BMT

To Dr. Gilda Cardenosa for giving me many gifts and lessons, the most treasured one: allowing genuine love and compassion for our patients to be the guides of our actions. Thank you for inspiring me.

RD

Teaching Files are one of the hallmarks of education in radiology. There has long been a need for a comprehensive series of books, using the Teaching File format that would provide the kind of personal consultation with the experts normally found only in the setting of a teaching hospital. Lippincott Williams & Wilkins is proud to have created such a series; our goal is to provide residents, fellows and practicing radiologists with a useful resource that answers this need.

Actual cases have been culled from extensive teaching files in major medical centers. The discussions presented mimic those performed on a daily basis between residents and faculty members in all radiology departments.

The format of this series is designed so that each case can be studied as an unknown, if desired. A consistent format is used to present each case. A brief clinical history is given, followed by several images. Relevant findings, differential diagnosis, diagnosis, discussion of the case, questions for further thought, reporting responsibilities and "what the treating physician needs to know" follow. Answers to the questions conclude each case. In this manner, the authors guide the reader through the interpretation of each case, with a strong emphasis on critical thinking.

We hope that this series will become a valuable and trusted teaching tool for radiologists at any stage of training or practice, and that it will also be a benefit to clinicians whose patients undergo these imaging studies.

—*The Publisher*

Bill Hanafee and I had the good fortune of Ruby Richardson of J.B. Lippincott asking us to do our first book, *Computed Tomography of the Head and Neck*, published in 1982. Almost 30 years later, the fifth and by far the most comprehensive project the Lippincott Williams & Wilkins team has helped us produce, *Head and Neck Radiology* by Mancuso and Hanafee, was released to the public in September 2010. This Teaching File book is a companion to that major work and is planned to coordinate with the rich educational and clinical care content and emphasis of the "big book."

All of the production groups over the years have been consummate professionals dedicated to delivering the best-quality resource to help care for patients with head and neck diseases. A special thanks this time around to Ryan Shaw and Charley Mitchell for developing and guiding this project to its most meaningful conclusion.

This work clearly would not have been possible without two other people. Kelly Paulling, my assistant, was truly extraordinary in helping with the manuscript and illustration preparation as well as countless logistical issues. The second, Chris Sistrom, M.D., Ph.D., developed information technology (IT) tools at the University of Florida College of Medicine that allow for extraordinarily efficient collection and transfer of images from our teaching file repository to this and other educational resources. Also, the online tool for computed tomography and magnetic resonance imaging protocols made available in searchable form at *www.xray.ufl.edu* and reflected in Appendixes A and B of the text are a tribute to his dedication and ingenuity. Those tools and the logistical setup of the IT workflow through our computer system that Chris created made the production process more efficient than I could ever imagine.

Many thanks to these folks and the many others on the team, including my neuroradiology colleagues who picked up my clinical slack from time to time, who made this almost 5-year project possible.

AAM

It has been an honor to work with my teacher and mentor Dr. Mancuso. I would like to sincerely thank Dr. Ronald Quisling, Professor and Section chief, Dr. Jeffery A Bennett, Fellowship director and Dr. Jimmy Johnson, Assistant Professor of Neuroradiology Division at University of Florida for their encouragement and support during this project.

SB

The following 164 cases are examples drawn from a comprehensive core curriculum in head and neck radiology. The crossover areas between traditional neuroradiology and ENT imaging such as neuro-ophthalmology, skull base pathology, and cranial nerve assessment are covered thoroughly. Diseases that might be of primary interest to oral and maxillofacial surgeons are also presented.

The book chapters are organized by anatomic region, with each case in a chapter correlated to a specific chapter in Sections III through XVI of the core reference, *Textbook of Head and Neck Radiology* by Mancuso and Hanafee. **That specific chapter reference is displayed at the end of each case along with a secondary reference to the best correlating chapter on the pathology or pathophysiology related to the case as presented in Section II of the core text.** This organizational framework allows the reader or student to link the case to the more complete and fundamental anatomic, pathophysiologic, reporting, and clinical context knowledge presented in the core text. This will make study of the anatomy and pathology within the scope of the "head and neck" discipline about as efficient and complete as possible by way of this one-stop, comprehensive resource (assuming the core text is available).

Please realize that this book can be used as a guide in your daily practice of head and neck radiology as well as a study guide for examination preparation. In fact, the book is intended to move from the older-style "teaching file" type of resource emphasis on differential diagnosis as an endpoint of a case to an endpoint that emphasizes critical thinking and synthesis of that thought process with the clinical context. Hopefully, the reader's ability to synthesize imaging information, optimally structure report content, and act on the information in a manner required by the acuity of the clinical situation will be the main lessons learned in each case. "Making the diagnosis" remains an important but secondary concern. The goal is to communicate and contribute, as an expert in this imaging subspecialty might, to medical decision making.

To the ends just stated, the format in this edition has been changed to give greater emphasis to the discussion, and two other sections emphasizing clinical context have been added. Specific recommendations with regard to report content that are acuity, problem, and study specific have been added in a section called "Reporting Responsibilities." This edition also features another new section called "What the Treating Physician Needs to Know"—the intent of this section being to make known to the patient and treating medical provider the reasonable information yield of an imaging study in each clinical scenario given the study's risks and cost.

Each section in the individual cases presents a portion of the planning/diagnostic/consultation/reporting process which, when taken together, will help ensure accurate diagnosis and the best possible medical decision making and, hopefully, outcome. The rationale for each section's content is as follows.

CLINICAL HISTORY It is essential to put summary imaging findings and disposition in a clinical context. This discipline helps focus the remainder of the process. The information given is purposely typical of that available in an imaging request form. It is the authors' sincere desire that with computer physician order entry and linked electronic medical record information, such data, as part of a request for imaging consultation, will become much more comprehensive and appropriate. For now, this is what most of us are provided, so the cases are presented in that less than optimal mode.

FINDINGS The images are presented with a section composed of concise figure legends describing the important findings. This section might be covered over if the cases are to be taken as "unknowns."

DIFFERENTIAL DIAGNOSIS Based on the clinical presentation and imaging findings, a reasonable list of differential diagnoses will be presented. In several cases, there will be no differential consideration.

DIAGNOSIS A summary statement of the basic disease process and, sometimes, pertinent associated findings will help focus your understanding of the problem, as well as the implications for treatment, and a need for further diagnostic evaluation.

DISCUSSION There may be some intended redundancy from case to case in this section. The repetition will reinforce the need for logic and discipline in whatever interpretative method you choose for evaluating head and neck imaging studies.

The diagnostic process as presented in this section is, in most cases, anatomically driven at the outset. The disease extent and morphology are then factored together with clinically relevant issues. The reasons for reaching a particular diagnosis will be discussed, including arguments against the other differential possibilities when that is relevant. The differential diagnosis is, however, normally not the endpoint. One must also consider the impact of the information on patient care and comment and report appropriately for the acuity of the clinical situation on these issues in responding to the case material. A search for expected complications of the diagnosed disease or a suggestion for further study is just as relevant as producing an accurate diagnosis or differential diagnosis. This section, and the three that follow, will encourage such processes.

Questions for Further Thought

Questions presented may expand on the theme of the case, emphasize clinical context, or introduce new material.

Reporting Responsibilities

This new section will first describe the acuity of a given clinical case and the urgency of communication. The section will also summarize relevant information that would be beneficial to the clinician in managing the case, sometimes in combination with the following section, and that should appear in the formal radiology report. Such information will generally include description of the pathology, its extent and effects on adjacent structures, presence or absence of expected complications, and any other case-specific details. It might also include recommendations for further evaluation.

What the Treating Physician Needs to Know

This new section will list, in bulleted text, what information yield and direction the ordering provider may reasonably expect in execution of an appropriately focused imaging protocol, the written report, or as part of verbal consultation given the clinical context and imaging test at hand.

Answers

Learn More Box

The book chapters are organized by anatomic region, with each case in a chapter correlated to a specific chapter in Sections III through XVI of the core reference, *Head and Neck Radiology* by Mancuso and Hanafee. **That specific chapter reference is displayed at the end of each case in a "Learn More Box" along with a secondary reference to the best correlating chapter on the pathology or pathophysiology related to the case as presented in Section II of the core text.**

CONTENTS

CHAPTER 1

The Eye, Orbit, and Visual Pathways, Including Cranial Nerves III, IV, and VI

CLINICAL HISTORY *An adult with a history of recent eye trauma presenting with reduced visual acuity.*

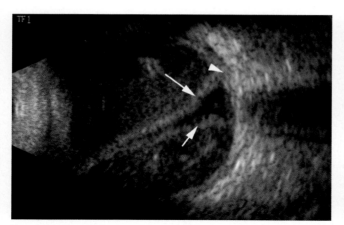

FIGURE **1.1A**

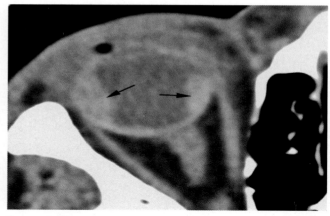

FIGURE **1.1B**

FINDINGS

Figure 1.1. Ocular membrane detachment extending to the point of penetration of the vortex veins lateral to the optic nerve head. The collections show internal reflections on (Fig.1.1A) ultrasound (US) and high density on (Fig.1.1B) non–contrast-enhanced computed tomography (CT).

DIFFERENTIAL DIAGNOSIS Serous choroidal detachment, hemorrhagic choroidal detachment, retinal detachment

DIAGNOSIS Hemorrhagic choroidal detachment

DISCUSSION Ocular membrane detachments and related fluid collections are named according to their location within the different retinal layers: hyaloid, subretinal, or choroidal detachment. Choroidal fluid collections accumulate in the suprachoroidal space, between the choroid and the sclera. A choroidal fluid collection is limited by the ciliary body anteriorly and extends to the level of the penetration of the vortex veins and the short posterior ciliary arteries posteriorly. It may be serous, exudate, or hemorrhagic. Subretinal hemorrhage is constrained by the anterior retinal attachment at the ora serrata and the posterior attachment at the optic nerve head.

The history of trauma and the imaging findings of choroidal fluid collections with internal reflections on US and high density on CT are the key to the diagnosis. Suprachoroidal hemorrhages are caused by the rupture of choroidal vessels, most commonly seen in the context of trauma, during or after eye surgery. Spontaneous choroidal hemorrhage is far less common.

US, usually performed by an ophthalmologist, may be the first and only imaging tool used. On CT and magnetic resonance imaging (MRI), a smooth lentiform collection is seen, not extending to the optic nerve head. On CT, the density of the collection is higher than that of the vitreous. MRI may show variable signal intensities according to the age of the hemorrhage.

Choroidal hemorrhage may occur spontaneously, but underlying primary ocular tumor or metastatic disease must be ruled out. Serous choroidal detachment may also show increased density on CT. On T2W magnetic resonance (MR), high signal intensity will be present, with T1 signal intensity either similar to the vitreous or slightly increased. This accumulation results from hypotony of the posterior chamber, due to increased vascular permeability caused by inflammation, or trauma.

Medical treatment will be given for any underlying cause and to prevent complications. In selected patients, drainage may improve outcome.

Questions for Further Thought

1. What are the causes of intraocular hemorrhage?
2. When should CT or MRI be performed in patients with ocular membrane detachments?
3. Name the retinal layers and potential spaces for the accumulation of effusion or hemorrhage.

Reporting Responsibilities

It is typically essential to directly and verbally report a detachment when it is first noted. This is especially true when the clinical circumstances are uncertain. This is true since many detachments require urgent care if a good visual outcome is the goal of treatment.

What the Treating Physician Needs to Know

• Describe the location and extent of ocular injury.
• Identify the type of detachment if one is present.
• Identify any underlying lesion.
• Evaluate for associated posttraumatic changes.

Answers

1. Intraocular hemorrhage may occur due to trauma; as a complication of intraocular surgery; or as a result of ocular disease, such as vascular, infectious, or tumoral pathologies.

2. US performed by skilled hands and in the correct clinical context may be sufficient for diagnosis and follow-up. Additional CT or MRI should be considered when some underlying causative pathology is suspected or to assess penetrating ocular trauma.

3. The sclera, the choroid, the retina (photosensitive inner layer and pigmented outer layer), and the hyaloid membrane comprise three potential spaces:

- Posterior hyaloid space (between the posterior hyaloid membrane and the inner retina)
- Subretinal space (between the inner or sensory and outer or pigmented retina)
- Suprachoroidal space (between the choroid and sclera)

LEARN MORE

See Chapters 45 and 10 in *Head and Neck Radiology* by Mancuso and Hanafee.

CASE 1.2

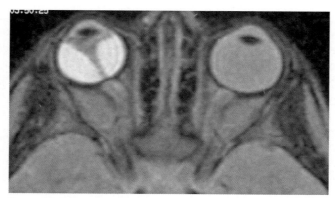

FIGURE **1.2**

FINDINGS

Figure 1.2. MR examination reveals unilateral microphthalmia. A dense tubular mass courses centrally from the lens to the optic nerve. The hyperintense signal of the vitreous chamber is suggestive of fluid or blood in the subretinal or subhyaloid space.

DIFFERENTIAL DIAGNOSIS Persistent hyperplastic primary vitreous (PHPV), closed-funnel retinal detachment

DIAGNOSIS PHPV

DISCUSSION Leukokoria is an abnormal white reflection from the retina seen on fundoscopy or flashlight photographs. It is a sign of ocular pathology of variable etiology. Retinoblastoma is the most common cause of leukokoria, but it may also be seen in several nonneoplastic diseases.

Imaging is performed to distinguish these nonneoplastic diseases from retinoblastoma.

Taking into account the age of the patient, sidedness (unilateral or bilateral), calcifications, and medical history, the list of differential diagnoses can be shortened.

The major causes of leukokoria in children under the age of 5 years are retinoblastoma, PHPV, Coat's disease, and retrolental fibroplasia or retinopathy of prematurity (ROP). Retinoblastoma most commonly presents as a unilateral calcified mass. Coat's disease is a unilateral exudative retinitis due to a vasculopathy of unknown etiology that generally presents later than 18 months of age. Diffuse calcification of the choroid may be present in 20% of patients during the chronic stage (>3 y). ROP usually affects both eyes in prematures who have received oxygen therapy. It is a fibroproliferative disease of underdeveloped retina and retinal vasculature causing retinal/vitreous fibrosis, hemorrhage, and scarring with calcifications. PHPV is a developmental disorder of the vitreous, typically unilateral and without calcifications before the age of 3 years.

Whereas retinal detachment is attached to the ora serrata, PHPV is always attached to the posterior capsule of the lens.

Question for Further Thought

1. What represents the retrolental soft tissue in PHPV?

Reporting Responsibilities

It is important to provide an accurate differential diagnosis of leukokoria and report based on the clinical "gravity" of the situation. Accurate direct communication may be the best course of action in many of these cases since there is sometimes a strong clinical impression existing that retinoblastoma is likely. If there is any chance of that being true, direct discussion is a good idea. This situation is more likely to arise when the imaging findings favor Coat's disease. The direct communication is most important to avoid even a remote possibility of an inappropriate enucleation.

What the Treating Physician Needs to Know

- Whether it concerns most likely a developmental disease or acquired disease
- What is the most likely diagnosis?
- If developmental, are there any associated abnormalities of the brain and face?

Answer

1. The retrolental tissue in PHPV is the result of scar formation along the center of the remnant of the primary vitreous and the hyaloid artery.

   In normal embryologic development, the primitive vitreous mesenchyme provides a matrix that later fills with a transparent gel, creating the secondary vitreous. The hyaloid artery, which perfuses the developing lens, regresses in the early part of the third trimester, leaving its embryonic remnant called the canal of Cloquet. If the primary vitreous does not resorb and the hyaloid artery does not regress, fibroproliferative tissue forms behind the lens, ultimately scarring the lens and opacifying the vitreous body and/or posterior chamber.

LEARN MORE

See Chapters 46 and 10 in *Head and Neck Radiology* by Mancuso and Hanafee.

CLINICAL HISTORY   *An elderly diabetic with visual loss.*

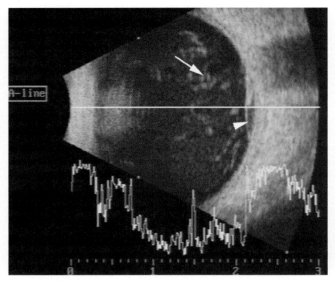

FIGURE **1.3A**

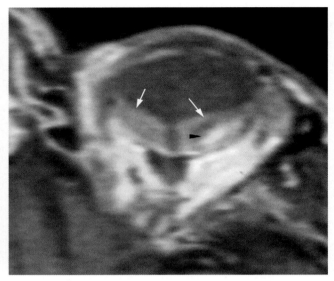

FIGURE **1.3C**

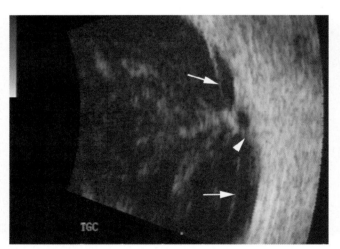

FIGURE **1.3B**

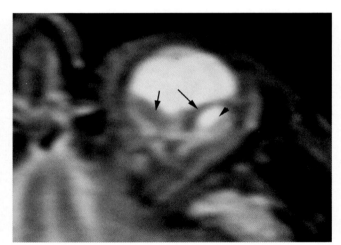

FIGURE **1.3D**

FINDINGS

Figure 1.3A. In dense vitreous hemorrhage (arrow), macular elevation (arrowhead) is a sign of underlying macular pathology.

Figure 1.3B. Traction over the macula is seen as a dome-shaped localized elevation of the macula (arrowhead) caused by the thick, attached posterior hyaloid (arrows). In dense vitreous hemorrhage, US is the only way to rule out macular elevation.

Figure 1.3C. T1W contrast-enhanced (CE) image showing enhancement of bilateral retinal detachments (arrows). In addition, there is a focal area of abnormality along the lateral aspect within that detachment (arrowhead).

Figure 1.3D. T2W images showing the chronic detachments and focal fluid collection. This was originally inter-

preted as a possible melanoma with secondary retinal detachment. However, the MR study showed that the focal abnormality was in fact not a mass due to melanoma but an evolving area of blood products.

DIFFERENTIAL DIAGNOSIS Macular degeneration with hemorrhagic retinal detachment versus hemorrhagic detachment with a subretinal mass

DIAGNOSIS Macular degeneration with hemorrhagic retinal detachment

DISCUSSION Senile macular degeneration is a common cause of visual loss in the elderly; however, it is typically a clinical diagnosis that seldom requires imaging by the diagnostic radiologist. It is a leading cause of loss of central vision, affecting 10% of the population over age 65 years and more than 25% of individuals over age 75 years. It is typically a disease of older adults that will be accelerated by risk factors that accelerate atherosclerotic vascular disease, such as hypertension and high cholesterol.

Macular degeneration is the result of chronic atherosclerotic changes in the choriocapillaris afferent vessels. This creates ischemic damage to the pigmented epithelial layer of the retina with thickening of Bruch's membrane and drusen (extracellular debris) deposition; in the wet version of macular degeneration, abnormal blood vessel growth occurs in the choriocapillaris, and effusions or hemorrhage may develop in the subretinal and/or subhyaloid space, as in this case. Detachments affecting the macula cause visual loss. These detachments, hemorrhages, and effusions with resultant inflammatory reparative vascularity may be visualized on imaging as uveoscleral thickening and contrast enhancement changes similar to uveoscleritis.

US does not have the resolution to exactly quantify the type of macular degeneration or to visualize the anatomy of the macula. US plays a role in ruling out the presence or absence of macular thickening or elevation. In dense vitreous hemorrhage, when fundus is not visualized, US is the only way to rule out macular thickening. The presence or absence of macular thickening helps prognostically and alerts the surgeon to the situation before a vitrectomy. US may also sometimes help to rule out macular traction from a thick posterior hyaloid. US does not directly help in the diagnosis of macular degeneration but helps to identify a macular problem with an opaque media.

An expanded choriocapillaris allows effusions and hemorrhages to develop in the subretinal space that lead to detachments and effusions with resultant inflammatory reparative vascularity. These changes may be visualized on contrast-enhanced computed tomography (CECT) and MRI as linear uveoscleral thickening and contrast enhancement changes similar to uveoscleritis and even focal mass lesions, which is the point of showing the images in this case. The findings may be complicated by intraocular bleeding in the subhyaloid and/or subretinal spaces that may further complicate the clinical and imaging evaluation.

Question for Further Thought

1. What is the difference between a rhegmatogenous and nonrhegmatogenous retinal detachment, and does this distinction have more to do with clinical rather than imaging evaluation?

Reporting Responsibilities

Any time potentially irreversible deterioration of vision occurs, the results of diagnostic testing should be communicated verbally to a knowledgeable health care provider who understands the urgency the implications of any positive imaging findings.

Findings of macular degeneration should be recognized as such, and care must be taken to not confuse these changes with intraocular masses. However, any detachment that is noted should be reported urgently as such, unless it is an obviously chronic condition, since it may not be known and might benefit from prompt treatment.

What the Treating Physician Needs to Know
- Whether degenerative changes of the eye are likely incidental or more important findings
- Whether abnormal findings in the eye such as localized enhancement, bleeding, or detachments are related to macular degeneration or some other disease process

Answer

1. Subretinal fluids are of two types. If the fluid is serous (clear subretinal fluid), then it is a rhegmatogenous detachment and always requires a surgical intervention. If the fluid is an exudate (dense subretinal fluid), there is a causative factor in the form of a thickened uvea secondary to uveitis or choroidal mass lesion.

   Collections within the subretinal space are constrained by the anterior retinal attachment at the ora serrata and the posterior attachment at the optic nerve head ending. As the volume of the subretinal effusion expands, the inner retinal surfaces begin to appose each other, creating a midline linear density extending from near the lens anteriorly to the optic nerve head ending posteriorly. Retinal detachments may actually fracture or break the continuity of the retinal surface, and this is referred to as a rhegmatogenous as opposed to nonrhegmatogenous retinal detachment; this distinction has more to do with clinical rather than imaging evaluation.

   Subretinal pathology cannot be directly visualized in an unbroken (nonrhegmatogenous) detachment. When an exophytic subretinal mass is suspected in the context of a nonrhegmatogenous detachment, direct funduscopic evaluation is precluded and imaging is likely to be necessary. The terms *endophytic* and *exophytic* refer to tumors arising from the retina or choroid, which project into the eye (endophytic mass) and can be directly visualized versus those that grow deep to the visualized retinal surface and potentially out of the eye (exophytic mass). This becomes particularly important in the diagnosis of retinoblastoma in children and uveal melanomas in adults.

> LEARN MORE
> See Chapter 47 in *Head and Neck Radiology* by Mancuso and Hanafee.

CLINICAL HISTORY *A 24-year-old man presenting with a swollen right eye after a blow on the eye during a hockey game.*

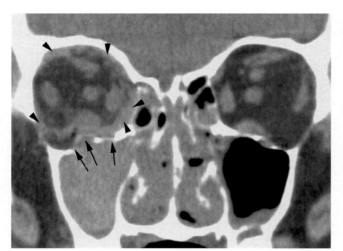

FIGURE **1.4A**

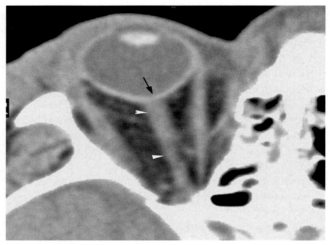

FIGURE **1.4B**

FINDINGS Coronal CT (Fig. 1.4A) shows a fracture of the orbital floor with upward displacement of bony fragments. The extraconal soft tissue swelling along the medial orbital wall and orbital floor represents a subperiosteal hematoma. The maxillary sinus is filled with blood, fluid, and mucosal thickening. On axial CT (Fig. 1.4B), proptosis due to the mass effect of the hematoma and bony fragments becomes apparent. The optic nerve is stretched, and there is some tenting of the globe at the attachment of the optic nerve.

DIFFERENTIAL DIAGNOSIS Not applicable

DIAGNOSIS Blow-in fracture of the orbital floor with secondary tension orbit

DISCUSSION The patient had suffered from blunt trauma to his eye during sports activities. A direct blow to the infraorbital rim probably caused torque to the zygomatic complex along with compressive forces to the rim; the transmitted energy resulted in an orbital floor injury with inward displacement of the fracture fragments. The same mechanism may occur after a blow to the supraorbital rim. Such blow-in fractures have a relatively high risk of injury to the ocular apparatus, such as lens luxation and retinal detachment or ocular motility problems. Accompanying intracranial traumatic effects may occur, particularly in supraorbital rim lesions.

If the fracture extends to the orbital apex, the optic nerve might become injured. Vision may also be compromised by a tension orbit, which is a situation where vision is threatened because of a mass effect in the orbit resulting in stretching of the optic nerve/sheath complex, eventually progressing to ischemic optic neuropathy in a rapid but unpredictable time course. The presented patient demonstrates relatively early tension orbit due to mass effect of bony fragments and an associated subperiosteal hematoma.

The referring service was immediately informed about this finding. The patient was monitored closely by visual acuity testing and pupillary response measurements. Since he showed progressive vision loss, the orbit was emergently decompressed. Vision was preserved in this young patient.

Questions for Further Thought
1. Describe imaging findings of tension orbit, and discuss the relevance of the findings.
2. What are possible causes of tension orbit?

Reporting Responsibilities
Reporting of orbital trauma should be escalated to urgent or emergent direct communication if:
- Tension orbit is established
- Compression of the optic nerve is present
- A foreign body is present

What the Treating Physician Needs to Know
- *Bony injury:* The category of fracture pattern, the complexity and displacement of the fracture, orbital apex injury
- *Soft tissue injury:* Intraorbital hematoma, orbital soft tissue herniation
- *Injury to the eye:* Lens dislocation, hemorrhage, intraocular gas, globe decompression
- *Injury to the optic nerve:* Compression, tension orbit
- *Intracranial injury:* Pneumocephalus suggesting a dural tear should be noted.
- If a foreign body is present

Answers
1. A procession of changes is seen in the development of tension orbit:

- A space-occupying process within the orbit
- Proptosis
- Stretching of the optic nerve/sheath complex
- Diminished diameter of the optic nerve/sheath complex

To this point, tension orbit is "incipient." Visual acuity, as well as pupillary response (looking for the development of an afferent pupillary defect), should be monitored at frequent intervals, and a team who might be needed to decompress the orbit should be made aware of a potential urgent or emergency procedure.

- Traction on the posterior aspect of the globe at the nerve globe junction will cause the posterior part of the globe to assume a cone-shaped or tented appearance.

By now, loss of visual acuity can be predicted with near certainty.

2. Any space-occupying lesion within the orbit may cause tension orbit: trauma, tumor, infection, and noninfectious inflammation.

LEARN MORE

See Chapter 48 in *Head and Neck Radiology* by Mancuso and Hanafee.

CLINICAL HISTORY *A patient with leukemia presenting with red, painful, proptotic eyes.*

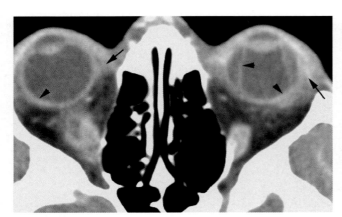

FIGURE 1.5A

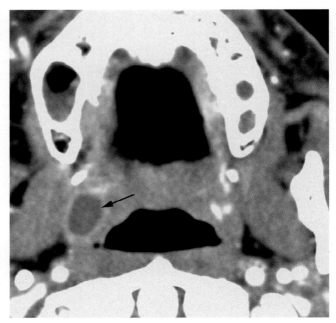

FIGURE 1.5C

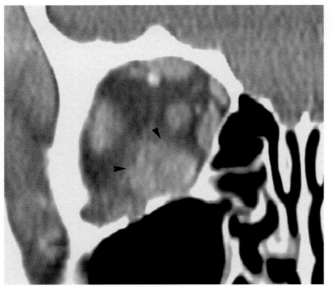

FIGURE 1.5B

FINDINGS On axial (Fig. 1.5A) and coronal (Fig. 1.5B) CT, there is bilateral scleral thickening and enhancement. On the left, associated inflammation of the periscleral soft tissues and choroidal detachment is seen. The right inferior rectus muscle is thickened, and the surrounding orbital fat is diffusely infiltrated. Axial CT at the level of the oropharynx (Fig. 1.5C) reveals a rim-enhancing collection in the right tonsil.

DIFFERENTIAL DIAGNOSIS Panoph thalmitis with choroidal detachment and tonsillar abscess: pyogenic or nonpyogenic bacterial infection, fungal infection

DIAGNOSIS Fungal infection involving the eye and orbit

DISCUSSION Fungal infection of the eye is most commonly seen in immunocompromised individuals. The most com-mon portal of entry is the paranasal sinuses, but it may also be the result of systemic involvement. Local and systemic signs may be insidious as a result of the immune status.

Orbital imaging findings of scleral and uveal thickening and enhancement, retinal detachment and effusion, periscleral edema, and involvement of an extraocular muscle with edema in the surrounding orbital fat are nonspecific findings and could be the result of viral, pyogenic, granulomatous, parasitic, fungal, or chronic inflammatory disease.

In this patient, however, the bilateral involvement and the concomitant tonsillar abscess point to systemic disease.

Ophthalmic fungal disease may show a rapidly progressive course. Visual outcome is usually poor, and the systemic form is frequently associated with a fatal outcome.

Question for Further Thought

1. List three ocular complications of scleritis.

Reporting Responsibilities

In case of endophthalmitis or panophthalmitis, direct communication with the treatment team is mandatory, with mentioning of the most likely causative pathology and complications that put the eye at risk.

What the Treating Physician Needs to Know

- Whether the disease is likely an infectious or inflammatory process
- Most likely diagnosis and full extent of disease
- Is there a local source of infection?

- Are there any complications, such as tension orbit, ocular membrane detachments, vascular thrombosis, or intracranial extension of disease?

Answer

1. Ocular membrane detachment, staphyloma, scleral perforation (rare)

> **LEARN MORE**
>
> See Chapters 49, 13, and 16 in *Head and Neck Radiology* by Mancuso and Hanafee.

CLINICAL HISTORY *A patient presenting with a very painful, swollen, inflamed left eye.*

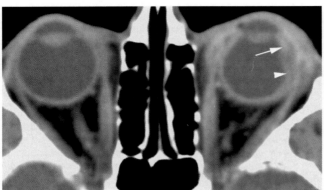

FIGURE **1.6A**

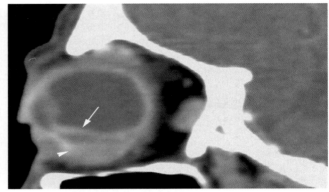

FIGURE **1.6C**

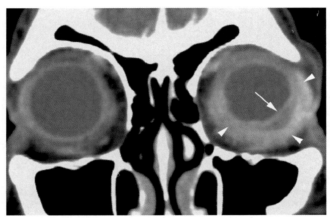

FIGURE **1.6B**

FINDINGS CECT shows marked enhancement of the uveal tract with focal enhancement in the region of the thickened ciliary body (see axial image in Fig. 1.6A). Associated detachment of the thickened choroid is best seen in its full extent on coronal CT (Fig. 1.6B). Obvious periscleritic edema is present, more lateral than medial (Fig. 1.6A) and most pronounced at the inferior of the globe (sagittal CT in Fig. 1.6C).

DIFFERENTIAL DIAGNOSIS Infectious or noninfectious inflammatory disease of the uveal tract with choroidal detachment

DIAGNOSIS Inflammatory keratoscleraluveitis with choroidal detachment

DISCUSSION The thickening and enhancement of the choroid, ciliary body, and/or iris is a manifestation of uveal tract infection. The uveal tract is the main vascular tissue in the eye, enveloping the eye with a slow-flow, highly vascular membrane. Both infection—transmitted by the blood supply—or vascular response to infection and inflammation that is triggered by immune complexes and/or associated with vasculitis are often initially and predominantly expressed in these structures. The imaging findings are nonspecific, and unless a source of the infection is demonstrated or evidence of bilateral disease pointing to a systemic process such as sarcoidosis or autoimmune disease is present, making a definitive diagnosis is not possible.

In this patient, the infection or inflammation also involves the sclera, cornea, and periscleral tissues with associated choroidal detachment (keratoscleraluveitis or endophthalmitis). No infectious agent could be identified. The patient was eventually successfully treated with steroids, and the final diagnosis was keratoscleraluveitis of uncertain inflammatory etiology.

Question for Further Thought

1. Name four systemic diseases that may affect the eye.

Reporting Responsibilities

In the case of endophthalmitis or panophthalmitis, direct communication with the treatment team is mandatory, with mentioning of the most likely causative pathology and complications that put the eye at risk.

What the Treating Physician Needs to Know

- Whether the disease is likely an infectious or inflammatory process
- Most likely diagnosis and full extent of disease
- Is there a local source of infection?

- Are there any complications, such as tension orbit, ocular membrane detachments, vascular thrombosis, and intracranial extension of disease?

Answer

1. Wegener's granulomatosis, sarcoidosis, rheumatoid arthritis, Behçet disease

> **LEARN MORE**
> See Chapters 50 and 13 in *Head and Neck Radiology* by Mancuso and Hanafee.

CLINICAL HISTORY *A patient presenting with eye injury after a car accident.*

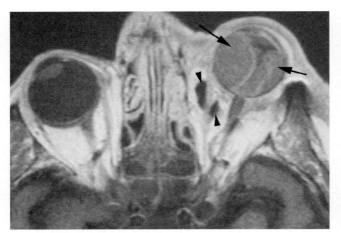

FIGURE **1.7A**

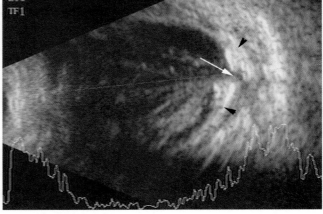

FIGURE **1.7C**

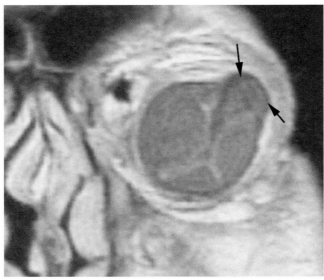

FIGURE **1.7B**

FINDINGS Axial T1W images show proptosis on the left. Within the globe ocular membrane, detachments extending to a point lateral to the optic nerve head (Fig. 1.7A) are present with related hyperintense collections. There is herniation of intraocular contents (Fig. 1.7B). Within the orbital fat, several signal voids are present. On US (Fig. 1.7C), scleral thickening and vitreous incarceration can be seen.

DIFFERENTIAL DIAGNOSIS Not applicable

DIAGNOSIS Traumatic eye injury with scleral tear and choroid detachment, intraorbital foreign bodies and/or gas

DISCUSSION Eye injury due to motor vehicle accidents may be caused by blunt and/or penetrating trauma. It may result in both bony and soft tissue injury. Foreign bodies,

usually glass, may remain embedded in the sclera and preseptal or postseptal soft tissues. Since both foreign bodies and gas show up as a signal void, MRI will not be able to differentiate such objects unless it shows a clear geometric configuration.

Scleral rupture may result either from elevation of the intraocular pressure due to a blunt force or from direct perforation by sharp penetrating trauma. Clinically, it can be hard to localize in a swollen injured eye. CT and MRI may show the scleral tear. On US, incarceration of the vitreous may point at the scleral disruption.

The capillary volume of the choriocapillaris is controlled largely by the intraocular pressure. Hypotony of the posterior chamber will allow the choriocapillaris to expand, and effusions will accumulate in the suprachoroidal space, causing choroidal detachment.

Question for Further Thought

1. Discuss the value of US, CT, and MRI in ocular trauma.

Reporting Responsibilities

Acute traumatic injuries to the eye should be communicated swiftly and directly, in particular:

- Injury of the eye of any type
- Retained foreign bodies
- Complications such as endophthalmitis or tension orbit

What the Treating Physician Needs to Know

- *Injury to the eye:* Lens dislocation, hemorrhage, detachments, intraocular gas, globe decompression
- Foreign body
- *Soft tissue injury:* Intraorbital hematoma, orbital soft tissue herniation
- *Bony injury:* If present, the category of fracture pattern, the complexity and displacement of the fracture, orbital apex injury

- *Injury to the optic nerve:* Compression, tension orbit
- Intracranial injury

Answer

1. US is generally the primary imaging modality unless it is technically not possible due to swelling and pain. It is helpful in demonstrating detachments and related fluid collections. It is especially useful to localize small anterior foreign bodies.

   CT can identify most clinically significant findings, such as ocular hemorrhage, scleral tear, ocular decompression, and tension orbit. It will demonstrate radiopaque foreign bodies. However, it is relatively insensitive to subtle injury in the anterior segment.

   MRI is usually used adjunctively in selected cases to look for retained foreign bodies or in case of delayed complications like orbital infection.

LEARN MORE

See Chapters 51 and 10 in *Head and Neck Radiology* by Mancuso and Hanafee.

CLINICAL HISTORY *A 56-year-old female presenting with blurred, distorted vision.*

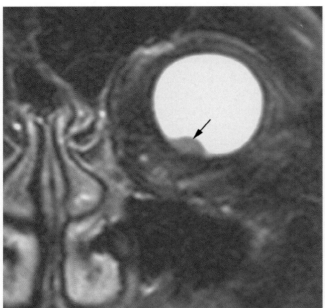

FIGURE **1.8A**

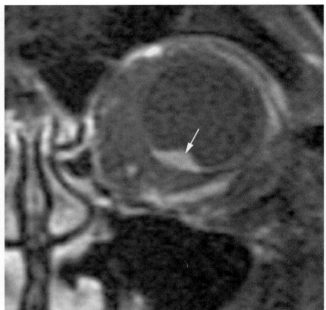

FIGURE **1.8C**

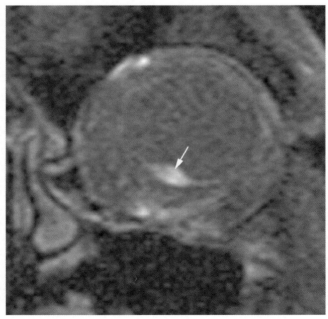

FIGURE **1.8B**

FINDINGS On coronal MR images, a choroidal lesion is present with slightly hypointense signal intensity on T2W imaging (Fig. 1.8A), slightly hyperintense signal intensity on fat-suppressed (FS) T1W imaging (Fig. 1.8B), and enhancement after contrast administration (Fig. 1.8C). The lesion is confined to the globe.

DIFFERENTIAL DIAGNOSIS Choroidal melanoma, choroidal hemangioma, choroidal nevus, lymphoma, leukemia, plasmocytoma, chorioretinal metastasis

DIAGNOSIS Choroidal metastasis

DISCUSSION An intraocular mass lesion may be caused by focal uveoscleritis, primary tumors (either benign or malignant), and metastases. Imaging features are often nonspecific, but taking into account the age of the patient and underlying conditions, the list of differentials may be shortened.

The presented patient had been diagnosed with breast cancer about a year prior to this MRI examination. Hematogenous spread of tumor cells will reach the eye via the short posterior ciliary arteries. Therefore, metastases are usually found in the posterior globe.

Like other ocular lesions, metastases may be associated with hemorrhagic detachments. The method of treatment will be decided by an oncologic team including an eye surgeon, medical oncologist, and radiation therapist. Decisions will be based on the extent of the ocular disease and ability to restore vision. The treatment strategy is linked to the treatment for the patient's underlying malignancy.

Questions for Further Thought

1. Which primary tumors metastasize to the eye?
2. Which imaging findings may help to differentiate ocular melanoma from metastasis?

Reporting Responsibilities

Ocular metastases may grow within weeks. Urgent reporting is necessary to ensure prompt treatment that might preserve vision.

What the Treating Physician Needs to Know

- Is the disease confined to the eye, or is there extraocular spread?
- Is there associated detachment?
- Is the disease multifocal and/or bilateral?
- Is there intracranial spread (along the optic nerve/sheath complex)?

Answers

1. Ocular metastases are usually from breast or lung cancer. Less common sites of origin are prostate, renal, thyroid, or gastrointestinal tumors. Extraocular melanoma may metastasize to the eye, and hematologic diseases may involve the globe.
2. Ocular melanoma has a typical appearance on US with low to intermediate internal reflectivity. In about a third of patients with metastasized disease, multifocal or bilateral involvement of the globe will be seen. Melanoma is typically a solitary lesion.

> ### LEARN MORE
> See Chapters 52 and 42 in *Head and Neck Radiology* by Mancuso and Hanafee.

CLINICAL HISTORY   *An infant with bilateral visual impairment and nystagmus.*

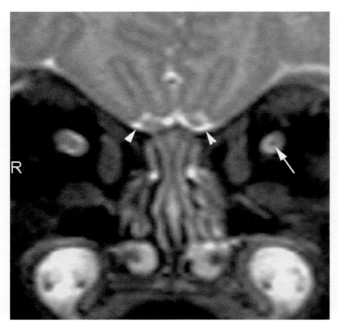

FIGURE **1.9A**

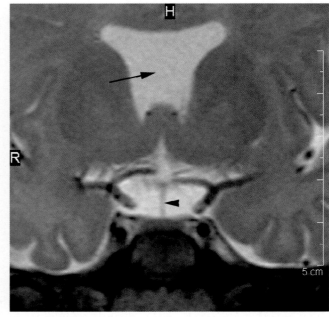

FIGURE **1.9C**

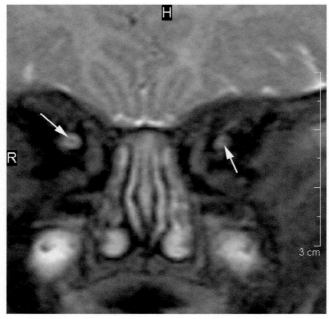

FIGURE **1.9B**

FINDINGS Coronal T2W images show thinning of the left optic nerve and segmental thinning of the right optic nerve. The olfactory structures including the olfactory tracts, olfactory sulcus, and gyrus rectus are normally developed (Fig. 1.9A,B). On an image slightly more posterior, a small pituitary stalk is seen, but the optic chiasm cannot be clearly visualized. The pituitary gland is present. The septum pellucidum is absent, and the lateral ventricles have a squared-off appearance with downward pointing at the inferior aspect (Fig. 1.9C).

DIFFERENTIAL DIAGNOSIS Septo-optic dysplasia (SOD)

DIAGNOSIS SOD

DISCUSSION SOD is one of the milder forms of brain and orbital developmental disorders (holoprosencephaly). There is a spectrum of anomalies that may affect the optic nerve, hypophysis, and forebrain. In SOD, the failure in brain development manifests with absence of the septum pellucidum and a particular shape of the lateral ventricles. The failure of brain development is associated with optic chiasm atrophy and optic nerve hypoplasia, which may be unilateral, bilateral, along the entire length, or segmental. The eye generally shows normal development. There may also be migrational abnormalities of the brain, such as heterotopia, cortical dysplasia, or schizencephaly, and abnormalities of the corpus callosum. The olfactory nerves and tract may be hypoplastic or absent. Pituitary developmental abnormalities may occur, and hypothalamic-pituitary dysfunction may lead to single or multiple endocrinologic deficiencies that may become lethal. Replacement therapy is indicated for these hormonal deficiencies.

Question for Further Thought

1. What is the normal size of the optic nerve?

Reporting Responsibilities

The imaging technique should be adequate to evaluate the optic nerves and chiasm, the pituitary gland, and the brain. In the case of severe pituitary dysfunction, the treating physician should be informed immediately about the diagnosis of SOD.

What the Treating Physician Needs to Know

- Are the optic nerves and chiasm hypoplastic?
- Is the septum pellucidum present?
- Are there any other (migrational) brain abnormalities?
- Is the pituitary gland and stalk normally developed?

Answer

1. In adults, the optic nerve normally measures 2.5 +/− 0.4 mm (two standard deviations). It may be slightly smaller in young children but should measure 2.9 mm^2 in cross-sectional area above the age of 1 year. The optic nerves are usually symmetric in size.

> LEARN MORE
>
> See Chapter 53 *Head and Neck Radiology* by Mancuso and Hanafee.

CLINICAL HISTORY *A young man who was involved in a motor vehicle accident developed decrease of visual acuity after admission in the emergency room.*

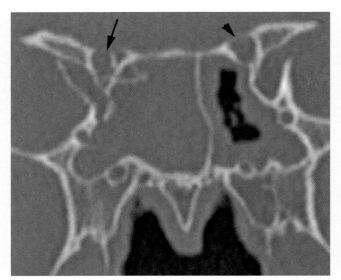

FIGURE **1.10A**

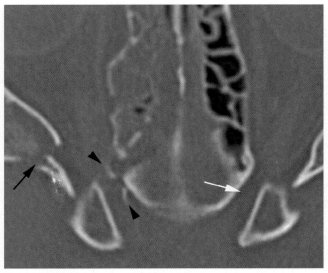

FIGURE **1.10B**

FINDINGS Coronal (Fig. 1.10A) and axial (Fig. 1.10B) CT show a comminuted fracture with displaced bony fragments within the right optic canal. The fracture also courses through the greater wing of the sphenoid, and the medial orbital wall is fractured and buckled (Fig. 1.10B). The sphenoid sinuses and the right ethmoid sinus are opacified, most probably with blood.

DIFFERENTIAL DIAGNOSIS Craniofacial trauma with optic canal fracture

DIAGNOSIS Craniofacial trauma with optic canal fracture

DISCUSSION Posttraumatic decreased visual acuity may be the result of direct or indirect injury to the optic nerve after blunt or penetrating trauma. Direct effects of trauma include compression, laceration, avulsion, or transsection of the nerve by a penetrating object, orbital or optic nerve sheath hematoma, or bony fragments. The mechanism of indirect trauma leading to optic neuropathy is most likely due to concussive and transiently compressive forces transmitted to the orbital apex and optic canal. Contusion and edematous swelling of the optic nerve within the narrow canal will likely cause ischemic injury to the nerve.

Extrinsic bony compression, as seen in the presented patient, will cause progressive vision loss. Decompressive surgery was considered. Unfortunately, the patient did not recover eyesight.

Questions for Further Thought

1. CT is the imaging method of choice for evaluation of blunt-force or penetrating orbital trauma. When should additional MRI be performed?
2. Is there a difference in treatment for direct optic nerve injury and indirect traumatic optic neuropathy?

Reporting Responsibilities

Direct communication of injury of the optic nerve or any other threat to vision is a medical urgency and sometimes an emergency.

What the Treating Physician Needs to Know

- Whether the optic nerve appears to be injured (compressed, lacerated, avulsed)
- Is the optic canal fractured?
- Is there a localized hematoma either of or outside the optic sheath?
- Is a foreign body present?
- Is there evidence of tension orbit?
- Is there a pattern of bony injury that might suggest indirect traumatic optic neuropathy?

Answers

1. MRI will more confidently show or exclude nerve/sheath laceration, nerve edema, and optic sheath hematoma. Causative bone fragments may not be identified by MRI.

2. Direct trauma to the optic nerve often requires surgical intervention: optic nerve decompression as long as the nerve is not transected, optic sheath fenestration, or removal of orbital hematoma.

Indirect trauma is less frequently treated surgically; steroids may be given.

LEARN MORE

See Chapter 54 in *Head and Neck Radiology* by Mancuso and Hanafee.

CLINICAL HISTORY *A 34-year-old female presenting with blurry vision followed by vision loss within 2 days and paresthesia and dysesthesia in the lower extremities.*

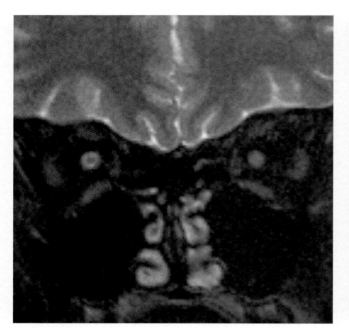

FIGURE **1.11A**

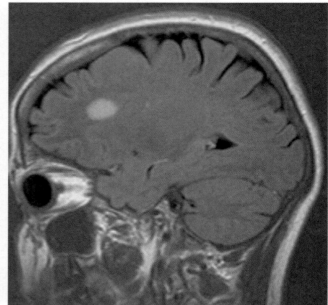

FIGURE **1.11C**

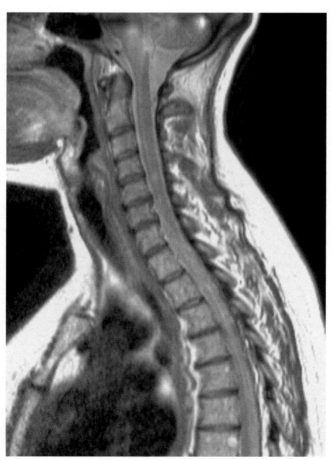

FIGURE **1.11B**

FINDINGS FS T2W imaging (Fig. 1.11A) of the optic nerve shows thickening and increased signal intensity of the left optic nerve. On a sagittal proton density image of the spine (Fig. 1.11B), small nodular lesions with high signal intensity are seen in the cervical spinal cord. Sagittal FLAIR image (Fig. 1.11C) shows one of three periventricular nodular white matter lesions.

DIFFERENTIAL DIAGNOSIS Optic neuritis in multiple sclerosis (MS), neuromyelitis optica (NMO; Devic disease), optic neuritis and transverse myelitis in collagen vascular disease (e.g., systemic lupus erythematosus [SLE], Sjögren)

DIAGNOSIS Optic neuritis in MS

DISCUSSION Acute optic neuritis can occur as an isolated, idiopathic event or may be linked to an autoimmune disease. The associated findings in the presented patient were suggestive of MS. Cerebrospinal fluid (CSF) analysis after spinal tap showed oligoclonal bands. The patient received corticosteroids and the vision improved. Six months after first admission, she presented with sensory and motor deficits of the left leg. Treatment with interferon was started for relapsing-remitting MS.

True NMO or Devic disease is a distinct disease entity. It is far less common and primarily affects females in their mid thirties. Imaging findings in these patients are unilateral or bilateral optic neuritis and longitudinally contiguous, extensive spinal cord lesions involving three or more segments. Brain lesions are rare at onset. During the course of disease, white matter lesions may evolve. Whether they are nonspecific or MS-like, they are usually asymptomatic. Recently, an NMO-specific autoantibody has been identified. This will bind selectively to the aquaporin-4 (AQP4) water channel, which is mainly present in the optic nerves, myelin, and within the brain in the periventricular region and in the hypothalamus. Thus, true NMO can be distinguished from MS based on clinical presentation, imaging findings, and serology and immunopathology studies.

Some collagen vascular disease, such as SLE and Sjögren syndrome have been reported to show imaging and serologic features similar to NMO.

Question for Further Thought
1. Why is it important to distinguish Devic syndrome from MS?

Reporting Responsibilities
Imaging findings in optic nerve and sheath inflammation and infection are most often nonspecific. Assessment for associated or underlying disease and complicating factors is mandatory. Direct communication at the time of initial suspicion of disease is often useful so that any delay in start of therapy can be avoided.

What the Treating Physician Needs to Know
- Whether the disease present is likely an infectious or inflammatory process
- Most likely diagnosis and full extent of disease
- Is an acute infection likely, and does the situation constitute an emergency relative to preserving the eye?
- Are any complications present outside of those related to the eye?

Answer
1. The differentiation is important because of differences in prognosis and treatment. NMO usually has a worse outcome with frequent and early relapses. It responds to immunosuppressive therapy and plasmapheresis, whereas MS patients will receive immune-modulating agents.

LEARN MORE
See Chapters 55 and 20 in *Head and Neck Radiology* by Mancuso and Hanafee.

CLINICAL HISTORY *A 24-year-old female presenting with progressive vision loss on the left. US examination showed thickening of the optic nerve.*

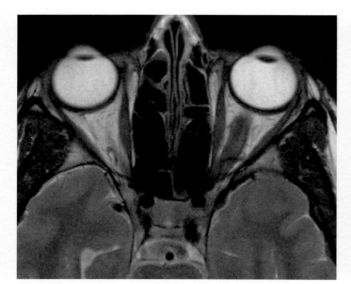

FIGURE **1.12A**

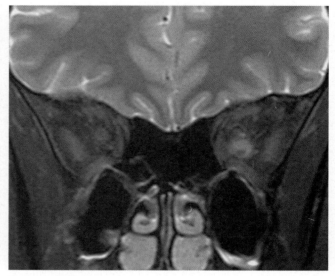

FIGURE **1.12C**

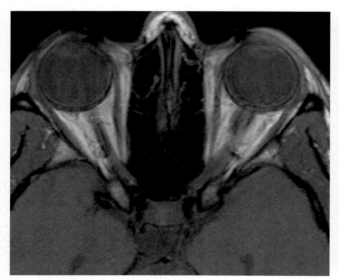

FIGURE **1.12B**

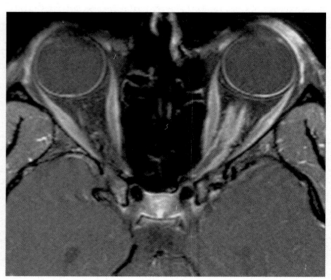

FIGURE **1.12D**

FINDINGS On axial T2W (Fig. 1.12A) and T1W images (Fig. 1.12B), the optic nerve/sheath complex appears thickened. A coronal FS T2 image (Fig. 1.12C) shows a lesion encasing and compressing the optic nerve. This lesion shows homogenous enhancement on a T1W FS CE image (Fig. 1.12D) with extension into the optic canal.

DIFFERENTIAL DIAGNOSIS Optic nerve meningioma, leukemia, idiopathic orbital inflammatory syndrome (IOIS also known as pseudotumor)

DIAGNOSIS Optic nerve sheath meningioma

DISCUSSION A primary optic nerve sheath meningioma (OSM) arises from the arachnoid surrounding the optic nerve in the orbital or intracanalicular segment. This patient is rather young for an OSM outside the context of neurofibromatosis type II. These tumors are mostly seen in middle-aged and older women.

Patients typically present with progressive vision loss. A slow onset of symptoms associated with optic nerve head atrophy and large atypical vessels on the optic nerve head at funduscopy make up a classic triad of findings in optic sheath meningiomas.

Exophthalmos, headache, ptosis, and diplopia may also be present.

The patient shows typical MRI findings of an enhancing lesion growing concentrically along the optic sheath. On CT, microscopic calcifications can increase the density of the lesion. Gross linear, diffuse, patchy, or nodular calcifications may be present along and/or within the mass. Linear calcification or linear enhancement is referred to as the "tram tracking sign." Adjacent bone may be hyperostotic due to reactive changes and/or be infiltrated.

A similar imaging pattern may be seen in leukemia or pseudotumor. However, combined with clinical data, there is little doubt about the diagnosis. Optic nerve involvement in leukemia implies central nervous system (CNS) disease and usually occurs in the late stages of disease. Patients with pseudotumor typically present with painful vision loss.

Questions for Further Thought
1. What are the treatment options for OSM?
2. What are the considerations for treatment choice?

Reporting Responsibilities
A compressive lesion causing visual loss should be promptly communicated, since treatment may preserve vision that might otherwise be lost.

What the Treating Physician Needs to Know
- Can a lesion be identified that is compressing or involving the optic nerve and causing the vision loss?
- If a lesion is present, what is the extent of tumor relative to the optic canal and optic chiasm, and is there spread approaching or crossing the midline?
- Is there any bone involvement?

Answers
1. Observation, radiation, and surgery
2. Vision and tumor extent. If there is stable, acceptable vision loss without threat of the opposite optic nerve or significant intracranial extension, OSM can be observed. Surgical treatment is generally reserved to manage tumors that have already caused the involved eye to be blind. Radiotherapy may be used to stop or slow progression of tumors threatening the optic chiasm. It is also used following surgical removal when a gross total resection cannot be accomplished with acceptable morbidity.

> ### LEARN MORE
> See Chapters 56 and 31 in *Head and Neck Radiology* by Mancuso and Hanafee.

CLINICAL HISTORY *A 42-year-old male with vision loss and decreased color vision accompanied by pain.*

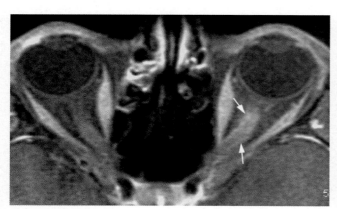

FIGURE **1.13A**

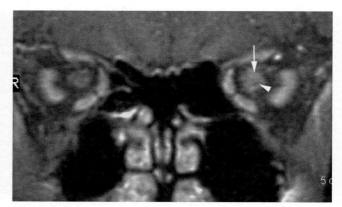

FIGURE **1.13B**

FINDINGS Axial (Fig. 1.13A) and coronal (Fig. 1.13B) CE T1W MR images with fat suppression show indistinctness and enhancement of the optic sheath extending into the surrounding orbital fat. There seems to be some enhancement of the optic nerve as well when comparing to the left optic nerve on the coronal image.

DIFFERENTIAL DIAGNOSIS Infectious perineuritis (viral, bacterial, fungal, parasitic) autoimmune-based inflammatory neuritis (e.g., SLE, sarcoidosis, Wegener's granulomatosis), IOIS (pseudotumor)

DIAGNOSIS IOIS (pseudotumor)

DISCUSSION Pseudotumor is a noninfectious inflammatory process of unknown etiology. IOIS may present as a localized perineuritic form. These patients typically present with a unilateral painful vision loss. An afferent pupillary defect will often be present.

Imaging findings are nonspecific: enlargement and enhancement of the optic sheath and or nerve may be seen in acute inflammatory or infectious disease.

IOIS is a diagnosis of exclusion. Other diseases have to be ruled out first. Bilateral involvement of the optic nerve raises the likelihood of a systemic process. In such cases, accompanying systemic signs and symptoms may point out the diagnosis (e.g., involvement of joints in autoimmune diseases or pulmonary involvement in sarcoidosis). Laboratory tests might support Wegener's granulomatosis with a positive cANCA, sarcoidosis with a positive angiotensin converting enzyme (ACE) or autoimmune disease based on an appropriate immune panel result. Imaging of infectious perineuritis has no distinguishing features unless a source of infection is seen outside the nerve/sheath complex (e.g., foreign body or paranasal sinus disease).

If IOIS is strongly suspected, a therapeutic trial of corticosteroids may be given. Biopsy may be necessary to rule out other causes of perineuritis.

Question for Further Thought

1. Which other regions may become involved with pseudotumor?

Reporting Responsibilities

Any time potentially irreversible deterioration of vision is occurring, the results of diagnostic testing should be communicated verbally to a knowledgeable health care provider who understands the urgency and the implications of any positive imaging findings. Some more specific circumstances are as follows:

- Virtually all cases suspicious for perineuritic IOIS are also suspicious for infection, and one has to rule out causative pathology such as sinonasal infection or an intraorbital foreign body.
- Complications such as tension orbit, vascular thrombosis, ocular detachments, or intracranial involvement of disease must be directly and rapidly communicated with the treatment team.

What the Treating Physician Needs to Know

- Whether the disease is likely an infectious or inflammatory process
- If inflammatory, is it likely pseudotumor?
- Full extent of disease

Answer

1. In the head and neck region, the orbit is by far the most involved region. Besides the perineuritic location, as shown in this patient, it can present as predominantly

periscleritic, myositic, lacrimal, or a more diffuse form. The actual distribution of the disease often spills over from one of these predominant sites to other areas, including the orbital apex and cavernous sinus.

Pseudotumor may also be located in the parapharyngeal and submandibular spaces, larynx, maxillary sinus, and oral cavity.

LEARN MORE

See Chapters 57 and 18 in *Head and Neck Radiology* by Mancuso and Hanafee.

CLINICAL HISTORY *A 41-year-old female presenting with dry eyes, diplopia, and temporary vision loss on the right. The patient suffered from heat intolerance, nervousness, insomnia, and hair loss. CT images are shown below:*

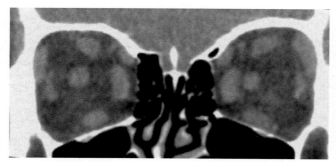

FIGURE **1.14A**

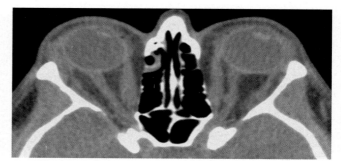

FIGURE **1.14C**

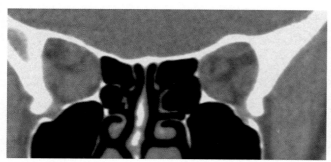

FIGURE **1.14B**

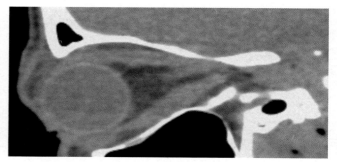

FIGURE **1.14D**

FINDINGS Coronal (Fig. 1.14A,B), axial (Fig. 1.14C), and sagittal (Fig. 1.14D) CT images show bilateral proptosis and asymmetric thickening of extraocular muscles with sparing of the tendons. There is edema and vascular congestion in the intraorbital fat. On the right, there is obliteration of the fat pad around the optic sheath near the orbital apex.

DIFFERENTIAL DIAGNOSIS Graves' dysthyroid ophthalmopathy (GDO), lymphoma, granulomatous diseases (Wegener's granulomatosis, sarcoidosis)

DIAGNOSIS GDO

DISCUSSION Graves disease is the most common cause of hyperthyroidism. It is caused by a B and T lymphocyte reaction to thyroid-stimulating hormone (thyrotropin) receptors (TSHRs). In the thyroid, this leads to hyperstimulation of the gland and, therefore, a reduced thyroid-stimulating hormone level. Orbital fibrocytes of the extraocular fat and connective tissue (like the thyroid gland) also have a high expression of TSHR. The resulting lymphocyte and macrophage reactive process affects the extraocular soft tissues—most dramatically, the extraocular muscles.

The patients usually present with bilateral proptosis, leading to dry and irritated eyes. The thickening of the muscles may cause disturbed eye movements and compression of the optic nerve at the orbital apex.

Either CT or MRI without contrast suffices when the clinical decision making strongly supports GDO. In the presented patient, the diagnosis is based on the signs of hyperthyroidism, confirmed by endocrinologic testing, and the typical imaging features.

Imaging in the acute/subacute stage typically shows vascular congestion and edema of the orbital fat. The volume of the orbital fat is usually increased, although it may also appear decreased due to the thickening of the muscles. The proptosis of GDO is proportional to the extent of muscle mass expansion and/or intraorbital fat volume. Muscle thickening may cause obliteration of the fat planes around the optic sheath in the orbital apex. The more effacement is seen, the greater the risk for optic neuropathy. The temporary vision loss on the right side in this patient was probably due to some nerve compression by muscular hypertrophy aggravated by inflammatory changes. Other possible findings in neuropathy are hydrops of the optic nerve and dilatation of the superior orbital vein due to vascular congestion. Enlargement of the lacrimal gland may also occur.

In the chronic stage of disease, the muscles will become atrophic, fat replaced, and fibrotic. Treatment consists of correction of the thyroid dysfunction. In the acute phase, steroids and immunosuppressives may be given to reduce the inflammatory reaction. Surgical intervention may become necessary to correct optic neuropathy, muscle dysfunction, or lid lag.

Question for Further Thought

1. Increased orbital fat content is not specific for GDO, name three other causes for increased orbital fat content.

Reporting Responsibilities

The diagnosis is usually expected, and routine reporting suffices. This may not be the case if the disease is unilateral; in those instances, direct communication might be useful to firmly establish GDO as the most likely diagnosis. The need for urgent direct communication escalates if the study suggests a significant chance of compressive optic neuropathy and/or the clinical situation includes an optic neuropathy. An alternative diagnosis also usually requires direct verbal communication.

What the Treating Physician Needs to Know

- Extent of proptosis
- Whether there is evidence of acute phase disease such as orbital fat edema or whether the disease is likely in its later fibrotic phase
- If there is evidence of compressive optic neuropathy
- If not GDO, other possible diagnostic alternatives

Answer

1. Increased orbital fat content may also be seen in obesity, diabetes, and prolonged corticosteroid use.

LEARN MORE

See Chapters 58 and 20 in *Head and Neck Radiology* by Mancuso and Hanafee.

CLINICAL HISTORY *A middle-aged female presenting with intermittent proptosis.*

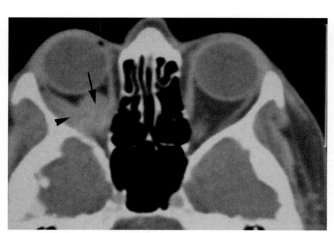

FIGURE **1.15A**

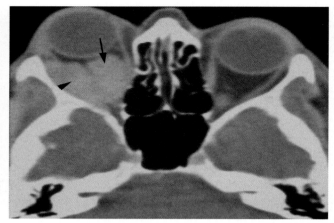

FIGURE **1.15B**

FINDINGS Two well-defined, enhancing, intraorbital lesions are seen on the right on CECT (Fig. 1.15A). One lesion is fusiform and located along the course of the lateral rectus muscle. The other one is an ovoid intraconal mass. Because the proptosis was intermittent, the CT study was repeated during Valsalva's maneuver (Fig. 1.15B). Whereas the lateral lesion shows considerable dilatation, the intraconal one is less altered in size. Also note the marked proptosis in (Fig. 1.15B).

DIFFERENTIAL DIAGNOSIS Orbital varix in association with a vascular malformation

DIAGNOSIS Orbital varix in association with a cavernous venous malformation

DISCUSSION Orbital varix and cavernous venous malformation, also known by the less correct terminology as cavernous hemangioma, are slow-flow malformations consisting of dilated venous space in a fibrous and muscular stroma.

The diagnostic clue for orbital varix is enlargement during increased venous pressure that can be provoked during crying, Valsalva's maneuver, or holding the head in a gravity-dependent position. Therefore, imaging—either MRI or CT—should be performed during Valsalva or in prone position whenever there is clinical suspicion of a varix. It will show a strongly enhancing tubular or tortuous vein with dynamic size variation correlated to venous pressure.

Orbital varix is an uncommon lesion that may present at any age. It may be congenital, idiopathic or posttraumatic,

associated with a cavernous vascular malformation, or secondary to an arteriovenous (AV) fistula.

This patient had an associated cavernous venous malformation (also referred to as hemangioma), which is the most common vascular orbital tumor in adults, usually presenting between the second and fourth decade of life. Typical imaging features are a markedly enhancing, well-circumscribed lesion, sometimes showing a pseudocapsule. Changes in venous pressure typically do not affect their size.

Phleboliths may be seen in both venous and cavernous malformations. Both lesions will be observed unless pain or functional compromise requires treatment.

Question for Further Thought

1. Name four possible complications of vascular malformations.

Reporting Responsibilities

When a vascular lesion is suspected, the referring physician should be informed about the risk of bleeding during a potentially planned intervention (biopsy). If there is threat to vision due to the size of the lesion or complications, immediate communication is required.

What the Treating Physician Needs to Know

- Likely nature of flow dynamics in a vascular lesion
- In case of varix, whether it represents an isolated varix or one with an associated vascular malformation
- Complications

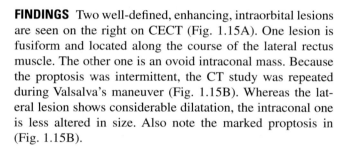

Answer

1. Vascular malformations may bleed, thrombose, become infected, or show a local immune response to viral or other upper respiratory tract infections.

LEARN MORE

See Chapters 59 and 9 in *Head and Neck Radiology* by Mancuso and Hanafee.

CLINICAL HISTORY *An elderly patient presenting with painful, unilateral proptosis and ocular dysmotility.*

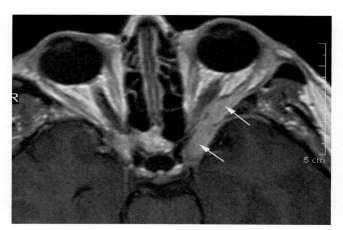

FIGURE **1.16A**

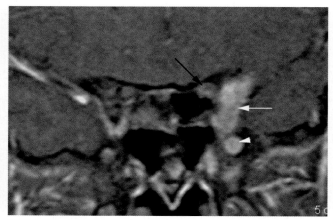

FIGURE **1.16C**

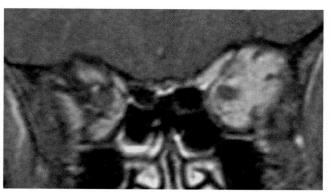

FIGURE **1.16B**

FINDINGS Axial CE T1W MR image (Fig. 1.16A) and coronal CE T1W images with fat suppression (Fig. 1.16B,C) show proptosis on the left due to an infiltrating mass involving the muscle cone and extending into the orbital apex, orbital fissure, and anterior aspect of the cavernous sinus. There is also enhancement of the second branch of the trigeminal nerve and of the optic nerve sheath within the optic canal (Fig. 1.16C).

DIFFERENTIAL DIAGNOSIS Lymphoma with neurotropic behavior, granulomatous disease, metastatic disease with perineural spread, malignant fibrous tumor, orbital pseudotumor

DIAGNOSIS Lymphoma with neurotropic behavior

DISCUSSION Painful proptosis may be the presenting symptom in inflammatory processes, pseudotumor, or malignant tumors of the orbit. Proptosis is related to the size and firmness of a lesion. Since almost all malignant tumors are firm, proptosis is often the presenting feature in these patients. Orbital pain is often present in malignancies and is the most distinguishing factor from benign tumors.

The imaging features of the unilateral mass in this elderly patient do not allow differentiating tumoral from inflammatory disease or pseudotumor. The final diagnosis of lymphoma was made after a biopsy.

Orbital lymphoma is a relatively common cause of proptosis. It is usually a B-cell non-Hodgkin type. Orbital lymphoma is often part of a systemic disease state. Therefore, one should look for evidence of bilateral or extraorbital involvement, including intracranial localizations.

Question for Further Thought

1. Name possible localizations of lymphoma in the orbit.

Reporting Responsibilities

Any orbital mass thought to be malignant should be discussed with the referring physician—in particular, in the case of compressive optic neuropathy or aggressive behavior. The precise localization and tumor spread and the likelihood of being related to systemic disease should be mentioned.

What the Treating Physician Needs to Know

• If the tumor is arising in the muscle cone

- Full extent of disease, including the relationship to the optic nerve/sheath complex and possible threat to vision
- Whether the tumor is solitary or multiple or bilateral to suggest systemic disease
- Whether there are any findings outside the orbit that might help identify the origin of the lesion
- Most likely diagnosis
- In case of suspected malignancy, whether the exam included a survey of regional lymph nodes

Answer

1. Lymphoma may occur anywhere in the orbit. It has a predilection for the lacrimal gland and will typically involve the entire gland. Lymphoid tissue in the subconjunctiva may give rise to an isoated preseptal lymphoma. Retrobulbar intraconal, extraconal, muscular, or transcompartmental involvement may be seen. Perineural disease is an uncommon but important mode of spread of lymphoma. Orbital lymphoma does usually not invade the bone.

LEARN MORE

See Chapters 60 and 27 in *Head and Neck Radiology* by Mancuso and Hanafee.

CLINICAL HISTORY *A young adult presenting with downward and inward proptosis of the left eye.*

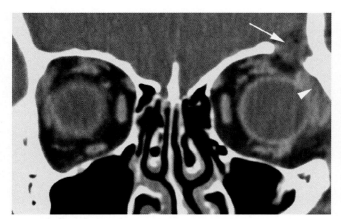

FIGURE **1.17A**

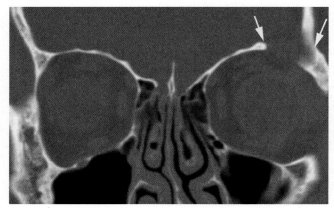

FIGURE **1.17B**

FINDINGS A partially fatty and partially solid or cystic lesion is noted in the upper outer quadrant of the left orbit on CT (Fig. 1.17A). The lacrimal gland seems enlarged but was in fact only displaced and not involved by the lesion. In bone window (Fig. 1.17B), a well-defined focal defect in the lateral orbital roof, suggestive of a very slow growth pattern, is seen in (Fig. 1.17B).

DIFFERENTIAL DIAGNOSIS Complex dermoid cyst

DIAGNOSIS Complex dermoid cyst

DISCUSSION Based on the clinical presentation, this patient was suspected to have a mass lesion arising from the lacrimal gland. Imaging revealed a lesion in the upper outer quadrant containing fat. This finding is indicative of a dermoid cyst.

A dermoid cyst is the result of congenital inclusion of epidermal and dermal elements as suture lines close during embryonic development. Within the orbit, they are most commonly seen at the frontozygomatic suture. Although typically a lesion of childhood, causing a painless mass, they may appear and grow at any age. If located deep, they will be detected only after growth leading to mass effect.

The imaging appearance varies greatly with the tissue content: They may be cystic or show mixed density or signal intensity. Only in about 40% to 50%, fatty tissue or a fat–fluid level, typical of dermoid, is present. Unlike sebaceous cysts, which also contain fat, they are not attached to the skin but tethered to the periosteum. Associated bony changes such as scalloping, thinning, focal dehiscence, and sclerosis are common. Extension of the mass through a bony suture may cause a dumbbell appearance.

Treatment consists of complete surgical resection.

Question for Further Thought

1. Describe the imaging features of a complicated dermoid cyst.

Reporting Responsibilities

Detailed description of the location and extent of a dermoid cyst will guide surgical approach and prevent incomplete resection. These are of no significant threat and may be reported routinely. If findings suggest a lesion of more aggressive pathologic potential such as Langerhans cell histiocytosis (LCH), direct communication is wise.

What the Treating Physician Needs to Know

- Whether or not the lesion is arising from the lacrimal gland
- Likely diagnosis and full extent of disease—in particular, bone involvement and extraorbital extension
- Any threat to vision

Answer

1. A dermoid cyst may rupture spontaneously or after trauma. The lesion will show irregular margins and enhancement with pronounced inflammatory changes in the surrounding tissues.

LEARN MORE

See Chapters 61 and 8 in *Head and Neck Radiology* by Mancuso and Hanafee.

CLINICAL HISTORY *A bone marrow transplant patient presents with a fever and signs of sinus disease.*

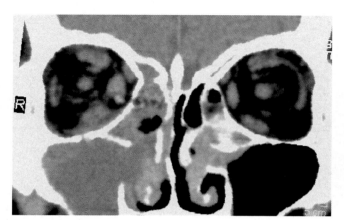

FIGURE **1.18A**

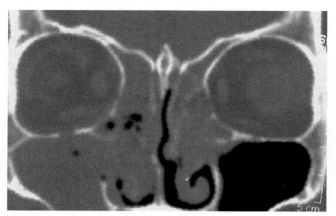

FIGURE **1.18B**

FINDINGS Coronal sinus CT (Fig. 1.18A) shows an opacified ethmoid and right maxillary sinus. There is also subtle erosion of the infraorbital canal in comparison to the uninvolved left side. Soft tissue setting (Fig. 1.18B) reveals some infiltration of the extraconal fat along the orbital floor.

DIFFERENTIAL DIAGNOSIS Postseptal orbital cellulitis—likely an aggressive infection, recurrent leukemia, posttransplantation lymphoproliferative disorder

DIAGNOSIS Postseptal orbital cellulitis due to invasive fungal sinusitis

DISCUSSION Given the context of sinusitis in an immune-suppressed patient, the presented imaging features are highly suggestive of invasive fungal disease. It may also be seen in diabetics and occasionally in frail elderly with normal immune status. This aggressive form of fungal disease, usually aspergillosis or mucormycosis, tends to be angioinvasive—in particular, arterial invasive. It will involve vascular bundles coursing through foramina such as the infraorbital canal, thereby spreading disease on both sides of a bony wall or septum, sometimes without frank bone erosion. Perivascular infiltration of the fat bordering such canals will lead to early diagnosis. If not treated properly and in time, fungal disease may rapidly spread intraorbitally and intracranially.

Diffuse inflammatory reaction may be accompanied by soft tissue or bone necrosis.

Treatment should be targeted on both local control of the infection and removing the source of infection.

Questions for Further Thought
1. How does fungal disease manifest in the immune-competent host with sinusitis?
2. What are some other relatively common conditions involving extraconal fat?

Reporting Responsibilities
Evidence of acute infections of the orbit must be urgently communicated directly to the treating physician with mentioning of the most likely causative pathology (e.g., sinonasal disease) and complicating factors (e.g., tension orbit).

What the Treating Physician Needs to Know
• Is the disease likely inflammatory or infectious?
• What are the most likely diagnosis and full extent of disease?
• Is there a local source of infection?
• Are there any complications: eye, optic nerve, cavernous sinus, intracranial?

Answers

1. In long-standing chronic sinusitis, dried-out secretions become a medium for fungal growth. This results in fungal colonization inciting chronic mucosal thickening. The relationship with the host is saprophytic.

2. Orbital pseudotumor and thyroid-associated orbitopathy are the two most common inflammatory conditions involving the extraconal space of the orbit, usually in association with involvement of the muscle cone. Secondary involvement of the extraconal space is seen from sinonasal and lacrimal gland disease or skull base osteomyelitis.

LEARN MORE

See Chapters 62 and 16 in *Head and Neck Radiology* by Mancuso and Hanafee.

CLINICAL HISTORY *A patient presenting with diminished visual acuity and an area of focal swelling over the left supraorbital ridge. The patient had suffered blunt-force frontal orbital injury several months earlier.*

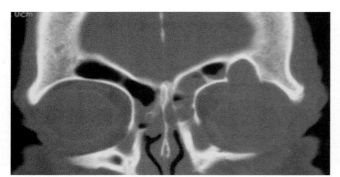

FIGURE 1.19A

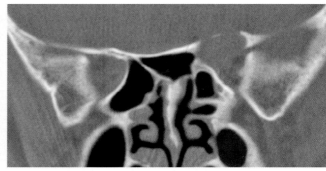

FIGURE 1.19D

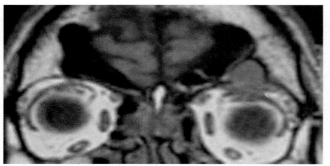

FIGURE 1.19B

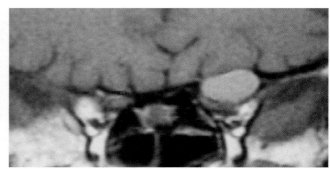

FIGURE 1.19E

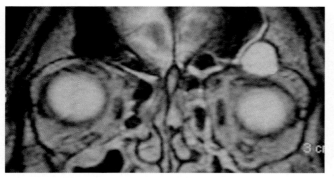

FIGURE 1.19C

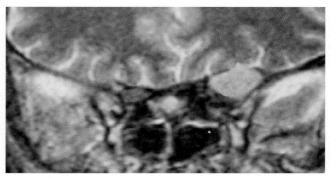

FIGURE 1.19F

FINDINGS The upper row of images (Fig. 1.19A–C) shows a lesion causing bone remodeling of the left orbital roof. The lesion signal characteristics on T1W (Fig. 1.19B) and T2W (Fig. 1.19C) MR images are consistent with slightly proteinaceous fluid. On the lower row of images (Fig. 1.19D–F), a similar lesion is seen at the orbital apex. The higher signal intensity on T1 (Fig. 1.19E) is compatible with highly proteinaceous fluid or blood. The cyst causes severe compression of the optic canal and nerve.

DIFFERENTIAL DIAGNOSIS Traumatic hematocyst

DIAGNOSIS Traumatic hematocyst

DISCUSSION Intraorbital hematomas may develop into hematic cysts. The presented patient had a history of blunt trauma to the orbit. This must have led to a subperiosteal hematoma at the time. Hematomas may resorb, but they can also become persistent. If so, cholesterol clefts will be formed within the hematoma and a granulomatous reaction to blood product debris will develop around the hematoma. This chronic inflammatory response and internal rebleeding may give cause to a slowly growing mass, eventually causing remodeling and sometimes dehiscence of adjacent bone. The pattern of bone expansion will help to differentiate a hematic cyst from a meningocele. Hematic cysts will only become symptomatic when large enough to cause proptosis, ocular dysmotility, or decreased visual acuity. This may be months to years after the initial trauma.

Question for Further Thought

1. Name three nontraumatic causes of intraorbital hematomas.

Reporting Responsibilities

A delayed posttraumatic complication putting the optic nerve at risk should be communicated urgently; otherwise, reporting may be routine.

What the Treating Physician Needs to Know

- Whether or not bony injury is present
- Is there posttraumatic soft tissue injury or herniation?
- Are any foreign bodies present?
- What is the status of the orbital apex and optic nerve?

Answer

1. Anticoagulation, coagulopathies, ruptured vascular malformation

LEARN MORE

See Chapters 63, 10, and 11 in *Head and Neck Radiology* by Mancuso and Hanafee.

CASE 1.20

CLINICAL HISTORY *A patient presenting with facial pain in the distribution of cranial nerve V1 on the left.*

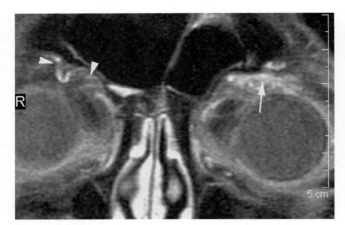

FIGURE **1.20A**

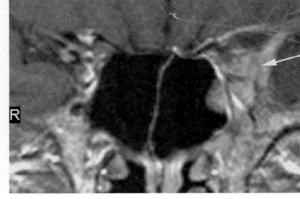

FIGURE **1.20C**

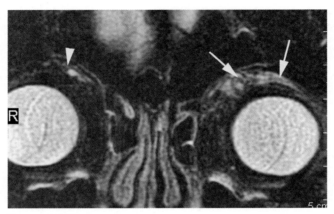

FIGURE **1.20B**

FINDINGS On coronal T2W MRI (Fig. 1.20A), subtle infiltration of the extraconal fat is seen along the supraorbital neurovascular bundle. Postcontrast FS T1W images (Fig. 1.20B,C) show enhancement following the course of the neurovascular bundle and extending into the orbital fissure.

DIFFERENTIAL DIAGNOSIS Inflammatory or neoplastic infiltrative process: pseudotumor, lymphoproliferative disease, perineural tumor spread, metastatic disease

DIAGNOSIS Perineural tumor spread along cranial nerve V1 in a patient with a history of skin cancer

DISCUSSION The extraconal space is often involved in orbital disease, but it is usually not the site of disease origin. A thorough evaluation of related or underlying disease in the surrounding structures such as the sinonasal region, lacrimal gland, skull base, or meninges may reveal the causative fac-

tor. The location and extent of disease may also be of considerable help in the differential diagnosis. Bilateral disease is suggestive of systemic disease. Spread along neurovascular bundles is typically seen in fungal disease in immunocompromised patients but may also be the result of tumor spread or perineural growth from adenoid cystic carcinoma, squamous cell carcinoma (SCCa), sarcoma, or neurotropic lymphoma.

Good medical history taking is important to further interpret such imaging findings.

The presented patient had a skin cancer removed 1 year before the MR examination, and perineural tumor spread to the first branch of the trigeminal nerve was confirmed.

Questions for Further Thought

1. Describe the imaging features of perineural tumor spread.
2. What conditions may mimic perineural tumor spread?

Reporting Responsibilities

For any extraconal orbital mass, the precise location and extent must be described. The most likely diagnosis should be established, and any threat for compressive optic neuropathy or aggressive behavior suggestive of malignancy should be reported verbally and urgently.

What the Treating Physician Needs to Know

- If the tumor is arising in the extraconal compartment
- Whether the tumor is primarily in the extraconal fat, subperiosteal, or coming from bone or surrounding structures such as the sinuses, nasal cavity, or lacrimal gland
- Full extent of disease and most likely diagnosis

- Does the situation constitute an emergency relative to preserving vision?

Answers

1. Obliteration of the tissue planes around the neurovascular structures, enlargement and/or enhancement of the nerve, erosion of the bony canal or foramen
2. Enhancement of the normal perineural vascular plexus, neuritis (e.g., viral or postradiation therapy)

LEARN MORE
See Chapters 64 and 24 in *Head and Neck Radiology* by Mancuso and Hanafee.

CLINICAL HISTORY *An adult with a slightly tender, firm orbital mass.*

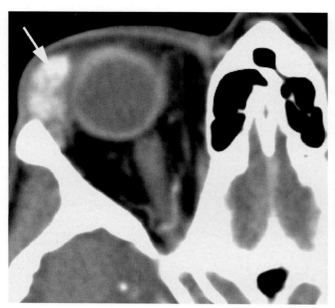

FIGURE **1.21A**

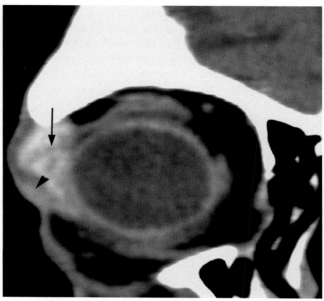

FIGURE **1.21B**

FINDINGS Axial (Fig. 1.21A) and coronal (Fig. 1.21B) CECT images showing a swollen lacrimal gland with fairly marked intrinsic contrast enhancement (arrows in both A and B) and abnormal but less-enhancing tissue surrounding the gland (arrowhead in Fig. 1.21B).

DIFFERENTIAL DIAGNOSIS Infectious dacryoadenitis, noninfectious inflammatory conditions including the autoimmune Sjögren and Graves diseases, sarcoidosis, Wegener's granulomatosis, and the Langerhans and other histiocytoses including Rosai-Dorfman, xanthogranulomatous disease, and Erdheim-Chester disease.

Lymphoma and epithelial or rare vascular tumors might also be included as well as vascular malformations. Lymphoepithelial cysts are associated with HIV.

DIAGNOSIS Lacrimal gland form of IOIS, also known as pseudotumor

DISCUSSION IOIS is an acquired immune-based process that lacks systemic involvement. It is a sporadic disease with no known predisposing factors. Although not as common as thyroid ophthalmopathy, it is one of the more frequent causes of orbital disease and is diagnosed in approximately 5% of these cases.

Orbital pseudotumor is the most common unilateral, noninfectious inflammatory condition that involves the lacrimal gland. The lacrimal form of pseudotumor will most commonly involve the entire gland, eyelid, and adjacent extraconal fat.

Pseudotumor almost always presents as a unilateral swollen and painful orbital mass most typically in the upper outer quadrant when it is of primarily lacrimal origin. It may present acutely, in which case there is greater pain and redness, or it may present more chronically, in which case there may only be a painless superior temporal mass variably associated with fixation of the globe and/or its muscles. It is occasionally bilateral. The other noninfectious inflammatory diseases are more likely bilateral than pseudotumor and the degree of pain and swelling in the lacrimal gland region less. All disease may have associated conjunctivitis and a discharge. The eye may be displaced inferior and medially.

As just emphasized, the other noninfectious inflammatory conditions, including all of those named above in the Differential Diagnosis section, strongly tend to be bilateral. Tumors and other infiltrating processes can have an appearance identical with orbital pseudotumor. The age of the patient, bilateral findings, and/or associated systemic disease help to narrow the differential to IOIS versus one of several noninfectious inflammatory diseases, as well as lymphoma, in most cases. The clinical presentation of an acute, unilateral, painful swelling, possibly with proptosis, will almost always push the main diagnosis to pseudotumor or an infectious dacryoadenitis. If the presentation is a more chronic one with a unilateral painless superior temporal mass, the differential diagnosis centers between lacrimal gland tumor and pseudotumor.

Question for Further Thought

1. How might the definitive diagnosis of pseudotumor be confirmed in its acute and/or more chronic presentations?

Reporting Responsibilities

Many cases of orbital disease that are suspicious for an acute noninfectious inflammatory disease are also suspicious for infection or aggressive neoplasm; thus, direct communication with the treatment team is often appropriate. This becomes mandatory if an alternative causative pathology such as orbital abscess is discovered or if vision is threatened.

The report should endeavor to establish the etiology if it is not known and describe the full extent of the causative pathologic condition identified. Infectious inflammatory conditions should also be considered. It is particularly important to note one way or the other whether the disease is unilateral, bilateral, or multifocal. Also, a definitive statement should be made as to whether any adjunctive intracranial or other findings are present that would aid in the differential diagnosis or present a less risky site for tissue sampling other than the orbit.

What the Treating Physician Needs to Know

- Whether the disease is likely an infectious or noninfectious inflammatory process
- Most likely diagnosis and full extent of disease
- If infection is likely, is there a local source of infection?
- If the disease is an acute infection, does the situation constitute an emergency relative to preserving the eye function, such as when tension orbit is present?

- Are any complications present outside of those related to the orbit?
- If a noninfectious inflammatory disease, is it likely to be pseudotumor/IOIS?
- Are any foreign bodies present?

Answer

1. In the acute or subacute setting, the diagnosis of IOIS is typically made by a therapeutic trial of steroids or cyclophosphamide and/or biopsy, although sometimes antibiotics are given first to rule out an atypical presentation of orbital cellulitis or dacryoadenitis. Acute orbital pseudotumor will respond dramatically to steroids. If other noninfectious inflammatory disease is identified, steroid or immunosuppressive therapy may also be instituted so that in this regard responsiveness to these medical options is nonspecific in unilateral disease. Also, lymphoma may respond, at least initially, to such treatment.

    Biopsy is almost always considered in the chronic presentation because of the necessity to rule out a malignant tumor.

> ### LEARN MORE
> See Chapters 65 and 18 in *Head and Neck Radiology* by Mancuso and Hanafee.

CLINICAL HISTORY *An adult with a right orbital mass and facial pain.*

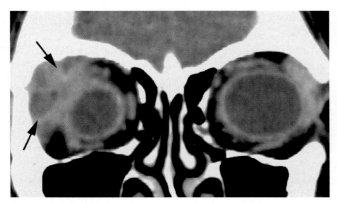

FIGURE **1.22A**

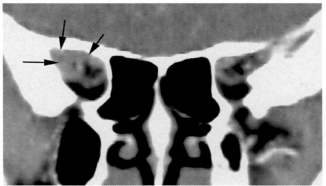

FIGURE **1.22B**

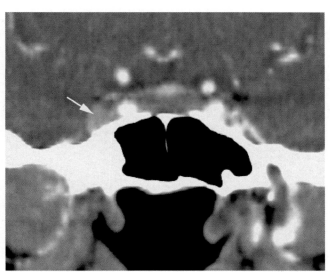

FIGURE **1.22C**

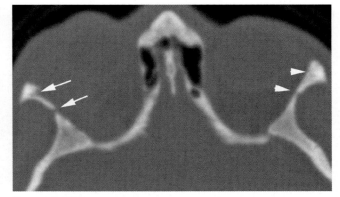

FIGURE **1.22D**

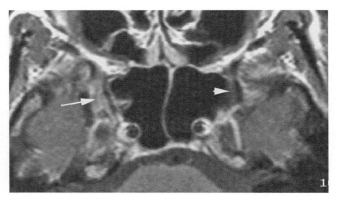

FIGURE **1.22E**

FINDINGS

Figure 1.22A. Coronal CT study shows the highly infiltrative mass in the lacrimal fossa (arrows).

Figure 1.22B. The mass is shown to infiltrate the posterior orbit near the orbital apex (arrows).

Figure 1.22C. Coronal reformations at the cavernous sinus show that the tumor has possibly extended through the superior orbital fissure, likely along V1 to the V2 and trigeminal ganglion region (arrow).

Figure 1.22D. There is erosion of the lateral orbital wall (arrows) compared to the left (arrowheads).

Figure 1.22E. CE T1W image shows that perineural spread along V2 (arrow) and proximally to at least the trigeminal ganglion is confirmed compared to the normal foramen rotundum region (arrowhead).

DIFFERENTIAL DIAGNOSIS Lacrimal gland origin adenoid-cystic carcinoma, lymphoma, perineural spread of skin cancer if an appropriate primary can be identified either by inspection or by history of removal of a skin lesion in the past

DIAGNOSIS Poorly differentiated adenocarcinoma of the lacrimal gland with perineural spread to at least the trigeminal ganglion

DISCUSSION Any orbital mass or disease process may be approached by first establishing whether it is preseptal or post-septal. If postseptal, it should be established that the disease process arising is primarily intraconal or extraconal or that it is transcompartmental. This case considers a lacrimal gland tumor that by anatomic definition is both preseptal and post-septal and extraconal, at least in origin. These tumors, when malignant, may spread across the other orbital compartments and become transcompartmental.

The lacrimal gland may be thought of as a minor salivary gland when considering the likely etiology of a unilateral tumor. Approximately 50% of lacrimal gland tumors are malignant, as in this case; of these, most are epithelial and the remainder are mainly lymphoproliferative tumors. Mucoepidermoid, adenoid cystic, and less well differentiated adenocarcinomas are the more common lacrimal gland malignancies. The remaining tumors include B-cell lymphomas, metastases (usually from breast or lung cancers), and more rare forms of carcinoma or vascular tumors such as hemangioendothelioma or hemangiopericytoma. Bilateral tumor involvement is almost always due to lymphoma, although that tumor may be unilateral or so asymmetric that it appears to be unilateral. When bilateral findings are present on imaging studies, sarcoidosis or other systemic disease also become reasonable considerations. In this setting, laboratory testing might support Wegener's granulomatosis with a positive cANCA, sarcoidosis with a positive angiotensin-converting enzyme (ACE), or autoimmune disease based on an appropriate immune panel result.

Benign mixed tumors are the most common benign intraglandular tumor. Dermoid cysts may present as lacrimal gland lesions, although they arise from intraorbital inclusions of ectodermal elements. Orbital nerve sheath tumors presenting in the lacrimal fossa region are rare outside of those related to neurofibromatosis type 1.

Questions for Further Thought

1. How are lacrimal gland neoplasms typically treated?
2. What imaging-derived factors may greatly alter the approach to treatment?

Reporting Responsibilities

Any lacrimal gland region mass thought to be malignant should be discussed with the ordering health care provider unless it is already known that malignancy is present. If there is a threat of compressive optic neuropathy or very aggressive behavior that suggests a malignant tumor, reporting should be escalated to very urgent unless this threat has been already established.

The report must emphasize—at the time of first discovery—that even though a mass appears benign, a primary or metastatic malignant tumor can appear benign and serial studies must be done to confirm a benign rate of progression if observation is the chosen form of management rather than removal.

What the Treating Physician Needs to Know

- If the tumor is arising from the lacrimal gland
- Is the tumor a solitary finding, or are there multiple or bilateral tumors to suggest a systemic disease?
- Are there any findings outside of those related to the lacrimal gland mass that might contribute to the diagnostic or therapeutic process?
- Most likely diagnosis and full extent of disease—for instance, whether the tumor is primarily remaining in the extraconal fat or if it involves bone or shows perineural spread. Has the lesion become transcompartmental, and does it threaten the optic nerve/sheath complex?
- Does the situation constitute an emergency relative to preserving the vision?

Answers

1. Benign and malignant epithelial neoplasms must be removed, en bloc with a cuff of surrounding normal tissue for adequate diagnosis and treatment. Radiation may be added depending on imaging and postoperative pathologic findings.
2. Bone destruction and perineural spread are very useful but uncommon clues of probable malignancy that have tremendous potential to alter the surgical and/or overall treatment plan.

LEARN MORE
See Chapters 66 and 22 in *Head and Neck Radiology* by Mancuso and Hanafee.

CLINICAL HISTORY *CT of a newborn presenting with bilateral palpable masses in the inferior medial aspect of the orbit and some upper airway noisiness.*

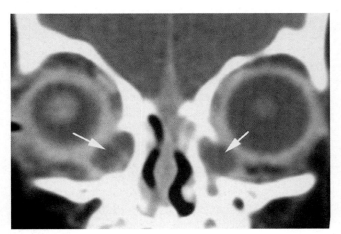

FIGURE **1.23A**

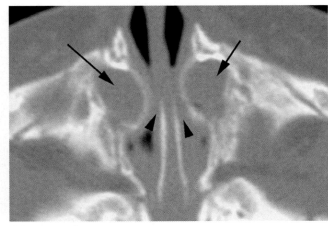

FIGURE **1.23C**

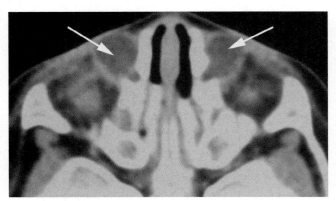

FIGURE **1.23B**

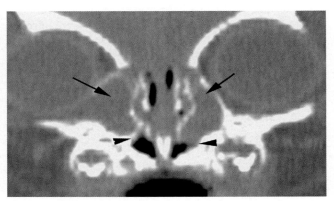

FIGURE **1.23D**

FINDINGS Coronal (Fig. 1.23A) and axial (Fig. 1.23B) sections show bilateral distention of the lacrimal sacs (arrows in A through D). Correlating bone window images (Fig. 1.23C,D) show the chronically enlarged nasolacrimal canals (arrows). The canals are obstructed at their outlet to the nasal cavity under the inferior turbinate (arrowheads).

DIFFERENTIAL DIAGNOSIS None by imaging

DIAGNOSIS Developmental dacryostenosis with secondary nasolacrimal mucoceles

DISCUSSION Developmental abnormalities of the orbit and nasolacrimal apparatus may be isolated findings. Nasolacrimal apparatus anomalies are not often associated with other findings involving the eye or orbit and not usually part of syndromes and other more generalized genetic errors.

Any orbital mass or disease process may be approached by first establishing whether it is preseptal or postseptal. Nasolacrimal apparatus problems are generally preseptal in

their manifestations. Most of these, such as absence of the valves of Hasner and those of the puncta and canaliculi, do not come to imaging, even dacryocystography.

Dacryostenosis/atresia is a spontaneous and very common anomaly. It is only rarely syndromic or associated with other conditions, although it might be present in patients with midface anomalies and clefts. In this condition, the end of the nasolacrimal duct beneath the inferior turbinate fails to completely canalize. This can result in essentially a "mucocele" or "amniocele" (in utero) of the sac and duct. High-grade obstruction can lead to marked enlargement of the canal, which, if bilateral, can actually occlude the nasal aperture. This may be associated with nasolabial cysts.

Questions for Further Thought

1. What are two more common causes of upper airway obstructions in a neonate related to facial development?
2. What is another cause of upper airway obstruction related to craniofacial development?

Reporting Responsibilities

These are typically routine studies that may be reported routinely. Direct communication is rarely required unless there is a superimposed infection or in the rare circumstance of bilateral disease that has progressed to obstruct the nasal aperture region.

What the Treating Physician Needs to Know

The report should clearly identify that this is an obstructed system and exclude an obstructing mass with as high a degree of confidence as possible:

- Confirmation of the diagnosis of dacryostenosis
- Confirmation that there is no obstructing mass
- Whether there are associated anomalies or if there is an alternative consideration

Answers

1. Choanal atresia is the most common form of infantile upper airway obstruction that comes to advanced imaging. Nasal aperture stenosis is not really common, but it is the next most likely to come to advanced imaging.
2. Encephaloceles of the anterior and central skull base may present as airway obstruction in the neonate.

LEARN MORE

See Chapter 67 in *Head and Neck Radiology* by Mancuso and Hanafee.

CLINICAL HISTORY *A young adult with swelling and pain in the inferior medial orbital region due to secondary acquired nasolacrimal duct obstruction (SALDO). Other history withheld.*

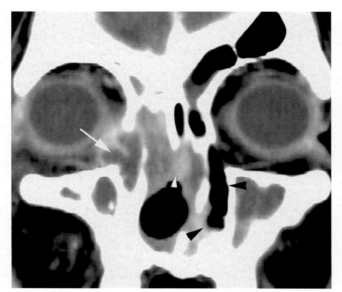

FIGURE 1.24A

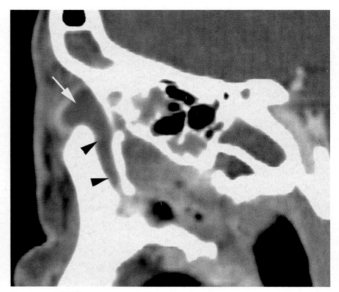

FIGURE 1.24C

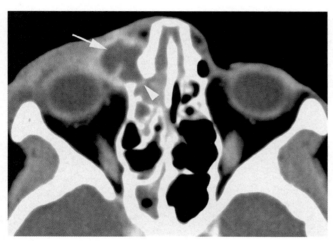

FIGURE 1.24B

FINDINGS

Figure 1.24A. CECT shows that the lacrimal sac is distended with a likely fluid collection (white arrow). There is extensive disease within the nasal cavity (white arrowhead). The nasal cavity disease also causes at least partial obstruction of the nasolacrimal duct on the left (black arrowheads).

Figure 1.24B. Axial section clearly shows that the disease presenting on the face is centered in the lacrimal sac (arrows) and that it erodes the lacrimal bone (white arrowhead).

Figure 1.24C. Sagittal reformation shows the extent of disease in the lacrimal sac (arrow) as well as in the nasolacrimal duct/canal (arrowheads) and nasal cavity.

DIFFERENTIAL DIAGNOSIS SALDO with infection due to Wegener's granulomatosis, sarcoidosis, or other rarer nasal cavity disease

DIAGNOSIS SALDO with secondary bacterial infection in a chronic cocaine abuser with cocaine-related nasal cavity disease

DISCUSSION Any orbital mass or disease process—in this case, an infection—may be approached by first establishing whether it is preseptal or postseptal. Nasolacrimal drainage apparatus problems are generally predominantly preseptal in their manifestations. Most of these infections do not come to imaging since they are caused by self-limited viral infections or easily treated bacterial infection. This case considers nasolacrimal drainage apparatus inflammatory processes and those arising in this location that might spread across the orbital compartments and related spaces.

SALDO may be due to an unknown infectious or noninfectious inflammatory process. This can also be caused by dacryoliths, tumor, radiation therapy, systemic and topical medicines, trauma, and a host of other etiologies.

Noninfectious inflammatory diseases may be local or related to systemic disease. Practically the only specific ones that involve the nasolacrimal system with any significant incidence are sarcoidosis and Wegener's granulomatosis. Primary acquired nasolacrimal duct obstruction (PANDO) is an idiopathic inflammation, and fibrosis may cause stenosis or obliteration of the nasolacrimal duct; its specific etiology is not known.

Infections, like noninfectious inflammatory conditions, may be local or related to systemic disease. Most of these conditions arise within the nasolacrimal system, with less due to secondary spread from conditions of the sinonasal region and lacrimal gland.

Infections are a common cause of SALDO. Also, infections of the lacrimal drainage system often develop in cases of PANDO and other noninfectious inflammatory causes of SALDO. These infections may be local or related to systemic disease. Most are low-grade bacterial infections from organisms such as Bacteroides, Actinomyces, and Chlamydia. Pyogenic and granulomatous (including tuberculosis [TB] and syphilis) bacterial and fungal (Candida, Aspergillus, and Nocardia being most common) infections are all possible etiologies. Immunocompromised and diabetic patients are at higher risk for some chronic bacterial or fungal infection, although these infections or colonization likely occur more frequently without those underlying disease states. Viral infections are primarily herpes varieties.

These conditions produce inflammation and various degrees of obstruction of the lacrimal drainage system. This may eventually lead to fibrosis and chronic obstruction. There may be a secondary abscess or osteomyelitis. Stones may develop in the drainage system and be a contributing factor in both recurrent disease and obstruction.

Imaging in this case strongly suggested an underlying and causative noninfectious etiology based on the pattern of disease in the nasal cavity leading to the nasolacrimal duct obstruction. Laboratory testing might support Wegener's granulomatosis with a positive cANCA, sarcoidosis with a positive ACE, or autoimmune disease based on an appropriate immune panel result. Biopsy may be necessary to exclude lymphoma or other tumors in such a situation, although in this case, it was the history that made the situation clear.

Questions for Further Thought

1. How do the nasal septum findings in particular affect the consideration of possible etiology?
2. On this particular part (anterior inferior at and just behind the nasal vestibule) of the nasal septum, what is a primary etiologic consideration?

Reporting Responsibilities

Virtually all cases suspicious for an acute infectious etiology call for direct communication with the treatment team. This becomes mandatory if there is clear evidence of abscess or any threat to vision.

The report should endeavor to establish the etiology if it is not known and describe the full extent of the causative pathologic condition if identified. In more chronic circumstances, noninfectious inflammatory conditions (previous Discussion section) should also be considered.

Chronic infectious disease usually requires only routine reporting. Direct communication is occasionally required when a mass lesion likely to be cancer is discovered or an abscess or osteomyelitis is demonstrated.

The report should clearly identify that this is an obstructed system and exclude an obstructing mass with as high a degree of confidence as possible.

What the Treating Physician Needs to Know

- Confirmation that the disease is primarily of the nasolacrimal drainage system and if there likely is obstruction
- If there are any clues to specific etiology
- Likely level of obstruction
- Whether there are complicating factors outside of the system that require treatment or further evaluation
- Whether there is an obstructing mass

Answers

1. The nasal septal perforation in particular brings diseases associated with vasculitis into the differential, including Wegener's granulomatosis, sarcoidosis, and cocaine abuse.
2. This particular part of the septum is where cocaine is typical "pinched" when snorted and really brings that possibility to the forefront. Wegener's granulomatosis and sarcoidosis tend to involve the nasal septum more in the nasal cavity than the nasal vestibule.

> LEARN MORE
> See Chapters 68 and 13 in *Head and Neck Radiology* by Mancuso and Hanafee.

CLINICAL HISTORY *An adult patient with a subcutaneous mass, somewhat painful and inflamed appearing, presenting in the inferior and medial portion of the orbit.*

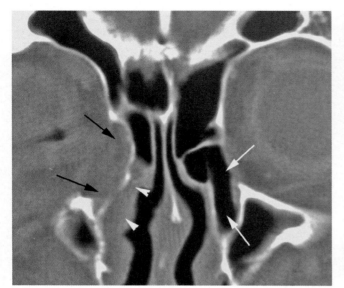

FIGURE 1.25A

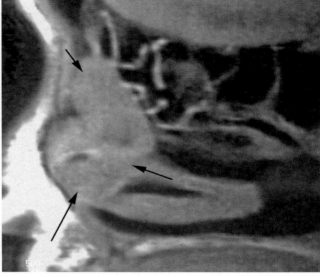

FIGURE 1.25D

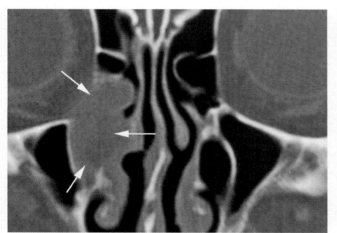

FIGURE 1.25B

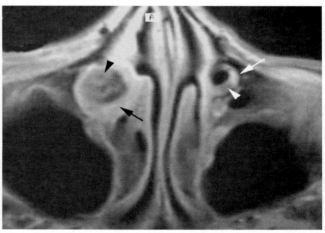

FIGURE 1.25E

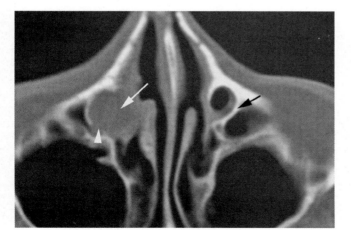

FIGURE 1.25C

FINDINGS

Figure 1.25A. There is an abnormal mass in the lacrimal fossa region (black arrows) that seems to be contiguous with abnormal tissue in the nasal cavity (arrowheads). Compare to the normal nasolacrimal sac and duct region on the opposite side (white arrows).

Figure 1.25B. A section slightly posterior to that in (Fig. 1.25A) shows that the mass conforms to the anatomy of a distended nasolacrimal sac and duct (arrows).

Figure 1.25C. Axial sections confirm that the mass is within the nasolacrimal drainage system (white arrow) and erodes bone (white arrowhead) compared to the normal side (black arrow).

Figure 1.25D. T1W MRI section on the same patient shows a mass extending along the nasolacrimal drainage system. The mass appears to likely be largely solid.

Figure 1.25E. T1W CE image shows that the mass has a complex central portion (black arrowhead) and a thick very enhancing wall (black arrow). Compare the normal nasolacrimal mucosa (white arrowhead) on the opposite side as well as the integrity of the lacrimal bone (white arrow) with that on the affected side.

DIFFERENTIAL DIAGNOSIS Chronic dacryocystitis with "mucocele" of the lacrimal sac and nasolacrimal duct

DIAGNOSIS Adenocarcinoma of the nasolacrimal sac and duct. There was inflammation, as well as tumor, present.

DISCUSSION Any orbital mass or disease process may be approached by first establishing whether it is preseptal or postseptal. Nasolacrimal drainage apparatus problems are often preseptal in their clinical manifestations. Many of these patients do not come to imaging, but almost all persistent mass lesions will come to MR and/or CT imaging. This case considers nasolacrimal drainage apparatus abnormality that was due to both tumor and related obstructive inflammatory changes.

SALDO is almost always due to an infectious or noninfectious inflammatory process; however, this can also be caused by tumor intrinsic or extrinsic to the lacrimal drainage system. PANDO is a diagnosis that can be made only after tumor and other etiologies of the obstruction are excluded.

Primary tumors of the lacrimal drainage system are rare. The benign squamous cell papilloma is most common of these rare lesions, and primary SCCa is the most common malignancy. Lymphoma may arise primarily in the lacrimal drainage system, although this also a rare event. The lacrimal sac and duct are far more likely to be involved secondarily by skin and sinonasal malignancies than by cancers arising within the sac or duct themselves. Eyelid tumors and skin cancers may involve the puncta and canaliculi.

Occasionally, tumors and other conditions within bone such as fibrous dysplasia will obstruct the lacrimal drainage system.

Questions for Further Thought

1. What class of organism might cause chronic dacryocystitis in a diabetic that might not be so common an etiology in a nondiabetic patient?
2. What are the neurovascular bundles at risk for perineural spread in these cancers?

Reporting Responsibilities
These are usually routine studies that may be reported routinely. If tumor is not the primary working diagnosis, then direct communication is wise if a likely tumor is identified. The report should clearly identify the following:

• Whether this is a tumor arising from or secondarily involving the lacrimal drainage system
• Full extent of soft tissue abnormalities including whether the orbital septum or postseptal structures are likely involved
• Extent of bone involvement if such is present
• Whether perineural spread is demonstrated and, if so, its full extent
• Whether there is regional metastatic adenopathy

What the Treating Physician Needs to Know
• Extent of the tumor as described in the Reporting Responsibilities section
• If there are any clues to specific etiology
• Whether there are potential complicating factors outside of the lacrimal drainage system that require treatment or further evaluation

Answers
1. Fungal infection
2. Primarily, the medial infraorbital distal branches where they lie deep to the superficial musculoaponeurotic system adjacent to the lower nasolabial fold

LEARN MORE
See Chapters 69 and 21 in *Head and Neck Radiology* by Mancuso and Hanafee.

CLINICAL HISTORY   *A patient with extensive orbital cellulitis at physical examination, with the extent relative to the orbital septum uncertain.*

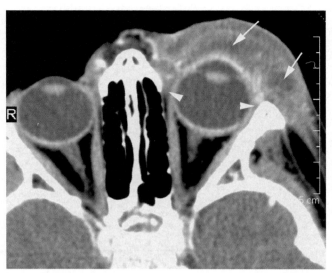

FIGURE **1.26**

FINDINGS

Figure 1.26. CECT shows very extensive soft tissue swelling limited by the attachments of the orbital septum (arrowheads) in an early suppurative stage (arrows).

RELEVANT ANATOMY   Orbital septal attachments

DIFFERENTIAL DIAGNOSIS   Abscess versus cellulitis and preseptal versus preseptal and postseptal

DIAGNOSIS   Extensive preseptal cellulitis—early suppurative stage eventually evolving to a pyogenic eyelid abscess. The source was uncertain.

DISCUSSION   Any orbital mass or disease process may be approached by first establishing whether it is preseptal or postseptal. Preseptal problems most commonly arise from the skin, eyelids, lacrimal gland, and nasolacrimal drainage apparatus—all of which are components of the preseptal space. Most of these problems do not come to imaging. This case considers a preseptal inflammatory process that arises from sources other than the lacrimal gland and nasolacrimal drainage system and has the potential to spread across the orbital compartments and related spaces.

The inflammation by definition will be anterior to attachments of the orbital septum and involving structures related to the eyelid such as the palpebral ligaments, tarsal plates, and the lacrimal sac. Swelling of preseptal soft tissues and obliteration of fat compared to the opposite side may be obvious. It is important to search for subtle elevation of the periosteum, especially along the medial orbital wall. There may be associated abscess and osteomyelitis.

Spread of lesions to postseptal spaces may be direct, via veins as with infectious thrombophlebitis and along nerves for instances in cancers. Postseptal spread will manifest as alterations of the usual appearance of intraorbital fat. If phlebothrombosis is present, it may progress to involve the major orbital veins; the veins will increase in size, and an intraluminal clot may become visible. Edema of the intraorbital fat is a generic finding and may be seen in venous congestion, thrombosis, increased venous pressure associated with regional AV fistulas, or cellulitis. Edema may also be associated with a neoplasm.

Most preseptal soft tissue infections are due to acute preseptal cellulitis due to a bacterial skin and eyelid infection. Infection may also be secondary to trauma or seen as a surgical complication. Preseptal infections with other organisms are typically secondary to viral, bacterial, and parasitic infections arising from the sinonasal region, lacrimal gland, and lacrimal drainage system.

Preseptal inflammation that mimics acute infections may also be due to insect bites and toxic exposures. It may also be due to relative nonspecific conditions such as angioneurotic edema and more rare conditions such as Kimura disease.

Questions for Further Thought

1. What is a common source of postseptal cellulitis and abscess?
2. What is the bony posterior medial attachment of the orbital septum at and just below the level of the medial eyelid canthus?

Reporting Responsibilities

Virtually all cases suspicious for an acute infectious etiology call for direct communication with the treatment team. This becomes mandatory if there is clear evidence of abscess, causative sinonasal pathology that might be treated surgically, or any threat to vision.

The report should endeavor to establish the etiology if it is not known and describe the full extent of the causative pathologic condition if identified. In more chronic circumstances, noninfectious inflammatory conditions should also be considered.

Chronic infectious disease usually requires only routine reporting. Direct communication is occasionally required when a mass lesion likely to be cancer is discovered or an abscess or osteomyelitis is demonstrated.

What the Treating Physician Needs to Know

- Confirmation that the disease is primarily of the preseptal soft tissues
- Likely diagnosis and if there are clues to aid in identifying the source of the type of inflammation/infection
- Is there a likely postseptal, lacrimal gland, nasolacrimal, or sinonasal origin?

- Is there postseptal extension?
- Whether there are complicating factors within or beyond the preseptal soft tissues that require treatment or further evaluation
- Whether there is a mass rather than an inflammatory condition or a mass complicated by inflammation

Answers

1. Pyogenic sinusitis, most typically frontoethmoidal
2. The posterior lacrimal crest

LEARN MORE

See Chapters 70 and 13 in *Head and Neck Radiology* by Mancuso and Hanafee.

CLINICAL HISTORY *An adult patient with a mass and no obvious cutaneous lesion in the nasolabial fold region.*

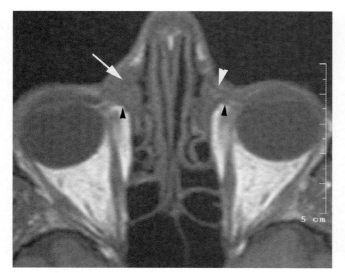

FIGURE **1.27A**

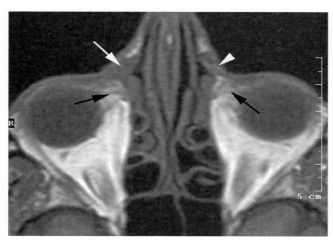

FIGURE **1.27B**

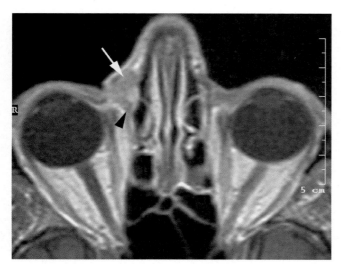

FIGURE **1.27C**

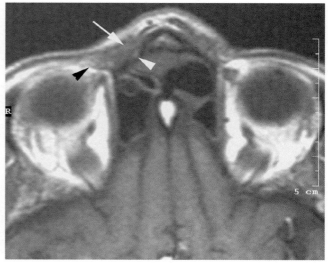

FIGURE **1.27D**

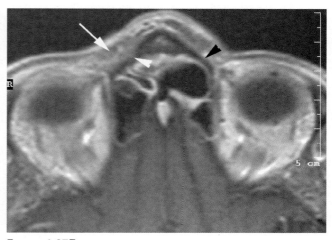

FIGURE **1.27E**

FINDINGS

Figure 1.27A. T1W image without contrast shows thickening of the preseptal soft tissues (white arrow) compared to the normal opposite side (white arrowhead). The mass is limited posteriorly by the attachment of the orbital septum (black arrowheads).

Figure 1.27B. T1W image without contrast again shows the infiltrating preseptal mass (white arrow) compared to normal preseptal soft tissues on the opposite side (white arrowhead). Note the attachment of the orbital septum on both sides (black arrows).

Figure 1.27C. CE T1W image slightly more superior than that in (Fig. 1.27B) and about the same level as (Fig. 1.27A) shows preseptal mass (white arrow) at the posterior lacrimal crest (black arrowhead).

Figure 1.27D. Non–contrast-enhanced T1W image more superior than those previously seen and along the region of the nasal process of the frontal bone. The preseptal tumor (white arrow) appears to be invading the nasal process of the frontal bone (white arrowhead). It still is constrained by the attachments of the orbital septum superiorly (black arrowhead).

Figure 1.27E. CE T1W image confirming likely invasion of bone (white arrowhead) compared to the cortical bone on the other side (black arrowhead) by the tumor spreading within the preseptal soft tissues (arrow).

RELEVANT ANATOMY The orbital septum at its attachments, especially medially to the posterior lacrimal crest

DIFFERENTIAL DIAGNOSIS Tumors in the preseptal area arise from the nasolacrimal apparatus, the conjunctiva, the adjacent facial skin, or structures of the eyelids. These are almost always carcinomas of cutaneous, adnexal, or glandular origin. Lymphoma of the conjunctiva or eyelid may occur, and if the disease is bilateral, this becomes likely. Inflammation is usually apparent clinically and not imaged. Localized bony abnormalities such as fibrous dysplasia can mimic subcutaneous cancer.

DIAGNOSIS Carcinoma arising in the preseptal soft tissues invading the medial aspect of the orbital septum and bone

DISCUSSION Any orbital mass or disease process may be approached by first establishing whether it is preseptal or postseptal. Preseptal problems most commonly arise from the skin, eyelids, lacrimal gland, and nasolacrimal drainage apparatus— all of which are components of the preseptal space. Most of these problems do not come to imaging. This case considers a preseptal subcutaneous malignant tumor that does not arise from the nasolacrimal drainage system and has the potential to spread across the orbital compartments and related spaces as well as invade bone; these factors are important determinants of the treatment plan.

Tumors may be of local origin or related to systemic disease. Practically, the preseptal space is only infrequently secondarily involved in systemic malignancies such as lymphoma or metastatic disease. Primary benign and malignant tumors arise in the skin and eyelid, with others due to secondary spread from conditions of the sinonasal region, lacrimal gland, and lacrimal drainage system.

The lesions by definition will be anterior to or involving attachments of the orbital septum and involving structures related to the eyelid such as the palpebral ligaments, tarsal plates, and the lacrimal sac. Swelling of preseptal soft tissues and obliteration of fat compared to the opposite side may be obvious. Spread of lesions to postseptal spaces may be direct, via vessels, or along nerves. Postseptal spread will manifest as alterations of the usual appearance of postseptal intraconal and/or extraconal fat. It is important to search for subtle erosion of bone, especially along the orbital septum attachments. Subtle bone erosion should always be confirmed by very

high resolution CT examinations since invasion will markedly alter the treatment approach in most patients. Moreover, MRI can never be used to completely exclude bone invasion when tumor is adjacent to bone.

Questions for Further Thought

1. Does the mass involve the orbital septum?
2. Does the mass extend to the postseptal soft tissues?
3. What neurovascular bundle(s) is/are at risk as perineural conduits?
4. What regional nodes are at risk?

Reporting Responsibilities

These are usually routine studies that may be reported routinely. If tumor is not the primary working diagnosis, then direct communication is wise if a tumor is identified. The report should clearly identify the following:

- Full extent of soft tissue abnormalities, including whether the orbital septum or postseptal structures are likely involved
- Presence and extent of bone involvement
- Whether perineural spread is demonstrated and, if so, the full extent
- Whether there is regional metastatic adenopathy
- Are their findings that suggest this is a systemic malignancy, such as lymphoma, an alternative inflammatory process, or a benign lesion mimicking a malignant tumor presentation?

What the Treating Physician Needs to Know

- Confirmation that the disease is primarily of the preseptal soft tissues
- Likely diagnosis and if there are clues to aid in identifying the source or type of tumor
- Is there a likely postseptal, lacrimal gland, nasolacrimal, or sinonasal origin?
- Extent of the tumor as described in the Reporting Responsibilities section

Answers

1. Yes. The septum is clearly involved to its attachment on the posterior lacrimal crest.
2. No. There is no evidence of direct or perineurovascular spread to infiltrate postseptal structures.
3. The supraorbital and infraorbital bundles as part of the ophthalmic and maxillary divisions of the trigeminal nerve are at risk.
4. The facial lymph nodes (infraorbital most likely), parotid, and level 1 are all at some risk.

> **LEARN MORE**
>
> See Chapters 71 and 21 in *Head and Neck Radiology* by Mancuso and Hanafee.

CLINICAL HISTORY *An adult patient presenting with ophthalmoplegia and facial pain.*

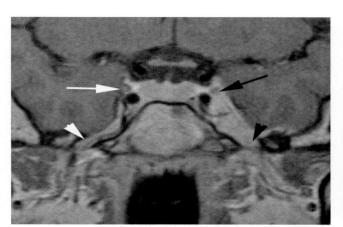

FIGURE **1.28A**

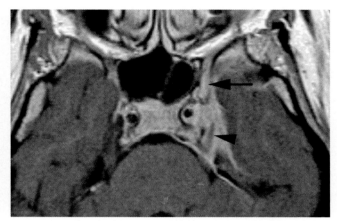

FIGURE **1.28B**

FINDINGS

Figure 1.28A. T1W CE image shows infiltration of the cavernous sinus and paracavernous region on the left side with involvement of V3 on the left (black arrowhead) compared to the normal on the right (white arrowhead). On the right side, cranial nerve III (white arrow) appears normal; that on the left appears compressed and perhaps abnormally enhancing in part (black arrow).

Figure 1.28B. T1W axial section shows the marked thickening of the V2 branch (arrow) within the foramen rotundum and shows cranial nerve III surrounded by abnormal enhancing tissue.

DIFFERENTIAL DIAGNOSIS Cavernous sinus thrombosis (bland and infectious). Infections may be local or related to systemic disease. These conditions may be due to secondary spread from eye, optic nerve and sheath, and extraconal and preseptal compartments or from sinonasal disease such as pyogenic sinusitis or rhinocerebral mucormycosis or other fungal infection.

Systemic diseases include but are not limited to sarcoidosis, Wegener's granulomatosis, and Langerhans cell histiocytosis (LCH).

DIAGNOSIS Tolosa-Hunt syndrome (THS)

DISCUSSION The noninfectious inflammatory conditions, including pseudotumor (idiopathic or nonspecific orbital inflammatory syndrome) and the related THS, commonly involve the cavernous sinus. Other noninfectious inflammatory diseases may be local or related to systemic disease. These include the granulomatoses and histiocytoses that may present and appear identical with pseudotumor (IOIS) or lymphoma. These diseases include but are not limited to sarcoidosis, Wegener's granulomatosis, and LCH.

Infections may also be local or related to systemic disease. These conditions may be due to secondary spread from eye, optic nerve and sheath, and extraconal and preseptal compartments or from sinonasal disease such as pyogenic sinusitis or rhinocerebral mucormycosis or other fungal infection.

THS, or cavernous sinus "pseudotumor," is an acquired immune-based process that lacks systemic involvement. This is probably a variation of IOIS that involves the orbital apex and cavernous sinus region. It is a diagnosis of exclusion. The process is unilateral in most cases. In bilateral cases, it is often asymmetric. Bilaterality raises the likelihood of an alternative diagnosis of systemic disease such as lymphoma or sarcoidosis.

Spread to the superior orbital fissure and orbital apex to or from the cavernous sinus is possible. It is probably reasonable to lump the steroid-responsive nonspecific granulomatous inflammation of the cavernous sinus into the generalized category of IOIS/pseudotumor. Continued spread to the middle and posterior cranial fossa is also possible.

On both CT and MRI, the inflammatory morphology appears as an indistinct, contrast-enhancing, infiltrating process involving the cavernous sinus, trigeminal cistern, and overlying dura and possibly leptomeninges often with contiguous disease at the orbital apex and superior orbital fissure. Circumferential narrowing of the anterior genu and clinoidal segments of the carotid may be seen on any vascular imaging study.

THS is usually iso- or slightly hyperintense to skeletal muscle on T2W images, the relatively low signal intensity probably being related to its fibrous and collagenous component and dense cellularity. Unfortunately, tumors and other infiltrating processes can have an identical appearance.

The other noninfectious inflammatory diseases may have a few distinguishing features from THS that might be helpful in the differential diagnosis. Associated sinonasal and intracranial findings as seen on parts of those structures included in the field of view may help with the differential diagnosis.

Questions for Further Thought

1. How might you tell a viral trigeminal neuritis from THS?
2. How might leptomeningeal involvement alter the differential diagnosis?
3. What is perhaps the most important consideration when such disease morphology is present? What should be done to raise or lower the degree of confidence in excluding that diagnostic possibility?

Reporting Responsibilities

Many cases of cavernous sinus disease that are suspicious for an acute noninfectious inflammatory disease are also suspicious for infection or aggressive neoplasm; thus, a direct communication with the treatment team is often appropriate. This becomes mandatory if there is clear evidence of compressive optic neuropathy or alternative causative pathology, such as orbital abscess or aggressive sinonasal infection, or a complicating factor such as optic nerve compression is discovered.

The report should endeavor to establish the etiology if it is not known and describe the full extent of the causative pathologic condition identified. Infectious inflammatory conditions should also be considered and carefully excluded with as high a degree of confidence as possible. The rationale, or perhaps some of the process used to exclude infection, is best documented in the report. Unfortunately, it is difficult to totally exclude fungal infection on the basis of imaging findings alone.

The report should recognize whether a complication such as vascular thrombosis or intracranial involvement of the disease process beyond the cavernous sinus region is present.

What the Treating Physician Needs to Know

• Whether the disease is likely an infectious or inflammatory process

• If inflammatory, is it likely pseudotumor/THS?
• Is an acute, subacute, or chronic infection likely, and does the situation constitute an emergency relative to preserving eye function?
• Most likely diagnosis and full extent of disease
• Is there a local source of infection?
• Are any complications present outside of those related to the cavernous sinus?

Answers

1. In viral infections, there is a distinctly perineural spread with disease localizing along the trigeminal nerve and its rootlets in the trigeminal cistern—a pattern that may aid in the differential diagnosis.
2. Diffuse or even relatively localized leptomeningeal involvement is typically not present in THS but is seen in systemic or mainly CNS noninfectious inflammations such as sarcoidosis, Wegener's granulomatosis, and LCH; and infections such as TB and other meningovascular infections as well as lymphoma or other tumors exhibiting meningeal dissemination.
3. Consider the cavernous sinus changes might be related to isolated fungal infection. Use the imaging study to identify a local source such as the sphenoid sinus or posterior nasal cavity that infiltrates the pterygopalatine fossa region to access the cavernous sinus.

> ### LEARN MORE
> See Chapters 72 and 18 in *Head and Neck Radiology* by Mancuso and Hanafee.

CLINICAL HISTORY *An adult patient with atypical facial pain and slowing developing ophthalmoplegia.*

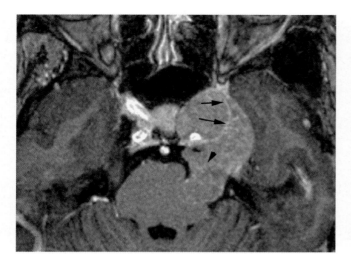

FIGURE **1.29A**

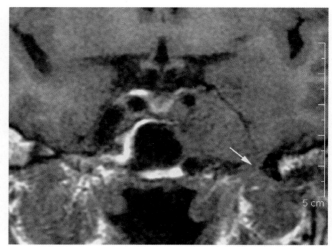

FIGURE **1.29C**

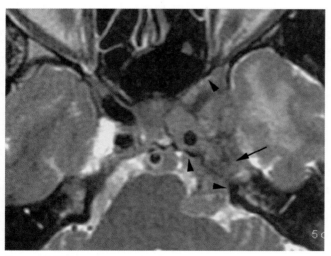

FIGURE **1.29B**

FINDINGS

Figure 1.29A. T1W CE image shows the lesion growing possibly through the petroclival tunnel toward the root entry zone of cranial nerve V on the pons (arrowhead). The tumor appears to be growing on both sides of enhancing dura (arrows).

Figure 1.29B. T2W image shows the mass to have a possible intraosseous component likely along the petrous apex and multiple areas of extension that suggest a dural growth vector (arrowheads).

Figure 1.29C. Noncontrast T1W image suggests growth across the foramen ovale (arrow).

DIFFERENTIAL DIAGNOSIS Nerve sheath tumors, metastases, lymphoma, eccentric parasellar extension of pituitary adenoma, hemangiopericytoma, slow-flow vascular malformation ("hemangioma")

DIAGNOSIS Atypical (rhabdoid) meningioma

DISCUSSION The point of origin of these lesions may be within or adjacent to the cavernous sinus. They are typically well circumscribed; thus, an infiltrative morphology suggests an alternative diagnosis of inflammatory or malignant pathology. A benign tumor arising in the cavernous sinus other than a meningioma or neurogenic tumor is very unusual.

Meningiomas are by far the most common tumor of the cavernous and paracavernous region. Occasionally, very eccentric pituitary adenomas can mimic a meningioma.

A benign neurogenic tumor of the cavernous sinus arising from a nerve other than cranial nerve V is rare. Various benign bony origin conditions of central skull base bone origin may secondarily involve the cavernous sinus.

Developmental masses that may primarily arise in the cavernous sinus region or involve it secondarily include dermoid and epidermoid cysts and vascular malformations most commonly, but less optimally, referred to as hemangiomas; the latter are rare but can mimic a meningioma.

Meningiomas of the cavernous sinus are most commonly based along its outer dural wall. Because the cavernous sinus dura forms the diaphragma sellae medially and also folds inward to form the dural membrane separating the pituitary fossa from the cavernous sinus, meningiomas can arise from these structures as well. This results in several different growth patterns: (1) meningiomas projecting external to the cavernous sinus from its outer dural reflection; (2) those arising from the diaphragma sellae that project into the suprasellar space, possibly impinging on the optic chiasm;

and (3) those arising from the internal dural reflection that remain within the cavernous sinus or the sella. Meningiomas characteristically grow on both sides of the dural membrane of origin. These features help to differentiate cavernous meningiomas from other intracavernous masses, such as nerve sheath tumors, metastases, aneurysms, and parasellar extensions of pituitary adenomas.

Facial pain of trigeminal origin is a common feature of benign or malignant cavernous sinus tumors. This may be typical trigeminal neuralgia or atypical facial pain. Involvement of all three divisions of the trigeminal nerve strongly points to the cavernous sinus as a source of pathology. Trigeminal nerve involvement may cause paresthesias and numbness as well as pain.

Ocular motility disturbance with diplopia and pupillary dysfunction is common due to cranial nerves III, IV, and VI involvement. Rarely, the diplopia is painful. A Horner syndrome may be present, or the pupil may be fairly nonreactive if both the sympathetic and parasympathetic portions of cranial nerve III are involved. Decreased visual acuity is possible.

Questions for Further Thought

1. What important search pattern must be covered even if a cavernous sinus mass appears to be a meningioma?
2. Name three developmental masses that one might encounter in or around the cavernous sinus and what may be a severe complication of one of them.

Reporting Responsibilities

Many cases of cavernous sinus disease that are suspicious for a benign tumor may, on the basis of imaging, become suspicious for a low-grade infection, low-grade malignant neoplasm, perineural cancer spread, or a vascular lesion; thus, a direct communication with the treatment team is often appropriate. This becomes mandatory if there is clear evidence of causative pathology that might result in sudden deterioration such as aneurysm or if a potentially malignant tumor is discovered.

The report should endeavor to establish the etiology if it is not known and describe the full extent of the causative pathologic condition identified. Inflammatory, vascular, and malignant conditions should also be considered in every case, if only to be excluded with confidence. Such exclusions are best documented in the report to ensure they have been considered.

What the Treating Physician Needs to Know

- If the specific diagnosis of benign tumor of the cavernous sinus can be confirmed
- If not a benign tumor of the cavernous sinus, what is the most likely diagnosis?
- If a benign tumor is present, the full extent of disease—intracranial, extracranial, and within or as it affects bone
- Specific anatomic relationship to surrounding anatomic structures, especially the carotid artery
- Whether the lesion has an extent beyond the cavernous sinus that would allow for safe imaging-guided percutaneous biopsy
- Best surgical approach based on the extent of disease
- Whether complicating factors are present such as rupture of a dermoid cyst

Answers

1. Perineural spread of cancer to the cavernous sinus must not be mistaken for a benign lesion—check the peripheral course of all divisions of cranial nerve V in all cases to exclude such a possibility with the highest degree of confidence.
2. Dermoid or epidermoid cyst, teratoma, slow-flow vascular malformation. A severe complication would be rupture of a dermoid or epidermoid cyst with secondary chemical arachnoiditis.

LEARN MORE
See Chapters 73 and 31 in *Head and Neck Radiology* by Mancuso and Hanafee.

CLINICAL HISTORY *An elderly adult patient with facial pain and numbness of all divisions of the trigeminal nerve. Remote history of skin cancer removal.*

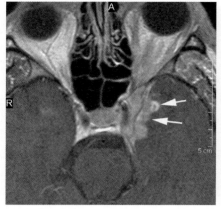

FIGURE **1.30A**

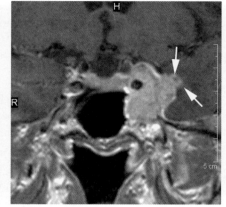

FIGURE **1.30B**

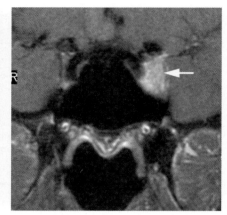

FIGURE **1.30C**

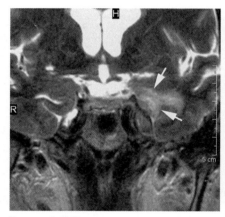

FIGURE **1.30D**

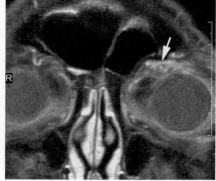

FIGURE **1.30E**

FINDINGS In (Fig. 1.30A–C), CE T1W images show an infiltrating mass in the cavernous sinus, where it invades across the lateral dura of the cavernous sinus to invade the brain. The brain involvement is confirmed by the T2W image showing brain edema in (Fig. 1.30D). In (Fig. 1.30E), the process infiltrates the superior and medial margins of the orbit potentially along the supratrochlear and supraorbital neurovascular bundles. Findings are indicated by arrows in each figure.

DIFFERENTIAL DIAGNOSIS Lymphoma/leukemia, meta-static disease, perineural spread from a primary orbital can-cer or sinus cancer, idiopathic (nonspecific) orbital inflam-matory syndrome (pseudotumor)

DIAGNOSIS Perineural recurrence of forehead SCCa along the first division of the trigeminal nerve to the trigeminal ganglion and cistern from which it invades adjacent brain.

DISCUSSION The central point of cavernous sinus malig-nant tumors may be within or adjacent to the cavernous sinus.

These malignancies are typically of an infiltrative morphol-ogy that may alternatively suggest an inflammatory etiology. Malignant tumors arising primarily in the cavernous sinus other than lymphoma are very unusual. Malignancies of the cavernous sinus are most often due to contiguous spread from the nasopharynx, sinuses, and nasal cavity either directly or perineurally, although metastasis to the cavernous sinus may be bloodborne or spread via the CSF and meninges. Perineural spread may also arise from sites geographically more remote such as the skin, as in this case. Pituitary malignancies are rare; however, when they occur, they spread directly to the cavernous sinus.

Contiguous direct cavernous sinus spread is most common in nasopharyngeal and sinonasal cancers. Direct invasion occurs via skull base erosion or through the foramen lace-rum. Perivascular spread along the carotid artery may cause such invasion without bone destruction. Perineural spread is usually seen along branches of the trigeminal nerve (V2 and V3) when the tumor involves the infratemporal fossa or masticator space.

It is extremely important to understand that a cavernous sinus malignancy might actually be due to retrograde perineural spread along branches of the trigeminal nerve from very distal and diverse sites. This is most common in skin cancer, and that pattern is the point of emphasis of this case. Skin cancers, parotid cancer, and rare neurogenic malignancies may also reach the trigeminal ganglion and cistern by way of connections between the facial and trigeminal nerve peripheral and more central branches such as the auriculotemporal nerve and vidian/greater superficial petrosal nerve, respectively. Primary neurotropic lymphoma or a primary neurogenic malignancy may also rarely present most obviously in the cavernous region, as seen on imaging. This sometimes leads to the mistaken impression that the mass is a meningioma.

Various bony-origin primary tumors of central skull base bone origin in addition to bony metastases may secondarily involve the cavernous sinus. Bone tumors run the full gamut of tissues of origin found in bone: osteogenic, chondrogenic, and those of fibro-osseous origin. Most are benign, but a malignant version of these tumors is possible. Chordoma may present with cavernous sinus localization.

Pituitary malignancies are rare; however, when they occur, they spread directly to the cavernous sinus. An eccentric benign pituitary adenoma may mimic a malignant tumor.

Malignant mesenchymal lesions of the cavernous sinus are extraordinarily rare, but secondary involvement by rhabdomyosarcoma is not uncommon in sinonasal and nasopharyngeal primary tumors.

Metastases to the cavernous sinus from tumor elsewhere, such as breast, lung, or prostate, also can occur as a relatively common etiology for this disorder.

Relentlessly progressive facial pain of trigeminal origin is a common feature of cavernous sinus malignancies. This may be typical trigeminal neuralgia but is more usually atypical facial pain. Involvement of all three divisions of the trigeminal nerve strongly points to the cavernous sinus as a source of pathology. Trigeminal nerve involvement may cause paresthesias as well as pain. Headache is also a common complaint.

Ocular motility disturbance with diplopia and pupillary dysfunction are very common due to involvement of cranial nerves III, IV, and VI. A Horner syndrome or even a nonreactive pupil, if sympathetics and parasympathetics are involved, may be present.

In cases of particularly aggressive spreading pituitary tumors, the characteristic bitemporal defects visual field defects caused by such growth might also be present.

Questions for Further Thought

1. If there was no history of skin cancer, what would be the main clue that this is perineural spread from a cutaneous malignancy?
2. What is a strong factor against pseudotumor as a likely etiology in this case?

Reporting Responsibilities

Some cases of cavernous sinus infiltrating pathology that are suspicious for an aggressive neoplasm may be confused with infection or noninfectious inflammatory disease; thus, direct communication with the treatment team is most appropriate at the time of initial imaging. The report should endeavor to establish the etiology if it is not known and describe the full extent of the causative pathologic condition identified. If additional imaging might be useful or imaging directed tissue sampling is possible, such help should be offered.

This case specifically illustrates how any case of a suspected cavernous sinus malignancy should be considered a possible manifestation of retrograde perineural spread of tumor. Each potential neural and vascular route to the cavernous sinus should be specifically evaluated in every case to exclude that possibility and language included in the report that documents such a search.

If a possible malignant tumor is discovered, timely verbal communication of that finding should be considered mandatory. This also becomes essential if there is clear evidence of progressive ophthalmoplegia, optic neuropathy, or alternative causative pathology to tumor such as invasive fungal sinonasal infection. If an alternative etiology is discovered such as an aneurysm or dissection of the carotid artery that might have thromboembolic implications, then urgent, immediate verbal communication and proper documentation of such an etiology is necessary.

What the Treating Physician Needs to Know

- Whether the mass is likely a malignant lesion arising in or secondarily involving the cavernous sinus or inflammatory process
- If malignant, can the source be established as local direct extension, perineural or perivascular spread, or extension of meningeal tumor to involve the cavernous sinus?
- Full extent of disease
- Is there any other testing that might be useful in diagnosis or treatment planning?

Answers

1. The spread pattern along the course of the supraorbital neurovascular bundle and its branches
2. Brain involvement

> **LEARN MORE**
> See Chapters 74 and 24 in *Head and Neck Radiology* by Mancuso and Hanafee.

CLINICAL HISTORY *A 63-year-old female presenting with a right cranial nerve VI deficit.*

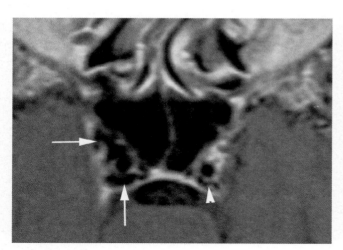

FIGURE **1.31A**

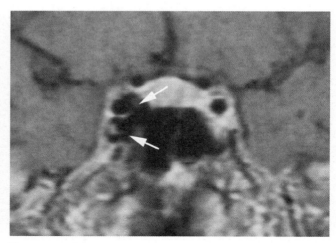

FIGURE **1.31B**

FINDINGS Axial (Fig. 1.31A) and coronal (Fig. 1.31B) T1W images. In (Fig. 1.31A), multiple nonenhancing defects are present in the right cavernous sinus region, perhaps with a serpiginous morphology (arrows), as well as on the opposite side (arrowhead).

DIFFERENTIAL DIAGNOSIS Exclude high-flow fistula and cavernous sinus thrombosis

DIAGNOSIS Low-flow (dural) cavernous carotid fistula (CCF)

DISCUSSION Symptoms of a CCF are most typically acute orbital injection, swelling, and proptosis. There may be pulsating exophthalmos and an orbital bruit in some cases of CCF. If complicated by cavernous sinus thrombosis, pain and ophthalmoplegia are also likely. In this case, there was only a cranial nerve VI palsy causing an ocular motility disturbance.

The two most common AV shunts involving the orbit are (1) high-volume, high-flow fistulas involving the cavernous segment of the internal carotid artery and the cavernous sinus and (2) low-volume, low-pressure dural AV fistulas or malformations involving the dural arteries of the cavernous sinus, as in this case. Transmitted arterial pressure in carotid cavernous and dural fistulas to the cavernous sinus reverses flow from the ophthalmic veins. This retrograde drainage may create orbital edema and injection of the conjunctiva. Another complication of cavernous AV shunts is cavernous sinus venous thrombosis.

The imaging features of dural fistulas are similar but usually less severe than those of CCF. This low-volume, low-pressure shunt can exhibit features of either small AV fistulas or even complex AV malformations. Dural sinus thrombosis is a common link in the mechanism of formation of dural fistulas. In some cases, the shunt occurs first and results in dural sinus stasis with thrombosis. In other cases, the dural sinus thrombosis occurs first and the dural fistula develops with neovascular growth into the thrombus. AV fistulas cause cavernous sinus stasis by balancing the pressure of afferent venous input from the orbit via superior ophthalmic veins, the dura of the anterior fossa via the superior clinoidal sinus, as well as from the sphenoparietal sinus. As the cavernous sinus outlets thrombose, back pressure occurs in the afferent vessels. Propagation of thrombus can occur as well into the temporal lobe veins, which drain into the sphenoparietal sinus, or into the orbital veins. The ultimate effect of the partial cavernous sinus thrombosis is to reverse flow in the orbit, which may cause the scleral injection, the orbital edema, and the proptosis. The development of these signs is more gradual because of the low-flow nature of these fistulas; thus, in some cases, like this one, only a cranial nerve VI deficit may be seen at presentation.

Questions for Further Thought

1. When might further imaging be necessary for diagnosis of a CCF?
2. How might a CCF be treated?

Reporting Responsibilities

A high-flow CCF must be discussed immediately since there can be a threat to vision the longer treatment is delayed.

A low-flow CCF should also be reported promptly and directly so that the circumstances of a causative infectious cavernous sinus thrombosis can be considered and excluded thus helping with a decision about whether antibiotics and/or anticoagulant therapy might be started to help avoid potential permanent ophthalmoplegia. In the case presented case, the results of a low flow CCF were called to the treating neuro-ophthalmologist.

What the Treating Physician Needs to Know

- Whether there is a vascular lesion of the cavernous sinus
- If so, what type?
- If there is a complicating factor such as cavernous sinus thrombosis
- Is the vascular lesion an immediate threat, such as that posed by an infectious or false aneurysm?
- If an alternative diagnosis is more likely
- Is there any other testing that might be useful in diagnosis or treatment planning?

Answers

1. The degree of vascular congestion and the degree of cavernous sinus and ophthalmic vein dilatation may determine whether dural fistulas can be detected by MR techniques or whether CT angiography or catheter angiography is required for confirmation. Catheter angiography remains a mainstay of diagnosis and is always a prelude to endovascular treatment. This study will most accurately depict the flow dynamics and angioarchitecture of the lesions as described in the previous section on pathophysiology of CCF. Newer 320 multidetector CT technology or its equivalent may nearly fully replace catheter angiography for diagnosis and therapy planning.

2. Carotid compression or observation may be the only treatment necessary in a low-flow CCF. Endovascular treatment may be required in a recalcitrant case. Septic cavernous sinus thrombosis (not a significant consideration in this case) requires immediate and aggressive antibiotic therapy. Cavernous sinus thrombosis may be treated with anticoagulants.

> ## LEARN MORE
> See Chapters 75 and 9 in *Head and Neck Radiology* by Mancuso and Hanafee.

CLINICAL HISTORY   *A 42-year-old female with slow onset of double vision.*

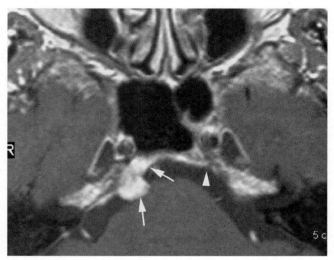

FIGURE **1.32**

FINDINGS

Figure 1.32. Contrast-enhanced magnetic resonance (CEMR) study shows an enhancing dural-based process (arrow) at the opening of Dorello's canal (arrowhead on normal side) as the cause.

DIFFERENTIAL DIAGNOSIS The cisternal segment may be involved by an aneurysm or extra-axial tumors—the most common, by far, being a meningioma and much less frequently a schwannoma. Schwannomas of cranial nerve VI are rare. Uncommon pathologies include dural and leptomeningeal chronic inflammatory diseases as diverse as sarcoidosis, Lyme disease, and chemical meningitis from a ruptured dermoid or rarely epidermoid cyst and infiltrating malignancies such as lymphoma and leukemia and meningeal carcinomatosis; these occasionally appear to be focal.

DIAGNOSIS Meningioma with involvement of cranial nerve VI at Dorello's canal

DISCUSSION MR, possibly including MR angiography, is the primary tool to investigate a possible structural cause for a cranial neuropathy that is likely to involve cranial nerves III, IV, or VI. CT may be used if the pathology might be of primarily bony origin or CT angiography might be required to more confidently exclude an aneurysm. MRI and MR angiography cannot be trusted to confidently exclude all conditions that may lead to these neuropathies, and adjunctive CT and CT angiography should be done whenever there is a strong suspicion of pathology in the face of a negative MR study.

Once a meningeal (dural, leptomeningeal, or both) lesion is identified, it is essential to determine whether this is secondary to a process arising primarily in bone or the meninges and then to establish whether the disease is multifocal of an isolated area of involvement. Isolated disease is most likely a meningioma but could be secondary to a bony abnormality, while multifocal disease will suggest a systemic disease, meningeal infection, or possibly a meningeal spreading malignancy.

In the evaluation of cranial neuropathies, diagnostic imaging, even performed optimally, sometimes fails to find a reason for the deficits even though significant pathology is present. In such a circumstance, if symptoms persist or progress, repeat studies are a reasonable part of the diagnostic strategy. Since diagnostic imaging can never exclude meningeal disease, lumbar puncture also becomes an important consideration in some cases when imaging is negative or suggests an inflammatory or euplastic etiology.

Questions for Further Thought

1. What segments of cranial nerve VI are involved?
2. How do you approach the systematic evaluation of a patient with a cranial nerve deficit?

Reporting Responsibilities

In general, the causative pathology producing such deficits should be discussed directly with the referring health care provider if the study is the initial one to demonstrate the disease. At the time of first imaging confirmation that disease is present, some of these diseases have the potential to progress rapidly. Facilitated communication may limit morbidity.

Special circumstances that require immediate direct communication with the referring treatment provider and documentation of that communication might include discovery of a vascular abnormality such as an aneurysm or CCF. A pupil-involving cranial nerve III palsy caused by aneurysm, with or without associated subarachnoid hemorrhage, is an emergency requiring immediate neurosurgical consultation. A likely cancer or inflammatory disease, such as aggressive fungal sinusitis that is likely to be rapidly progressive and threaten vision or other additional morbidity, should be communicated verbally.

It is important that the report contains a complete assessment of the extent of disease or tumor, including a statement of its relative significance to the diagnostic or therapeutic decision making at hand. These factors are suggested in the next section in summary form.

What the Treating Physician Needs to Know

- If there is a structural cause for the neuropathy
- Is more than one nerve potentially involved?
- What is the likely diagnosis?
- If there is an alternative explanation for the symptoms or signs of the neuropathy affecting the end organ of innervation
- Would additional imaging or possibly imaging-directed biopsy aid the diagnostic process?
- Degree of confidence of a negative study excluding significant causative pathology

Answers

1. The specific pathologies that involve atypical cranial nerve palsies are variable but can be grouped by three broad mechanisms of disease, including primary neurogenic tumors, pathology that causes a particular point of compressive neuropathy, and infiltrating or otherwise destructive neuropathies.

2. It is essential to first determine the specific localization of the offending pathology. This is logically and perhaps best approached by a systematic evaluation of the nerve from its brainstem origin to its end organ(s) that generate the signs and symptoms of disease. Following that, a morphologic evaluation of the disease process will almost always lead to a specific diagnosis or very short list of possibilities. The segmental evaluation of a cranial nerve from its nucleus in the brainstem, it course through the brainstem, its cisternal segment, its foraminal segment, and then it course to its site of end innervation is a useful framework for the interpretive discipline required.

> ### LEARN MORE
> See Chapters 76 and 31 in *Head and Neck Radiology* by Mancuso and Hanafee.

CLINICAL HISTORY *A 35-year-old female with chronic headaches and slow onset of visual problems and eventually documented visual field deficits.*

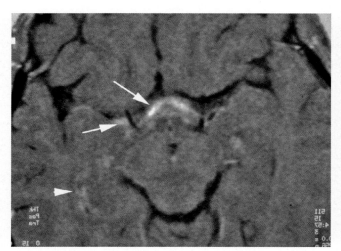

FIGURE 1.33A

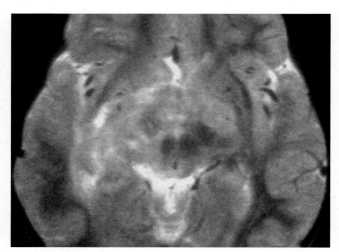

FIGURE 1.33B

FINDINGS In (Fig. 1.33A), there is a pia-arachnoid spread pattern (arrows) around the optic chiasm and in the basal cisterns and Virchow-Robin spaces (arrowhead) that perivascular spread pattern resulting the brain parenchymal changes seen in (Fig. 1.33B).

DIFFERENTIAL DIAGNOSIS A pia-arachnoid pattern in a patient with chronic complaints usually includes inflammatory conditions such as sarcoidosis, histiocytosis, TB, and neoplastic conditions including lymphoma/leukemia and carcinomatosis.

DIAGNOSIS Neurosarcoidosis manifest as a pia-arachnoid and parenchymal disease.

DISCUSSION Sarcoidosis is a systemic disease that may have more than one type of head and neck presentation, and it may mimic systemic disease such as Sjögren and lymphoma. It is likely an immunologic response to a mycobacterium infection, but this is not proven. In such a possible model of pathophysiology, it can reasonably be considered as an infectious disease or at least a "not obviously" infectious inflammatory disease. Depressed T- or B-cell function seems to be a predisposing factor in a significant percentage of patients. The disease is most prevalent in the southeastern United States and is most frequently seen in the 20- to 50-year age bracket.

Histopathology in sarcoidosis shows noncaseating granulomas. The diagnosis of sarcoidosis is made clinically by excluding other granulomatous processes while having the appropriately confirmatory laboratory studies, including a positive ACE test, Kveim test, and consistent histopathology. Imaging is supportive in most cases but in some circumstances may be the first study that actually suggests

sarcoidosis as a differential possibility because of the gross morphology and anatomic distribution of findings.

Neurosarcoidosis, in addition to affecting the visual pathways, will cause cranial neuropathies and more nonfocal intracranial symptoms as it spreads within the pia-arachnoid and along the dura. Brain and spinal cord involvement is likely due to a perivascular spread pattern; thus, it may mimic vasculitis, as seen in this case.

In CNS sarcoidosis, there will often be a clinical presentation dominated by visual problems, other cranial nerve deficits, and/or pituitary-hypothalamic dysfunction. The primary examination used for diagnosis should be CEMR, which will typically show excessive enhancement of the leptomeninges within basal cisterns and of cranial nerves. CEMR will also commonly show diffuse or multifocal dura enhancement. The meningeal findings are most easily and most often appreciated in the parasellar and suprasellar regions. This distribution of disease mimics meningeal disease due to meningeal carcinomatosis, leukemia, lymphoma, and Langerhans cell histiocytosis. Parenchymal brain involvement is usually via the perivascular spaces. Spinal cord involvement is uncommon.

Question for Further Thought

1. Does negative MRI or CT exclude a meningitic process?

Reporting Responsibilities

If the visual problem is chronic, there is often no immediate risk of further progression; however, whenever a compressive lesion is found, direct communication with the ordering provider is very wise. When the loss is acute, direct communication becomes essential whenever any compressive lesion disease process that is likely to be progressive is found.

It is important that the report contains a complete assessment of the extent of disease, including a statement of its relative significance to the diagnostic or therapeutic decision making at hand. These factors are suggested in the next section in summary form.

Often, no structural lesion is identified in a patient with a specific cranial neuropathy—in this case causing diminished visual acuity and/or visual field deficits. When the studies are negative, the patient may be reassured that there is no compressive lesion and further imaging may not be required. However, this may not create much peace of mind in someone who has lost part of his or her vision and is concerned about losing more. If the symptoms become progressively worse or an additional cranial neuropathy becomes suspect, the patient should be imaged again in follow-up.

What the Treating Physician Needs to Know

- If there is a structural, compressive cause for the diminished visual acuity or visual field deficit
- Is there likely a "medical condition" that would explain the deficit?
- Degree of confidence of a negative study excluding significant causative pathology

Answer

1. Imaging studies never exclude meningeal disease—that must be done by lumbar puncture and CSF analysis.

LEARN MORE
See Chapters 77 and 18 in *Head and Neck Radiology* by Mancuso and Hanafee.

CHAPTER 2

Sinonasal and Craniofacial Region, Including Cranial Nerve V

CASE 2.1

CLINICAL HISTORY *A 3-year-old boy presented with a swollen and tender mass over the bony brow and bridge of the nose. Selected images of postcontrast magnetic resonance imaging (MRI) are shown below:*

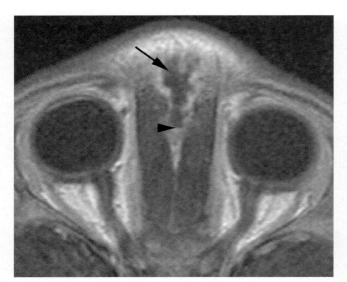

FIGURE **2.1A**

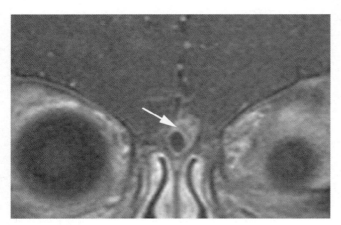

FIGURE **2.1B**

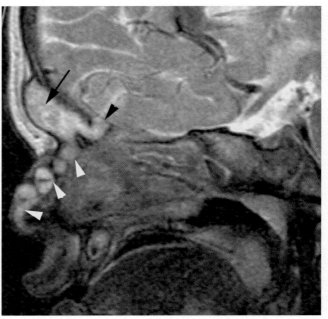

FIGURE **2.1C**

DIFFERENTIAL DIAGNOSIS If there is no skin pit, the clinical concern in infants and children typically will be encephalocele, ectopic brain tissue, dermoid, or venolymphatic malformation. Imaging will sort out those possibilities very rapidly. If infected, the main clinical concern will be a complicated sinonasal infection. Again, imaging will almost always leave no doubt about that differential possibility.

DIAGNOSIS Infected nasal dermoid cyst

DISCUSSION The development of skull combines that of the neurocranium, including its membranous and cartilaginous components; visceral cranium, including the maxilla, palate, and mandible; and development of sutures and related synchondroses.

The development of the face depends on five facial prominences. Neurogenic placodes form the olfactory, optic, and otic structures. The pharyngeal arches and pouches form the related structures of the pharynx.

All of this morphogenesis is under a high level of molecular regulation. This regulation modulates the behavior of genes that control systems such as the facial rhombomeres and neural crest elements. Errors in some of these systems result in specific known syndromes such as the Treacher-Collins syndrome (mandibulofacial dysostosis), Pierre Robin and DiGeorge syndrome, and hemifacial microsomia.

The migratory pathways of various germ cell layers cross each other during this extraordinarily complex process and are sometimes left or kept open along the way. This creates the opportunity for the formation of dermoid cysts and their

FINDINGS

Figure 2.1A. Contrast-enhanced (CE) T1W image shows an irregular, rim-enhancing and possibly infected cavity (arrow) extending posteriorly toward the expected position of the crista galli and foramen cecum (arrowhead).

Figure 2.1B. Coronal T1W image suggests intracranial extension at the posterior margin of this tract (arrow).

Figure 2.1C. Sagittal T1W image shows a larger, likely infected portion of the cyst and tract over the frontal bone (black arrow) and the tract extending within the soft tissues of the nose (white arrowheads) tracking back to the foramen cecum region (black arrowhead). However, the study strongly suggests that the process stops at the dural margin.

related tracts, meningoencephaloceles and the less common occurrence of abnormal brain tissue, endodermal remnants such as Rathke's cleft, or normal tissue such as the anterior pituitary lobe being left where it does not belong.

Nasal dermoid sinus cysts and tracts are common developmental anomalies of the face. Most present at birth and early childhood, but they may only become symptomatic in adulthood. They may present as an isolated cyst or with an opening to the skin. They most commonly appear as a midline nasal pit, fistula, or associated infected mass anywhere from the glabella to the nasal columella.

Dermoid cysts and their tracts may become intermittently inflamed and progress to abscess or osteomyelitis and rarely lead to meningitis or cerebral abscess. Connection with the central nervous system and associated congenital anomalies occur with a significant frequency. There is no known syndromic association of these anomalies.

Dermoid sinus tracts and cysts likely develop in the prenasal space, in theory when the dura protrudes through the fonticulus frontalis or directly into this space. The dural projection, which normally recedes, can retain an attachment to the epidermis and thereby trap ectodermal elements.

The role of imaging is to trace the tracts of these dermoid cysts to their proximal and distal points. This may include components in the soft tissues of the face, within or adjacent to the nasal cartilages and nasal septum, and through the anterior skull base through or in the vicinity of the foramen cecum.

Questions for Further Thought

1. What normal developmental spaces/canal exist in the anterior and central skull base that can lead to congenital masses in this region?
2. How is this condition treated?

Reporting Responsibilities and What the Treating Physician Needs to Know

- Exact extent of the dermoid cyst and related tract(s) and associated changes that may be due to infection or inflammation
- In particular, is there any intracranial or skull base attachment?
- Are there associated developmental abnormalities of the craniofacial region?
- Are there any other associated intracranial, craniofacial, or temporal bone abnormalities?

Answers

1. Transient spaces exist between the neural crest aggregates that form the skull base and nose. These spaces become the conduits for developmental midline nasal masses. The spaces are named the fonticulus frontalis, the prenasal space, and the foramen cecum.

The fonticulus nasofrontalis lies between the frontal and nasal bones. The prenasal space lies between the nasal bones, the precursor of the septum and nasal cartilages. These spaces typically fuse and ossify. When development is abnormal, dermoids, ectopic brain tissue, and encephaloceles result.

Similar important conduits in the central skull base include the intrasphenoidal synchondrosis and the craniopharyngeal canal.

The spheno-occipital synchondrosis base allows for growth of the skull base up to the time of skeletal maturity, typically in the mid teenage years. It is of only limited interest in congenital malformations.

The intrasphenoidal synchondrosis is in the midbody of the sphenoid bone just below the planum sphenoidale. It is opened at birth but closes to a sclerotic remnant that is barely visible by about 2 years of age. This can be a pathway of a central meningoencephalocele or site of ectopic brain tissue.

The craniopharyngeal canal extends from the roof of the nasopharynx to the floor of the sella during development. It is the pathway of migration for the endoderm Rathke's cleft and, therefore, the anterior pituitary gland remnants of both structures may be left anywhere along this migratory pathway. The tubular channel may persist indefinitely but is generally obliterated by bone that can be seen as a round sclerotic focus.

2. The patient was treated with antibiotics, and subsequent surgery was accomplished without an intracranial approach.

In general, nasal dermoids, gliomas, and encephaloceles are treated by complete surgical excision. Early surgical intervention is best so that the distortion of the developing face is kept to a minimum and local as well as intracranial infection is avoided. The entire lesion along with any tract must be excised in order to prevent recurrence. Imaging is critical to surgical planning to determine if there is an intracranial connection to the mass. Midline masses that have an intracranial connection will require a combined approach by a skull base team. The termination of stalk will always have to be traced to the skull base when it is any more than a fibrous residual.

LEARN MORE
See Chapters 79 and 8 in *Head and Neck Radiology* by Mancuso and Hanafee.

CLINICAL HISTORY *A 42-year-old female patient presented with spontaneous clear fluid discharge from left nose. After confirming that the discharge was cerebrospinal fluid (CSF), the patient was referred for imaging. Selected computed tomography (CT) and magnetic resonance (MR) images are shown below:*

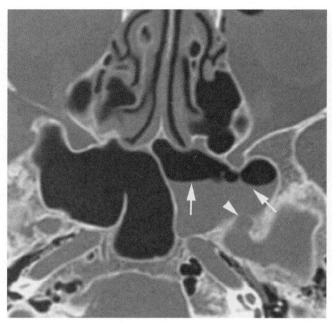

FIGURE **2.2A**

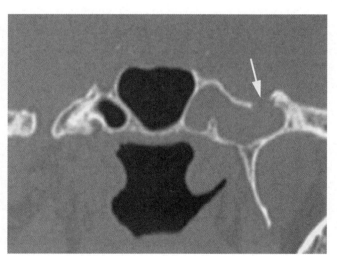

FIGURE **2.2B**

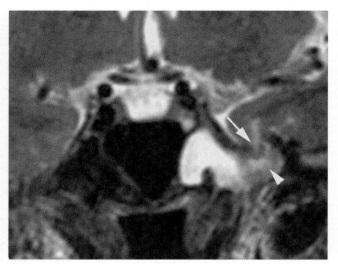

FIGURE **2.2C**

DIFFERENTIAL DIAGNOSIS None

DIAGNOSIS Sphenoid sinus defect causing CSF rhinorrhea and encephalocele

DISCUSSION Most cases of CSF rhinorrhea are due to defects in the cribriform plate. Another common area of such natural dehiscence is in the sphenoid sinus when the sinus development results in prominent lateral extension of its air cells such that the course of the maxillary division of the trigeminal nerve is along the sinus roof. The canal/groove for the nerve then provides an area of bony weakness. These natural areas of bony weakness are exposed to intermittent changes in pulsatile CSF pressure and perhaps the weight of the temporal lobe that likely cause further bony erosion over the long term. This leads to CSF leaks most commonly associated with at least some herniation of brain and meninges. Another cause of CSF leak from central skull base is arachnoid granulations aberrantly located over a pneumatized part of the skull rather than invaginated into the dura-covered peripheral intracranial venous drainage system. This creates bony weakness that when exposed to constantly pulsatile forces results in a defect that eventually produces a leak.

FINDINGS

Figure 2.2A. Axial CT section shows a sphenoid sinus fluid level (arrows) and a possible defect in the wall of the sphenoid sinus (arrowhead).

Figure 2.2B. Coronal image confirms a dehiscent sphenoid sinus roof lateral to the expected position of V2 (arrow).

Figure 2.2C. T2W MR image shows the inferior temporal lobe herniating into the defect (arrow), producing an encephalocele within the sinus lumen (arrowhead).

Questions for Further Thought

1. How was the clear fluid rhinorrhea confirmed as CSF in this patient?
2. What is role of nuclear medicine in CSF leaks, and how is the test performed?
3. What are the indications for CT cisternogram in patients with CSF leaks?
4. What treatment options do these patients have?

Reporting Responsibilities

CSF leaks may occur in settings of high or low acuity. In the setting of acute trauma, leaks are generally expected in severely injured patients; thus, direct communication is usually not necessary unless there is a defect that will obviously require surgical repair.

Direct communication is mandatory when the site may be a cause of ongoing or even recurrent meningitis and when a leak is caused by an encephalocele so that the surgeon does not inadvertently enter the meninges and brain.

What the Treating Physician Needs to Know

The report should generally cover the following issues, assuming a leak has been confirmed:

- Precise site and size of the bony defect(s) likely to be the site of leakage
- Degree of confidence in that localization
- Is there more than one possible site?
- Location of the leak site relative to known surgical landmarks such as the anterior and posterior ethmoid arteries
- Is there associated herniated brain and/or meninges?
- Is there any other testing that needs to be done to exclude herniated brain or meninges?
- Are there associated contributing or potentially complicating problems such as hydrocephalus, empty sella syndrome, or infection?

Answers

1. The nasal discharge was tested for beta-2 transferrin, which is a carbohydrate-free isoform of transferrin that is almost only found in the CSF. It is not found in blood, mucus, or tears, thus making it a specific marker of CSF.

2. Radionuclide cisternography is used to confirm or exclude a CSF leak in the face of recurrent meningitis or other suspicion of leak, if fluid cannot be collected. This technique is also valuable in the setting of questionable symptoms of continued leakage if fluid cannot be collected after a repair. While the radionuclide cisternogram is a very sensitive imaging test for confirming CSF leakage as a cause for rhinorrhea or otorrhea, it is much less definitive for precise localization. The technique involves the injection of radiotracer into the thecal space with pledget placement at the site of potential leak. The specific technique is as follows: Six cotton pledgets (1 cm²) are preweighed and labeled. Via lumbar puncture, 1 mCi of In-111 DTPA is then injected into the thecal space. The patient is scanned at 1 hour. If and when activity reaches the basal cisterns, a serum sample is drawn, and ENT is notified for pledget placement (typically six pledgets are placed, three on each side in the upper, middle, lower meatus). After 4 hours, the pledgets are removed; a serum sample is drawn, and SPECT scan of the head is obtained. The pledgets are weighed (preweight − postweight = weight of fluid in milliliters = grams). From the blood sample, serum activity in counts/seconds is determined. The pledget count rate is expressed as a ratio to that of serum. A ratio of greater than 1.5 above serum activity is considered an active leak. It is rare to see an active leak on the SPECT images; the pledget data are the key.

3. Defects leaking CSF can be detected by using careful multiplanar CT techniques without intrathecal contrast, at times combined with MR, about 90% to 95% of the time. Intrathecal contrast CT cisternography may help find the site of the leak in very complex or problem cases, such as those with multiple potential sites of leakage or when the surgical approach may be complicated, and when the leak is active. In the temporal bone, where fluid may not be available, testing for a leak with positive contrast CT cisternography makes more sense.

4. Bed rest, elevation of the head, avoidance of straining, and decreasing CSF pressure with the use of a lumbar drain are effective conservative options after blunt trauma or skull base surgery. Surgical repair is indicated for patients with traumatic CSF leaks who do not respond to conservative therapy and in almost all spontaneous leaks. CSF leaks may be repaired by intracranial, extracranial, and transnasal endoscopic repair. The endoscopic intranasal management of CSF rhinorrhea is the currently preferred method. In properly selected patients, it has a high success rate and less morbidity than other approaches. A fistula of the sphenoid sinus may be repaired with a graft via an intracranial, usually extradural, middle fossa approach and/or packing the sinus with fat and hydroxyapatite cement. In this patient, due to the encephalocele, an intracranial approach was used.

LEARN MORE
See Chapters 80 and 8 in *Head and Neck Radiology* by Mancuso and Hanafee.

CASE 2.3

CLINICAL HISTORY *A newborn boy presented with respiratory distress, feeding difficulties, and in whom it was difficult to pass nasogastric tube. CT images are shown below. (Please note that Fig. 2.3B is a normal CT shown for comparison.)*

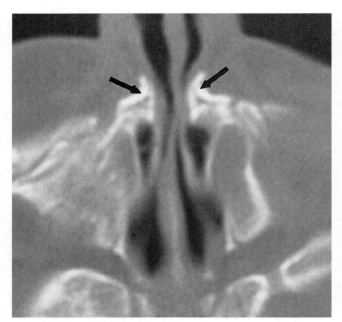

FIGURE 2.3A

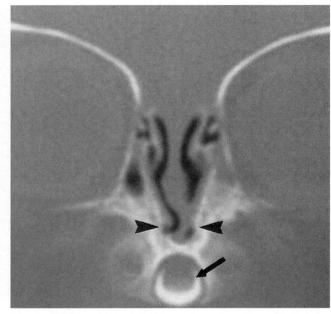

FIGURE 2.3C

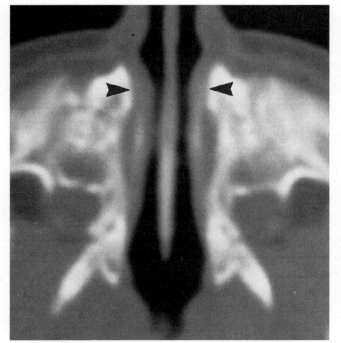

FIGURE 2.3B

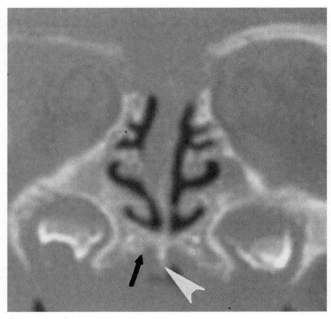

FIGURE 2.3D

FINDINGS

Figure 2.3A,B. Axial image in Fig. 2.3A through the lower pyriform aperture. The nasal process of the maxilla is medially displaced bilaterally (arrows) and thus narrows the pyriform aperture. This does not appear to be a true bone overgrowth but rather a medialization of normally configured structures; compare this appearance with that of the normal pyriform aperture in (Fig. 2.3B) in a different patient.

Figure 2.3 C. Coronal image through the pyriform aperture shows a single mega incisor (arrow) and severe narrowing of the inferior pyriform aperture (arrowheads).

Figure 2.3 D. Coronal image through the nasal cavity. Note the narrow palate (arrow) with an inferiorly projecting midline ridge (arrowhead).

DIFFERENTIAL DIAGNOSIS The clinical differential diagnosis is usually between choanal atresia and congenital nasal pyriform aperture stenosis (CNPAS). Otherwise, nasal obstruction in infants who come to imaging will be due to developmental masses such as an encephalocele or teratoma, nasolacrimal duct obstruction, venolymphatic or other vascular malformation, or even more rarely a tumor such as a chordoma or rhabdomyosarcoma. Imaging will sort out the differential definitively in virtually all cases.

DIAGNOSIS CNPAS

DISCUSSION The medial maxillary swelling forms the philtrum of the lip and the structures of the primary palate, including the four incisors. A deficiency in the size of the primary palate causes the changes seen in patients with CNPAS. A primary palatal deficiency also explains the abnormal incisors, narrow inferior portion of the nasal cavity, and triangular palate that are present. The deficient primary palate and palatal shelves may develop closer to the midline than normal where they may overlap and subsequently create a ridge along the inferior aspect of the palate seen in patients with CNPAS. This mechanism also explains the anterior narrowing of the nasal cavity and it being predominantly a medial to lateral phenomenon.

The clinical presentation is typical, as seen in this patient. If the patient presents within the first few months of life, it is usually triggered by an upper respiratory infection that further compromises an already narrowed nasal passage.

The diagnosis is made with CT of the nasal cavity. The average widths of the normal pyriform aperture at ages 0 to 3 months, 4 to 6 months, and 10–12 months are 13.4, 14.9, and 15.6 mm, respectively.

Patients with CNPAS have a pyriform aperture width of less than 8 mm compared to a normal of not less than 11 mm. This single measurement is the most useful for making the diagnosis of CNPAS. The height of the nasal cavity is essentially normal in patients with CNPAS. CNPAS, therefore, is an anomaly that narrows the entire nasal cavity, being most severe anteriorly and inferiorly. Adjunctive findings include a bony ridge along the inferior aspect of the palate and dental anomalies involving the incisors that are abnormally large and/or malpositioned.

Question for Further Thought

1. How is CNPAS treated?

Reporting Responsibilities
Conditions that affect the airway should always be reported promptly and directly to the health care provider or even emergently to a referral service that might need to manage the airway.

What the Treating Physician Needs to Know

- Is there a nasal cavity or nasopharyngeal obstruction?
- If so, is it due to choanal stenosis, CPNAS, or a mass of some sort?
- If it is a mass, does it have a possible intracranial or skull base attachment, or is there any further imaging required to define the nature of the mass?
- Is it an encephalocele or ectopic brain?
- Could it be a vascular malformation or tumor?
- If developmental in nature, are there associated abnormalities of the craniofacial region, and are there any associated intracranial abnormalities?

Answer

1. The prognosis for patients with isolated CNPAS is excellent. Most of these patients are treated conservatively with special feeding techniques until the nasal cavity grows, and, consequently, the obstruction is relieved.

LEARN MORE
See Chapter 81 in *Head and Neck Radiology* by Mancuso and Hanafee.

CASE 2.4

CLINICAL HISTORY *A 2-year-old boy presented with a slowly growing soft mass in the right submandibular region. He recently had a viral upper respiratory infection, during which this mass enlarged to the present size. He does not complain of pain or itching. Contrast-enhanced computed tomography (CECT) was performed, and selected images are shown below:*

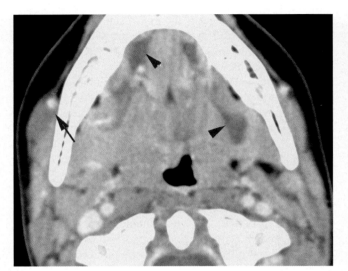

FIGURE **2.4A**

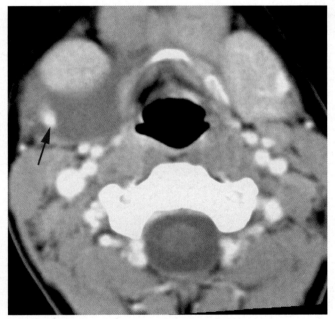

FIGURE **2.4B**

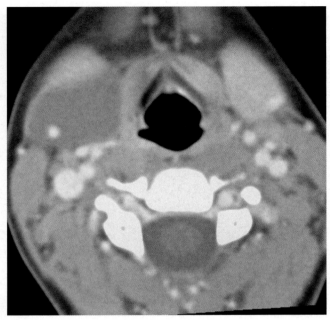

FIGURE **2.4C**

FINDINGS

Figure 2.4A–C. CECT images show a fluid density lesion insinuating around vessels (arrows in Fig.2.4A and B) and within existing spaces (arrowheads in Fig.2.4A and C).

DIFFERENTIAL DIAGNOSIS Branchial apparatus cyst if unilocular, epidermoid, ranula, and plexiform neurofibroma are the main differential considerations. This lesion was initially mistaken for a ranula. Imaging can easily differentiate these lesions.

DIAGNOSIS Lymphangioma of the floor of the mouth and the submandibular space

DISCUSSION Venolymphatic malformations arise as a result of a disordered connection between the lymphatic and venous systems. The lymphatic system develops from five primitive sacs that are derived from the venous system. If the lymphatic-venous connection fails, the accumulating lymph dilates the sacs and permeates the tissues.

It useful and necessary to lump all of the primarily lymphatic malformations into the category of venolymphatic malformation and drop the older terminology; doing so will demystify and simplify the subject somewhat and help in pathophysiology, clinical presentation, complications, and imaging appearance. All of these malformations ultimately derive from the venous system since the lymphatic system is a derivative of the venous system. Capillaries, veins, or cavernous remnants explain some enhancement. Rapid enlargement due to bleeding manifests on imaging studies as fluid–fluid levels and blood products. Since venolymphatic malformations contain lymph elements, they can also enlarge when a local immune response to viral or other infectious agents is mounted, as was the history in our case. The malformation itself might also become infected.

Venolymphatic malformations may be classified into three groups as suggested by the World Health Organization:

a. Lymphangioma simplex or capillary lymphangioma composed of thin-walled lymphatic spaces about the size of capillaries that occur in the orbit, lip, cheek, tongue, gums, and floor of the mouth where the tight connective tissue restricts the size of individual cystic spaces

b. Cavernous lymphangioma containing dilated lymphatic spaces intermixed with fibrous adventitia

c. Cystic lymphangioma or cystic hygroma composed of macrocystic lymphatic spaces measuring from millimeters to several centimeters in diameter. These tend to occur in regions where there is relatively loose areolar tissue, allowing the endothelial-lined spaces to expand and insinuate among the vessels, nerves, and muscles. Therefore, cystic hygromas are typically seen in the posterior triangle of the neck.

Syndromic associations of venolymphatic malformations include Turner, Klinefelter, and Noonan syndromes.

Questions for Further Thought

1. What is the role of imaging in venolymphatic malformations?
2. How are venolymphatic malformations treated?

Reporting Responsibilities

In general, vascular malformation is a primary differential diagnosis at the time of imaging, so no special communication is required.

Any time a vascular malformation places the airway at risk due to obstruction, communication with the referring treatment provider and documentation of that communication is necessary. If the malformation is complicated by infection, direct communication is also necessary. It is likely wise to directly communicate if there is evidence of recent bleeding into the malformation. Direct verbal communication is also wise when the diagnosis is not known since there may be excessive bleeding from planned tissue sampling or other operative intervention, sometimes as simple as a dental extraction.

What the Treating Physician Needs to Know

It is very important that the report contains a complete assessment of the nature and extent of the malformation, including all information that is relevant to treatment planning. This should include precise comments with regard to the following issues:

- Precise diagnosis and degree of confidence in the diagnosis
- Is there is an acute complication, and does the situation constitute an emergency relative to preserving some vital function?

- If significant diagnostic uncertainty exists, the odds that the condition may be a benign or malignant neoplasm as an alternative diagnosis
- Site of origin and all anatomic compartments or spaces involved, especially transcranial connections that might pose risk of an intracranial complication during attempts at ablation
- Likely nature of flow dynamics and if catheter angiography might be necessary for further clarification of that issue
- Relationship to osseous structures, particularly the alveolar ridges of the mandible and maxilla, and whether there is any associated skeletal dysplasia
- Other developmental abnormalities and the possibility of any syndromic associations

Answers

1. MR and CT easily demonstrate the full extent of venolymphatic malformations, which is not apparent on physical examination. MR is often more graphic in its presentation because of the excellent contrast between the static fluid-filled lesion and surrounding structures on heavily T2W images. Hemorrhage or infection can considerably alter the appearance of fluid. The insinuating growth pattern is almost always readily apparent on MR or CT and is the main finding that differentiates this condition from the differentials mentioned previously.

2. These lesions are usually treated surgically, but direct injection with sclerosing agents is a viable alternative for some patients. The aims are to relieve functional problems, such as with airway and feeding, while obtaining the best possible cosmetic result. Unfortunately, the lesions often do not lend themselves to easy gross total resection all of the time. They do not stay in the natural cleavage planes followed in classic surgical procedures, and they frequently wrap themselves around vital neurovascular structures. Those in the low neck may even extend into the brachial plexus and mediastinum or involve the chest wall. Islands of the malformation may be left behind purposefully so as not to sacrifice function. Repeated surgical procedures are not uncommon. Subtotal resection is more likely in the lymphangioma or combined varieties of venolymphatic malformations than in cystic hygromas but mainly depend on the location relative to critical neurovascular structures.

> **LEARN MORE**
> See Chapters 82 and 9 in *Head and Neck Radiology* by Mancuso and Hanafee.

CLINICAL HISTORY *A 43-year-old female patient presented 1 week after functional endoscopic sinus surgery (FESS) with recurrent sinus symptoms and double vision. A maxillofacial CT was performed, selected images of which are shown below:*

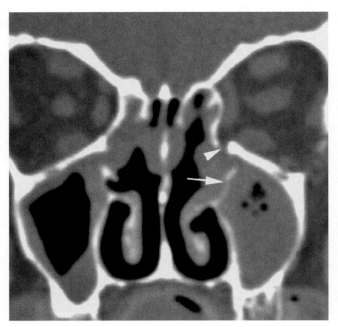

FIGURE **2.5A**

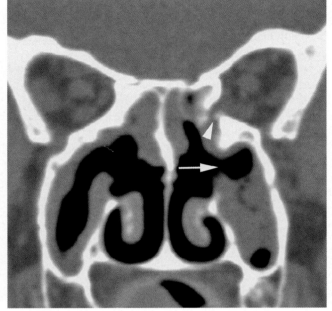

FIGURE **2.5B**

FINDINGS

Figure 2.5A. There was an incomplete resection of the uncinate process (arrow), and the orbit was entered with the microdebrider during surgery (arrowhead).

Figure 2.5B. A section somewhat more posterior shows that the patient had a fairly wide medial antrostomy but did not have a complete uncinectomy. Also, the orbital floor defect persists and the medial rectus muscle is adherent to the area of the defect, possibly injured, explaining the patient's double vision.

DIFFERENTIAL DIAGNOSIS Post FESS differential diagnosis is limited since the evaluation primarily centers on the effectiveness of the surgery and possibly complications. Thus, it would be limited to inadequate surgery and associated complications. Careful comparison with the preoperative CT would be very helpful.

DIAGNOSIS Inadvertent breach of the inferior medial wall of the left orbit leading to ocular muscle adherence and possible muscle injury causing double vision; incomplete uncinectomy and recurrent sinusitis.

DISCUSSION The fundamental assumption in FESS is that the surgical approach, to the extent possible, should preserve and enhance the normal patterns of mucociliary drainage, nasal airflow, and as much mucosa as possible. The context of the surgery might simply be restoration of normal drain-

age pathways, correction or repair of some congenital or acquired abnormality or extirpation of tumor, or complicated acute inflammatory disease. This case illustrates the importance of primary mucociliary drainage pathways. Although there was wide medial antrostomy, the patient experienced recurrent sinus symptoms perhaps because the uncinectomy was incomplete.

FESS should be a safe procedure. Anticipation of anatomic variants, such as a more medial than usual position of the medial orbital wall on the preoperative studies, might help to avoid the extremely unfortunate orbital entry and eye complications that occurred in this case.

Question for Further Thought
1. What is an Onodi cell, and what is its importance?

Reporting Responsibilities
In this case, the patient has suffered a significant complication that has long-term implications with regard to how normal ocular motility might be restored. There are also potential medicolegal implications of this complication. Such findings must be reported verbally and promptly, especially if the injury is new and there may be some benefit to early intervention.

Most sinus CT study reports are sent routinely unless there is a complex acute infectious complication of the disease that might have orbital or intracranial implications or a possible cancer is discovered. In the latter cases, timely direct verbal communication is wise.

What the Treating Physician Needs to Know

Sinus CT study performed for planning FESS:

- Extent of sinus development
- Extent of sinus disease so that it is clear if the pattern involves the frontal recess, osteomeatal, and/or posterior drainage pathways
- Extent of disease in the nasal cavity
- Anatomic variations that may be contributing to the disease patterns
- Clear statements of inclusion or exclusion of anatomic variants that might increase the risk of complications, including:
  - Anterior ethmoid artery being "on a mesentery"
  - Abnormally deep olfactory recess or reduced cephalocaudal dimension of the ethmoid complex
  - Findings suggestive of a possible anterior skull base encephalocele
  - Unusually medial position of the medial orbital wall or dehiscence or absence of the lamina papyracea
  - Protrusion of the optic nerve and/or the carotid artery into the sphenoid sinus and/or dehiscence of the bony covering over these neurovascular structures where they lie adjacent to the sphenoid or posterior ethmoid air cells or an Onodi air cell mimicking the sphenoid sinus

Sinus CT study performed for postoperative cases:

For reporting of diagnostic studies in a patient with recurrent or persistent symptoms, those studies being intended to find a cause and, if one is present, anticipated to form part of the basis of planning a repeat endoscopic sinus surgery (ESS), the following elements should be present:

- Does the study establish a likely cause for the recurrent or persistent symptoms?

- Is the recurrence due to the preexisting underlying condition, or is it the result of the prior surgery or due to conditions such as but not limited to:
  - Mobilization of the middle turbinate so that is has lateralized and assumed a position that results in obstruction to drainage
  - Inadequate uncinectomy—for instance, one that is placed too far posteriorly or causes lateralization of the residual uncinate
  - Sites of localized disease in unresected air cells
  - Cribriform plate injury or fractures of the junction of the vertical attachment of the middle turbinate with the lateral wall of the olfactory fossa such that CSF leakage may be present.

Answer

1. The most posterior ethmoid cell can pneumatize far laterally and superiorly to the sphenoid sinus. When such pneumatization occurs, the cells are referred to as sphenoethmoid cells or Onodi cells. Recognition of this anatomic variant can help the surgeon avoid injuring the carotid artery and the optic nerve. This variation, if not anticipated on preoperative imaging, can cause a surgeon to believe that he or she is in a posterior ethmoid air cell that should be well forward of the carotid artery and optic nerve rather than in an air cell that is as far posterior as the distal-most sphenoid sinus.

> ### LEARN MORE
> See Chapters 83 and 13 in *Head and Neck Radiology* by Mancuso and Hanafee.

CASE 2.6

CLINICAL HISTORY *A 10-year-old boy on antibiotics for acute sinusitis presents with redness and soft tissue swelling in the frontal region and new-onset headache. CT and MRI with contrast were performed. Selected images are shown below:*

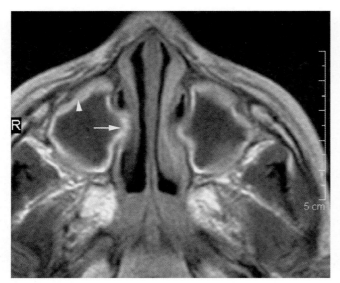

FIGURE 2.6A

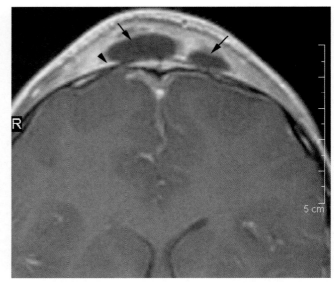

FIGURE 2.6D

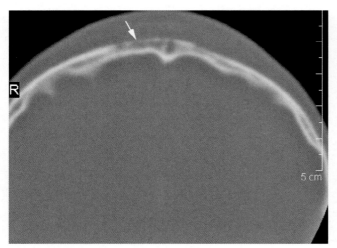

FIGURE 2.6B

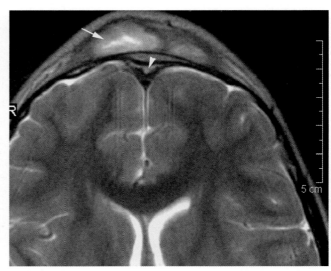

FIGURE 2.6E

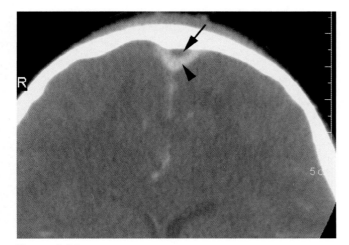

FIGURE 2.6C

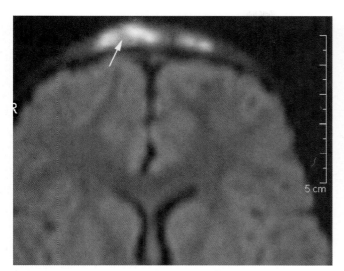

FIGURE 2.6F

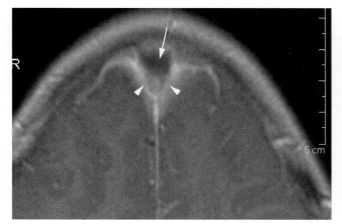

FIGURE 2.6G

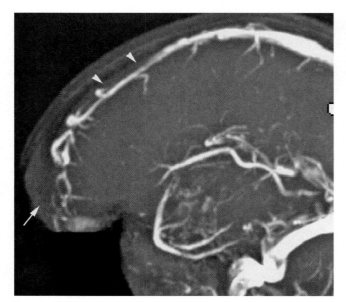

FIGURE 2.6H

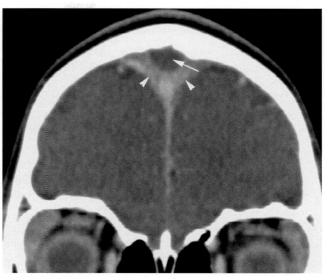

FIGURE 2.6I

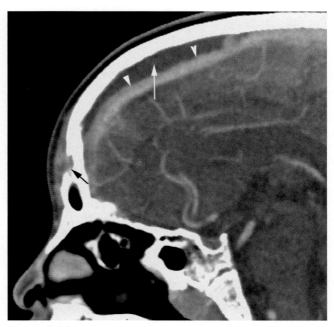

FIGURE 2.6J

FINDINGS

Figure 2.6A. The CE T1W image shows mucosal thickening in both maxillary sinuses (arrowhead) and the mucosa bulging the medial wall of the sinus (arrow), indicating that this purulent material in the sinus lumen is under pressure.

Figure 2.6B. A CT section just above the top of the frontal sinus shows erosion of the outer table of the frontal bone.

Figure 2.6C. A CECT section cephalad to that in Fig. 2.6B shows an epidural abscess (arrow) displacing the anterior-most portion of the superior sagittal sinus (arrowhead).

Figure 2.6D. The CE T1W image shows no obvious bone defect, but there are pockets of pus (arrows) within extensively swollen deep scalp soft tissues in the frontal region.

Figure 2.6E. T2W images show the bone to be intact. The scalp abscess shows findings suggesting relatively thick and purulent material (arrow). There is evidence of epidural abscess (arrowhead) displacing the superior sagittal sinus.

Figure 2.6F. Diffusion-weighted image shows restricted diffusion confirming abscess (arrow).

Figure 2.6G. CE T1W image correlating approximately with the CT image in (Fig. 2.6C) shows the epidural abscess that, in the absence of bone destruction, almost has to be due to thrombophlebitic spread from diploic vessels (arrow) displacing the superior sagittal sinus (arrowheads).

Figure 2.6H. MR venography shows the abnormality in the scalp (arrow) not obviously contiguous with the collection displacing the superior sagittal sinus (arrowheads). Again, this is a finding consistent with spread of disease within diseased veins.

Figure 2.6I. Coronal CT reformation shows the epidural abscess (arrow) and displaced superior sagittal sinus (arrowhead).

Figure 2.6J. Sagittal CT reformations confirm the area of scalp osteomyelitis (black arrow), which is barely contiguous with obvious sinus disease because the patient was partially treated and frontal sinus disease had largely resolved. The superior sagittal sinus is displaced (arrowheads) by the epidural abscess (arrow).

DIFFERENTIAL DIAGNOSIS The diagnosis of acute sinusitis is quite straightforward clinically. This patient's presentation and imaging essentially has no differential. The importance of imaging is to evaluate the extent of disease, detect clinically unsuspected complications, and identify possible structural etiology that may have predisposed the patient for such an episode.

DIAGNOSIS Acute sinusitis with extensive thrombophlebitic spread of disease to produce an epidural abscess as well as contiguous extension into the frontal subcutaneous tissues with deep scalp abscess formation

DISCUSSION Rhinosinusitis is the preferred term for this condition because the nasal mucosa is almost always simultaneously involved when sinusitis occurs. Approximately 0.5% to 2% of viral rhinosinusitis cases are complicated by bacterial superinfection. Patients with a history of allergy, occupational or vasomotor rhinitis, and anatomic obstruction such as septal deviation or nasal polyps will be predisposed to infections. The condition is also more common in patients with immune deficiency and ciliary motility disorders. This patient had no particular predisposing condition.

There was bone erosion of the anterior table of right frontal sinus with abscess formation in the deep scalp. However, no direct connection of the intracranial subdural emphyema and the infected sinus could be established. Many cases of extra-axial abscesses result from sinusitis. The spread to the epidural space may be direct through adjacent bone or via transdural veins—the latter occurring in this patient.

Other complications that can be seen with acute sinusitis are pre- and postseptal orbital cellulitis, subperiosteal and orbital abscess formation, cavernous and other dural venous sinus thrombosis, subdural empyema, meningitis, and brain abscesses.

Question for Further Thought

1. What is the pathophysiology of acute sinusitis?

Reporting Responsibilities

Direct communication is strongly recommended for all cases where imaging is done for the suspicion of complications of an acute sinusitis. This is mandatory if a complication is seen.

What the Treating Physician Needs to Know

The report should include the following information:

- Whether the findings are consistent with the clinical diagnosis of acute or subacute sinusitis or if there is a more likely alternative
- Clearly stated extent of disease and whether complications such as orbital involvement, vascular thrombosis, or intracranial extension of the disease are present
- Description of any coexisting anatomic finding or other disease that might be a contributing cause of the sinusitis

Answer

1. The coordinated action of the cilia of the columnar epithelial cell move the sinus contents toward the natural sinus ostia. Disruption of the ciliary function results in accumulation of sinus secretions and potentially infectious agents within the sinus.

Various conditions can affect the mucociliary function. This includes high airflow and cold air, toxins produced by microorganisms, environmental mediators of the inflammatory response, mechanical factors that impede transport of the mucosal blanket, primary ciliary dyskinesia and secondary ciliary dysfunction from chronic infections, and secondhand smoke exposure.

When the natural sinus ostia become obstructed, normal mucus drainage is impeded. The obstructed sinus environment becomes hypoxic and causes ciliary dysfunction and changes in mucus production, all of this further reducing normal mucus clearance. Uncomplicated acute bacterial sinusitis should be considered akin to an abscess or empyema since it is essentially a collection of pus under pressure. It is this fundamental situation that creates a potential for the orbital and intracranial complications. The intrasinus pressure encourages a retrograde thrombophlebitic spread of pus that is one mechanism causing the complications. It likely contributes to the pathophysiology of bone erosion and direct spread of disease beyond the bony sinus limits as well. Relieving this pressure by draining the causative sinus is a strategy aimed at the prevention and treatment for such complications. Such drainage also promotes the restoration of normal sinonasal mucociliary drainage by reversing some of the elements causing that dysfunction.

> ### LEARN MORE
> See Chapters 84 and 15 in *Head and Neck Radiology* by Mancuso and Hanafee.

CASE 2.7

CLINICAL HISTORY *A 52-year-old female patient presented with gradually progressive central headache radiating to the vertex. She has history of seasonal allergies and was used to recurrent and chronic episodes of sinusitis, but this headache has been bothering her more. No significant abnormalities were seen on examination. The patient was referred to imaging.*

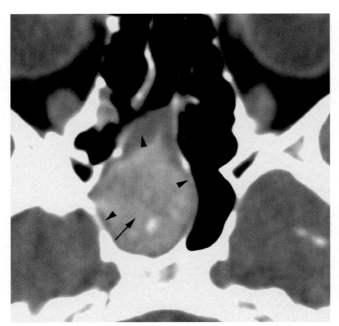

FIGURE 2.7A

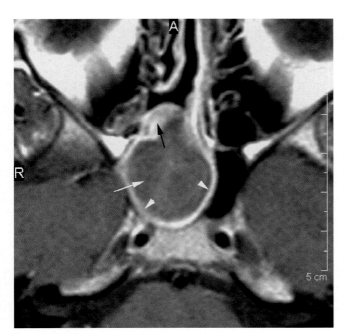

FIGURE 2.7B

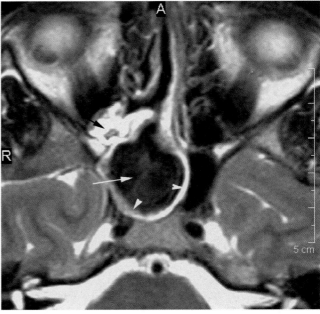

FIGURE 2.7C

FINDINGS

Figure 2.7A. The sinus contents bulge through the sinus ostium, and there is regressive remodeling of the sinus walls (arrowheads). The contents appear dense and likely desiccated with a central area of higher density (arrow).

Figure 2.7B. T1W CE MR shows the changes to be composed of relatively thin enhancing mucosa (white arrowheads) with somewhat thicker enhancing mucosa blocking the ostium (black arrow). The sinus contents appear of somewhat greater signal intensity than fluid (white arrow).

Figure 2.7C. T2W MR demonstrates the pathophysiology perhaps more graphically. The edematous mucosa within the sinus again remains relatively thin (arrows) with the polypoid mucosal thickening in the sphenoethmoidal recess and around the sphenoid ostium causing the primary obstruction somewhat thicker (black arrow). The T2W image provides a better idea of the desiccated nature of the luminal contents (white arrow) than the T1W image.

DIFFERENTIAL DIAGNOSIS None

DIAGNOSIS Chronic allergic rhinosinusitis with a secondary sphenoid sinus mucocele with likely fungal colonization

DISCUSSION Mucocele formation requires the obstruction of a draining ostium, complete opacification of a sinus, or individual air cell within a sinus complex. These conditions are most typically encountered in patients with chronic rhinosinusitis and especially those with nasal polyposis. A prior history of either trauma or previous sinus or facial surgery may also be encountered as a contributing etiologic factor. In fact, patients with chronic rhinosinusitis and nasal polyposis may have extensive mucoceles involving one or more sinus on either or both sides.

The mucoceles can be sources of significant consequences, including ocular motility disturbances, proptosis, hypertelorism, compressive optic neuropathy, and facial deformity, depending on the sinus involved. They may also become acutely infected, forming a mucopyocele that can lead to acute orbital and intracranial complications.

Questions for Further Thought

1. What is chronic rhinosinusitis?
2. How would this patient be treated?

Reporting Responsibilities

Direct communication is recommended for all cases where imaging is done for the suspicion of complications of a chronic rhinosinusitis. This is mandatory if a complication is seen.

What the Treating Physician Needs to Know

- Whether the findings are consistent with the clinical diagnosis of chronic rhinosinusitis or if there is a more likely alternative
- Full extent of the disease and description of any coexisting anatomic finding or other disease that might be a contributing cause of the chronic rhinosinusitis
- In isolated maxillary sinus disease, consider a dental origin.
- In isolated maxillary or sphenoid sinus disease, consider that there might be an obstructing nasal cavity mass other than inflammatory mucosal disease
- Whether there is a complication such as mucocele, orbital involvement, or intracranial extension, and if the situation constitutes an urgent medical situation that might require surgery
- Description of any anatomic variants that may affect an ESS approach to surgical decompression of the disease

Answers

1. Chronic sinusitis is considered when symptoms last longer than 12 weeks. They usually have associated nasal inflammation, and *chronic rhinosinusitis* is the preferred terminology. Chronic rhinosinusitis requires two or more of the following symptoms: mucopurulent drainage, nasal obstruc-

tion; or some combination of facial pain, pressure, and/or fullness, hyposomia, fever, cough, dental pain, and fatigue. There should also be confirmatory endoscopic inflammation and evidence of rhinosinusitis on imaging. Patients with a history of allergy, occupational or vasomotor rhinitis, nasal polyps, or anatomic obstruction such as septal deviation and concha bullosa will be predisposed to chronic infections. Rhinosinusitis is more common in immunodeficient patients, those with ciliary motility problems such as Kartagener syndrome, and those with mucous blanket problems such as patients with cystic fibrosis. Most chronic sinusitis is now thought to be noninfectious in etiology, although infection may have incited the process. Obstructed sinuses could also become secondarily infected. Common complications of chronic sinusitis are superimposed acute sinusitis and, in children, adenoiditis with secondary serous or purulent otitis media. Dacryocystitis and laryngitis may also occur as complications of chronic sinusitis in children. Other complications include osteomyelitis and mucocele formation. Orbital complications include pre- and postseptal cellulitis, subperiosteal abscess, orbital cellulitis, orbital abscess, and cavernous sinus thrombosis. Intracranial complications include meningitis, epidural abscess, subdural abscess, and brain abscess.

2. ESS would be required to remove the polypoid mucosa in the sphenoethmoid recess, open the sphenoid sinus ostium, and drain the mucocele. Other factors that decrease the mucociliary clearance, like additional polyps and anatomic variations, can also be addressed in the same setting. Postoperatively, the patient needs to be better managed medically with goals to improve mucociliary function and control of infection. This could be achieved by various treatment regimens that include the use of adequate antibiotic trial, intranasal corticosteroids, and saline irrigations. Sometimes, short courses of oral steroids, decongestants, topical vasoconstrictors, and mucolytics could be added. In this patient, identifying and treating the nasal allergy, if avoidance is not possible, is the key to achieving long-lasting relief. Smoking cessation is fundamental. Also, she will need short-term surveillance to ensure that the surgical drainage has been successful and that there is no recurrence of the mucocele.

LEARN MORE

See Chapters 85 and 16 in *Head and Neck Radiology* by Mancuso and Hanafee.

CLINICAL HISTORY *A 46-year-old male patient, a recent recipient of bone marrow transplant, presents with right-sided nasal discharge that he describes as dark colored. He also complains of mild right temporal region and neck pain. CT was performed, and selective images are shown below:*

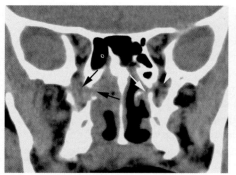

FIGURE **2.8A**

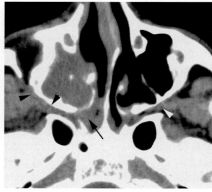

FIGURE **2.8B**

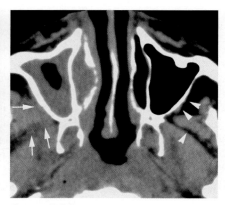

FIGURE **2.8C**

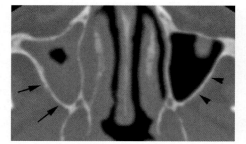

FIGURE **2.8D**

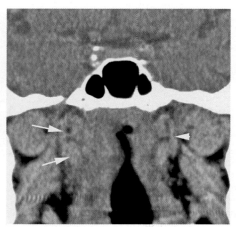

FIGURE **2.8E**

FINDINGS

Figure 2.8A. Coronal CT in an immunocompromised patient shows posterior nasal cavity disease extending through the sphenopalatine foramen into the pterygopalatine fossa (black arrows) as compared to the normal sphenopalatine foramen (white arrow) and fat within the pterygopalatine fossa (white arrowhead) on the left side.

Figure 2.8B. Axial section in the same patient seen in (Fig. 2.8A) shows the posterior nasal cavity disease infiltrating the pterygopalatine fossa (arrow) and extending along the retroantral fat pad (black arrowheads) compared to the normal tissue planes around the distal maxillary artery on the left (white arrowhead).

Figure 2.8C. There is continued spread of disease along the posterior superior alveolar branches of the distal maxillary artery and the maxillary artery (arrows) on the affected side compared to the normal structures on the left (white arrowheads).

Figure 2.8D. All of these findings are present without evidence of obvious bone erosion. Bone on the right side

appears only minimally irregular (arrows) compared to the bone on the unaffected side.

Figure 2.8E. This patient also had subtle asymmetry of the nasopharyngeal soft tissues confirmed to be an expression of infiltrating fungal disease in the nasopharynx spreading to the parapharyngeal space (arrows) with loss of normal tissue planes along the tensor muscle of the palate (white arrowhead shows the normal muscle on the left).

DIFFERENTIAL DIAGNOSIS In this setting, perhaps only lymphoma and posttransplant lymphoproliferative disorder (PTLD)

DIAGNOSIS Invasive fungal sinusitis

DISCUSSION The early detection of fungal sinus disease requires a high index of suspicion, depending on an understanding of its early spread patterns and that its invasive character may not be expressed as bone destruction in this early phase.

These infections are usually due to aspergillosis or mucormycosis and occur mainly in patients who are immunocompromised or diabetic. Ketoacidosis predisposes to mucormycosis because the acidic, glucose-rich environment favors fungal growth. This aggressive or fulminate fungal disease tends to be angioinvasive—in particular, arterial invasive; thus, diffuse inflammation may be accompanied by soft tissue and bone necrosis.

A hallmark of the disease is its predictable involvement of vascular bundles. In rhinosinusitis, the vascular pedicles and their ramifications at risk are those passing out of the sphenopalatine foramen into the posterior nasal cavity, those traveling in the infraorbital canal, and the posterior superior alveolar vessels that penetrate the posterior wall of the maxillary sinus. These vascular pathways allow disease to be on both sides of adjacent bone, sometimes without frankly destroying bone. The disease can then be recognized by perivascular infiltration of the fat bordering these bony channels as the vessels pass through surrounding fat pads en route to or from their respective foramina and canals. Regions important in the search for early imaging findings of invasive fungal rhinosinusitis include the fat pad of the canine fossa deep to the superficial musculoaponeurotic system (SMAS), extraconal fat along the orbital floor, the retroantral (retromaxillary) fat pad of the infratemporal fossa (as in this patient), and the fat of the pterygopalatine fossa. The disease may also begin in the lacrimal sac and the nasopharynx and initially be limited to those areas.

One of the hallmarks of such invasive fungal rhinosinusitis is also frank bone erosion, but the invasive soft tissue patterns without obvious bone invasion must be kept in mind, as early as possible, when trying to diagnose invasive fungal disease.

Complications include extension and involvement of the eye and orbit, cavernous sinus thrombosis, secondary extraaxial abscess, meningitis, and brain abscess.

Questions for Further Thought

1. Based on the imaging findings, can the risk of fungal sinusitis be stratified?
2. What is another infectious process that should be considered in the search pattern of immunocompromised patients sent for sinonasal evaluation?

Reporting Responsibilities

All cases of moderate or high risk where imaging is done for the suspicion of fungal sinusitis really call for direct, verbal communication with the treatment team if the study is positive or suspicious for an aggressive process. This becomes mandatory if there is clear evidence of an orbital or intracranial complication and newly discovered bone erosion since that can be a sign of an aggressive infection or other aggressive disease process such as cancer.

What the Treating Physician Needs to Know

The report should include the following information:

- Extent of disease and whether the findings are consistent with the clinical diagnosis of invasive fungal sinusitis

- Consider that a noninfectious inflammatory condition may be present if the pattern of disease suggests such an etiology.
- Clear statement of whether there are complications such as orbital involvement, vascular thrombosis, or intracranial extension of the disease

Answers

1. Based on the imaging findings, the risk of invasive fungal disease can be stratified for early diagnosis and triage.

Low risk:

- Scattered, bilateral sinus mucosal thickening of any degree without perivascular spread or bone erosion
- Localized sinus mucosal thickening without perivascular spread or bone erosion

Moderate risk:

- Unilateral posterior nasal cavity disease projecting toward the sphenopalatine foramen without perivascular spread or bone erosion
- Unilateral middle meatus and adjacent sinus disease without perivascular spread or bone erosion

High risk:

- Mucosal disease at any site that shows bone erosion or soft tissue necrosis
- Mucosal disease associated with loss of fat planes in the canine fossa deep to the SMAS, along the extraconal fat surrounding the infraorbital vascular bundle, along the retromaxillary fat pad, at the orbital apex or in the superior and inferior orbital fissure, and/or within the pterygopalatine fossa
- Infiltrating process in the nasopharynx, around the lacrimal sac, and/or anterior nasal septal swelling or necrosis

Low-risk patients are followed clinically and may be treated for viral or bacterial infections, or sometimes graft versus host reactions, and an otolaryngology consult is usually not obtained. Moderate- and high-risk patients receive nasal endoscopy by the otolaryngology service. Tissue sampling is obtained, if appropriate, in moderate-risk, and definitely high-risk, cases. These patients may be followed with CT if symptoms persist or progress even in the absence of endoscopic confirmation of fungal infection.

2. Pyogenic and/or fungal anterior nasal septal abscess may occur in this same group of patients, and the cartilage portion of the nasal septum should be a specific site of interpretive reference in all of these patients referred for sinonasal imaging with CT or MRI.

LEARN MORE

See Chapters 86 and 16 in *Head and Neck Radiology* by Mancuso and Hanafee.

CLINICAL HISTORY *A 35-year-old male patient presents with nasal irritation, stuffiness, recurrent nosebleeds, nasal crusting, facial pain, and hoarseness. He also recently developed a whistling sound with nasal breathing. Nasal endoscopy revealed septal perforation, significant nasal crusting, and few areas of necrosis. The right osteomeatal unit was deformed and scarred. CT images are shown below:*

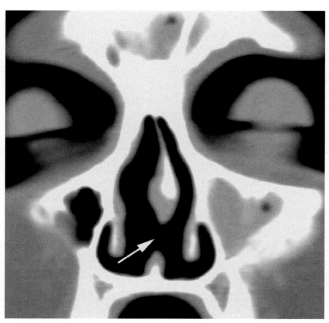

FIGURE **2.9A**

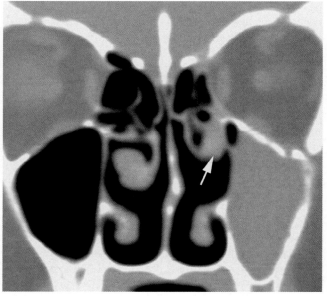

FIGURE **2.9B**

FINDINGS An anterior inferior septal perforation (arrow) is seen in (Fig. 2.9A). In (Fig. 2.9B), the middle turbinate has become scarred due to chronic nasal granulomatous changes and adherent to the lateral wall of the nasal cavity. The maxillary sinus is completely opacified due to the adhesive changes around its ostium (not shown). The images suggested chronic cocaine abuse, and this was eventually proven to be true.

DIFFERENTIAL DIAGNOSIS Wegener's granulomatosis, sarcoidosis, Langerhans cell histiocytosis, and Churg-Strauss syndrome

DIAGNOSIS Cocaine abuse

DISCUSSION Necrotic changes of the mucosa and septal perforation should lead one to think of the above differential. A history of cocaine use is obviously helpful but often not forthcoming until the pattern and extent of disease is firmly established. Sarcoidosis often presents as generalized mucosal thickening without clear evidence of aggressive behavior but can also present with changes nearly identical with those seen in cocaine abuse. Correlation with history, chest findings, and laboratory evidence of elevated angiotensin-converting enzyme levels help to confirm the diagnosis. Wegener's granulomatosis most commonly presents as a generalized necrotizing process in the nasal cavity and affecting the sinuses, with the appearance possible mimick-

ing sarcoidosis. The appearance is generally different from cocaine abuse, with more mucosal necrosis and bone loss. Levels of c-ANCA are elevated in Wegener's granulomatosis. Langerhans histiocytosis is typically not a disease of the sinuses and nasal cavity. Spread to those regions is usually from a contiguous site or a strategically placed bone lesion. Biopsy would be required for diagnosis of histiocytosis and other disease that can cause septal perforation, such as PTLD and lymphoma.

Question for Further Thought

1. What do posttreatment imaging findings reveal in these cases?

Reporting Responsibilities

All of the possibilities in the differential diagnosis at the time of first confirmation on imaging should be reported verbally to the referring provider since prompt confirmation of disease and therapeutic intervention in some of these diseases might be of benefit. The cocaine abuse risk should be reported verbally for obvious reasons of risk to the patient and others.

What the Treating Physician Needs to Know

- Whether the disease is likely an infectious or inflammatory process versus a neoplastic process
- Most likely diagnosis and full extent of disease

- Is there associated disease anywhere else in the craniofacial region that suggests a systemic process?
- Are there any complications within or outside of sinonasal region, such as those related to the orbit and brain?
- Direct communication is warranted if an acute inflammatory or neoplastic condition is suspected.

Answer

1. Some of the soft tissue changes may persist indefinitely and require serial imaging studies to differentiate persistent or recurrent disease from end-stage granulation tissue or more mature scar tissue. Nasal septal defects typically do not heal. Other bone loss may persist indefinitely. Reactive bone changes may become quite prominent in the absence of active disease.

> **LEARN MORE**
> See Chapters 87 and 15 *Head and Neck Radiology* by Mancuso and Hanafee.

CASE 2.10

CLINICAL HISTORY *A 25-year-old male patient presented to the emergency room after a fistfight. He was in pain, with bleeding from the nose and facial swelling. He also complained of clear fluid discharge from the nose. A maxillofacial CT was performed. Selected images are shown below:*

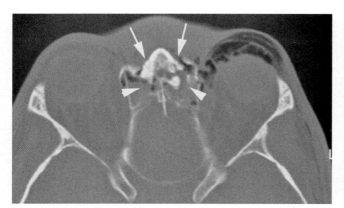

FIGURE **2.10A**

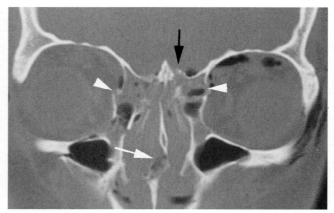

FIGURE **2.10C**

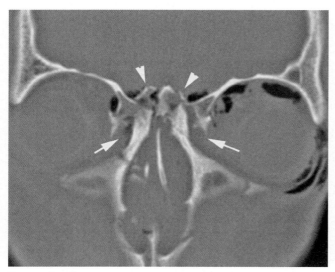

FIGURE **2.10B**

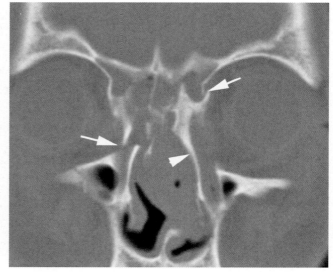

FIGURE **2.10D**

FINDINGS

Figure 2.10A. The nasal bones at their junctions with the frontal bones are driven posteriorly (arrows) with multiple fragments displaced into the expected position of the frontal recess (arrowheads).

Figure 2.10B. Coronal section shows the fracture fragments driven cephalad as well as posteriorly (arrowheads), resulting in pneumocephalus; the intracranial air confirms dural tears. While the more superior aspect of this fracture is severely comminuted, the intercanthal region has been left relatively intact (arrows).

Figure 2.10C. These fractures frequently result in disruption of the anterior skull base (black arrow) and CSF leakage. The medial orbital walls are spread laterally (white arrowheads), a reflection of the widening of the intercan-

thal distance. The nasal septum may be fractured, resulting in a septal hematoma (white arrow).

Figure 2.10D. There is disruption of the nasal and frontal bones with minimal, if any, comminution.

DIFFERENTIAL DIAGNOSIS None

DIAGNOSIS Naso-orbital-ethmoid (NOE) complex fracture

DISCUSSION NOE fractures usually result from central facial impact forces that exploit the differences between the stronger vertical struts and weaker horizontal struts, particularly when the applied force is directed in a more anterior to posterior orientation. The prominent position of the NOE complex anteriorly in the midface also makes it susceptible to injury.

These fractures may be simple or severely comminuted. The more simple fractures, if displaced, will typically show the nasal bones and frontal process of the maxilla to be telescoped posteriorly beneath the frontal bone. Comminuted fragments may spread medially into the nasal cavity, superiorly to the anterior cranial fossa, and laterally into the orbit. These patterns explain the association of NOE fractures, when due to high-energy impact, to be associated with CSF leak as well as brain and globe injuries.

Telescoping of the bones of the NOE complex between the ethmoidal labyrinths will increase the transverse distance between the medial orbital walls.

Other potential complications of NOE fractures are also predictable based on related anatomic relationships. Anterior skull base dural injury may result in CSF leak. Shearing of the traversing anterior and posterior ethmoid arteries may cause an orbital hematoma or impressive epistaxis. The optic canal is typically not directly involved by bony injury, but edema within the optic canal or free bone fragments may disrupt optic nerve perfusion.

Questions for Further Thought

1. How are NOE fractures classified?
2. What is telecanthus?
3. How do questions 1 and 2 relate to treatment?
4. What is a possible complication of frontal recess obstruction?

Reporting Responsibilities

Evidence of tension orbit, optic nerve injury, and foreign body or other coincidental findings like acute epidural hematoma would require urgent verbal communication directly with the health care provider.

In general, the report routinely should catalogue all details of the injury while anticipating possible complications. This would include bony injury; the basic pattern or category of the fracture pattern; and description of individual fractures with respect to their complexity, displacement, and comminution. With regard to the orbital injury, the report should contain details of the extent of orbital soft tissue herniation into adjacent sinonasal structures, the presence and location of intraorbital hematomas, and the status of the orbital apex with respect to both bone and soft tissue structures. Other complications such as entrapment of extraocular muscles, injury to nasolacrimal duct, neurovascular bundles, or medial canthal ligament disruption should be looked for and reported. With regard to the nasal cavity, anterior skull base, and cranium, if a blow-in fracture is present, the extent of injury, pneumocephalus suggesting dural tear, possibility of CSF leakage, and traumatic meningoencephaloceles should be noted in the report. A nasal septal hematoma should be excluded.

What the Treating Physician Needs to Know

- Is the face injured?
- Full extent of the injury and involved structures should be described.
- What complications might be anticipated based on the structures injured?
- Are there associated complications involving the eye, optic nerve/sheath complex, or foreign bodies?
- Is there a complicating infection?
- Are there any complications outside of those related to the face?
- Are there findings that suggest a risk of delayed complications?
- Are foreign bodies noted or suspected based upon the mechanism of injury?

Answers

1. The status of the central segment of bone left by a NOE fracture is the basis of the classification of fracture patterns for this type of injury. The Manson system classifies these fractures into three main groups: type I, where the fractured bony segment is large and the medial canthal tendon (MCT) insertion around the lacrimal fossa is intact; type II, where the buttress is comminuted with the MCT remaining attached to a small bone fragment; and type III, where the pattern cannot be diagnosed with imaging, requiring exploration to determine if the canthus is avulsed from the bone.

2. The eyelids consist of orbicularis oculi, tarsal plate, and suspensory ligaments. This apparatus attaches medially to both the anterior and posterior lacrimal crest via the MCT. Rupture or avulsion of the MCT (or its bony insertion) can also result in a greater intercanthal distance, known as telecanthus. Telecanthus requires four fracture sites, including the medial orbital wall, the nasomaxillary buttress and inferior orbital rim, the frontal maxillary junction, and the lateral nasal bone.

3. The main goal of surgery is to restore the anatomic position of the MCT and the displaced bony fragment(s) to which it may remain attached; this will prevent significant subsequent cosmetic and functional lid problems.

4. Frontal recess obstruction secondary to trauma could lead to chronic obstruction of the frontal sinus and a frontal sinus mucocele as a delayed complication.

LEARN MORE

See Chapter 88 in *Head and Neck Radiology* by Mancuso and Hanafee.

CLINICAL HISTORY *A 48-year-old male patient presented with left nasal obstruction for the last 3 months. CT and MRI were performed. Selected images are shown below:*

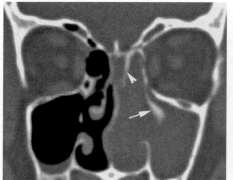

FIGURE **2.11A**

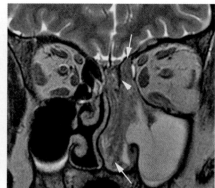

FIGURE **2.11B**

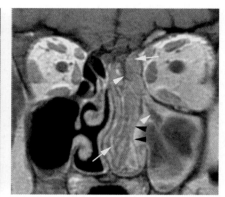

FIGURE **2.11C**

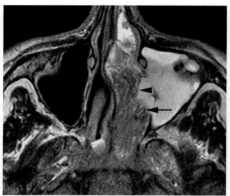

FIGURE **2.11D**

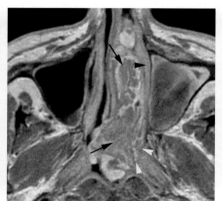

FIGURE **2.11E**

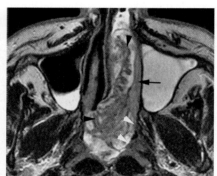

FIGURE **2.11F**

FINDINGS

Figure 2.11A. CT study shows a generalized opacification of the left nasal cavity and left maxillary sinus. There is bone loss as well as bone sclerosis. The medial wall of the ethmoid complex is much thicker than usual (arrowhead), as is the bone of the anteroethmoidal septum region (arrow).

Figure 2.11B. T2W MRI shows tumor, which appears to be somewhat papillary, growing all the way to the ethmoid roof (arrows). The thickened bone of the medial ethmoid wall can be anticipated (arrowhead) on the MR but not as definitively as on the CT in (Fig. 2.11A).

Figure 2.11C. CE T1W image to compare with (Fig. 2.11A) and (Fig. 2.11B). The papillary and "fronding" nature of the mass and its extension to the ethmoid roof are noted again (white arrows). The thickened ethmoid bony wall can be anticipated as well as the thickened antroethmoidal septum (white arrowheads). The bulging margin of the obstructed maxillary sinus contents forms an interface with the lateral aspect of the tumor (black arrowheads).

Figure 2.11D. Axial T2W images clearly show the frondlike nature of this papillary tumor (arrow) and clearly identify the interface between the tumor and obstructive sinus contents (arrowhead).

Figure 2.11E. T1W CE image to compare with (Fig. 2.11D). The papillary mass fills the nasal cavity and extends into the nasopharynx (arrows). It does not appear to invade the nasopharyngeal wall but clearly apposes that mucosa (white arrowheads). The same is true of the nasal cavity mucosa (black arrowhead).

Figure 2.11F. T2W image for comparison with other axial images shows the frondlike nature of the tumor (arrowheads) and a possible more solid attachment of the tumor along the lateral nasal cavity wall (black arrow). The interface with the nasopharyngeal wall is sharp (white arrowheads) and does not suggest invasion. Surgery showed the nasopharynx not to be invaded.

DIFFERENTIAL DIAGNOSIS Inflammatory polyps, benign minor salivary epithelial neoplasms, odontogenic tumors, squamous cell carcinoma (SCCa), olfactory neuroblastoma, and rarely sinonasal lymphoma. The diagnosis is suggested on imaging and confirmed by biopsy.

DIAGNOSIS Inverted papilloma

DISCUSSION Inverted papilloma is a descriptive term based on the microscopic appearance of the lesion. The neoplastic epithelium grows into the underlying stroma, causing the stroma to become heaped up over the epithelial nidus. Inverted papilloma, while usually benign, has malignant potential and must be treated like a low-grade malignancy. Of these lesions, 85% to 90% are histologically benign, but the remainder is associated with SCCa that may take an aggressive clinical course.

Inverted papilloma essentially is a lesion of the lateral nasal wall. Other sites of origin are unusual. The lesions are polypoid and more vascular than inflammatory polyps. The attachment to the lateral nasal wall may be discrete compared to the bulk of the tumor. Adjacent maxillary and ethmoid sinus involvement is common. Spread to the orbit and anterior skull base is unusual but does occur. Bone erosion is common but may appear more as remodeling, sclerosis, and dehiscence than aggressive erosion. Of particular interest is the appearance on T2W and contrast-enhanced magnetic resonance (CEMR) images; this lesion will often show an infolded frondlike general morphology that is not difficult to distinguish from standard inflammatory polyps. Lymph node metastasis and perineural spread only occur in a small subset of the 10% to 15% of cases with a complicating SCCa, which is mostly found coincidentally on histopathology within the confines of the papilloma.

Question for Further Thought

1. How is this condition treated?

Reporting Responsibilities

If the cancer is not known or there is an unanticipated finding in a known cancer such as intracranial extension, perineural tumor spread, or recurrence in a previously treated patient, then direct communication with the health care provider is recommended.

If an imaging study has been performed for a sinonasal mass based on clinical suspicion or for evaluation of a known cancer, the report should contain a complete assessment of the disease extent and all information that is relevant to treatment planning.

What the Treating Physician Needs to Know

- If the diagnosis is not known, whether the pathology is aggressive and whether cancer or some other aggressive disease process is more likely
- If the pattern of disease suggests a specific entity such as inverted papilloma
- If cancer is present, its full local extent; spread to critical contiguous sites (e.g., orbit, intracranial region, infratemporal fossa, and nasopharynx); perineural and/or perivascular spread; and likelihood of spread to cervical, facial, and/or retropharyngeal nodes.

Answer

1. Inverted papilloma is treated with surgery. The excision is best approached as an en bloc procedure with a margin of normal tissue even though the lesion is usually entirely benign. More limited resections can produce a high rate of recurrence. Lateral rhinotomy with medial maxillectomy and ethmoidectomy, including removal of the middle and inferior turbinates and all mucosa in the ipsilateral paranasal sinuses, results in a very low rate of recurrence. Rapid multiple recurrences with invasion of the sinuses, orbit, and cribriform plate should be treated as a low-grade malignancy, and the more radical en bloc should include suitable margins for a malignancy. Postoperative radiation therapy is usually added in such circumstances.

> **LEARN MORE**
>
> See Chapters 89 and 23 in *Head and Neck Radiology* by Mancuso and Hanafee.

CASE 2.12

CLINICAL HISTORY *A 19-year-old male patient presented with left facial pain for 2 months. He also noticed loosening of several of his left upper teeth. He has always been healthy, and he presented to his doctor very concerned. CT image is shown below:*

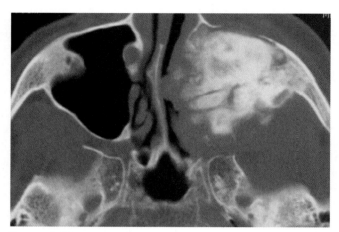

FIGURE 2.12

FINDINGS

Figure 2.12. Maxillofacial CT demonstrates a mass in the left maxillary sinus with osteoid matrix.

DIFFERENTIAL DIAGNOSIS The ossifying matrix of an osteogenic sarcoma may suggest a meningioma or even fibrous dysplasia as an initial diagnostic consideration. A juvenile ossifying fibroma of the maxilla may also raise the concern for a rare maxillary osteogenic sarcoma. Mucinous minor salivary gland cancers or metastases that calcify might mimic an osteogenic sarcoma.

DIAGNOSIS Spontaneous osteosarcoma of the maxilla

DISCUSSION Osteogenic sarcoma is the most common malignant primary tumor of bone. It most frequently occurs in the second decade of life. Predisposing factors include prior radiation, Paget disease, fibrous dysplasia, and chronic osteomyelitis.

Osteosarcoma is rare in the sinuses since the most commonly affected facial bone is, by far, the mandible. The maxillary is the most commonly affected sinus. Ethmoid and sphenoid bone osteogenic sarcomas are rare. Prior radiation treatments to the craniofacial region, especially in childhood, considerably raise the risk of this disease. In fact, sinonasal osteosarcoma is distinctly rare in the absence of a history of prior radiation. Most are high grade.

This histology was highly unusual in this patient, as he had no history of prior radiation or any other underlying condition.

Question for Further Thought

1. How is this condition treated?

Reporting Responsibilities

If the cancer is not known or there is an unanticipated finding in a known cancer, such as intracranial extension, perineural tumor spread, or recurrence in a previously treated patient, then direct communication with the health care provider is recommended.

If an imaging study has been performed for a sinonasal mass based on clinical suspicion or for evaluation of a known cancer, the report should contain a complete assessment of the disease extent and all information that is relevant to treatment planning.

What the Treating Physician Needs to Know

- If the diagnosis is not known, whether the pathology is aggressive and whether cancer or some other aggressive disease process is more likely
- If the pattern of disease suggests a specific entity such as an unusual bone or dental origin of the mass and/or a specific diagnosis
- If cancer is present, its full local extent; spread to critical contiguous sites (e.g., orbit, intracranial region, infratemporal fossa, and nasopharynx); perineural and/or perivascular spread; and likelihood of spread to cervical, facial, and/or retropharyngeal nodes.

Answer

1. If the lesion is contained within the sinus, the tumor is surgically excised usually along with adjunctive chemotherapy and radiation therapy. Preoperative chemotherapy is given to reduce the bulk of tumor if the lesion is large and has extended outside the sinonasal region.

LEARN MORE
See Chapters 90 and 38 in *Head and Neck Radiology* by Mancuso and Hanafee.

CASE 2.13

CLINICAL HISTORY *A 13-year-old girl from Guatemala presented with a left facial mass. The patient attained menarche 6 months ago and noticed slight facial swelling 2 months ago. Since then, the swelling has been rapidly growing. The parents were alarmed, and the girl was embarrassed to go to school. She also complained of dull pain and loosening of the left upper teeth. Selected images of maxillofacial CT are shown below:*

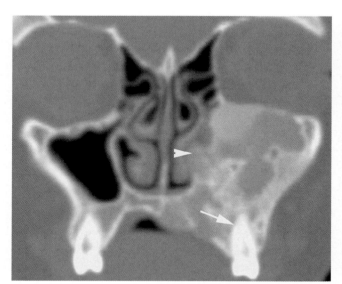

FIGURE 2.13A

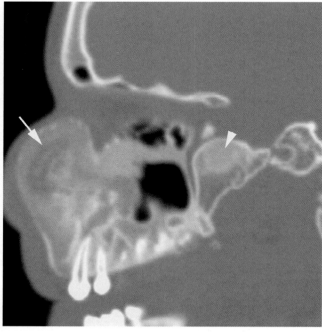

FIGURE 2.13C

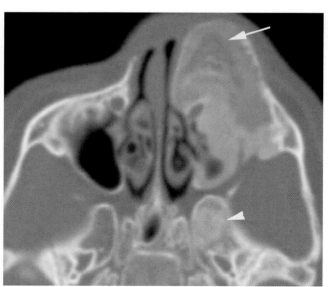

FIGURE 2.13B

FINDINGS

Figure 2.13A. A heterogeneously mineralized fibro-osseous mass involved the maxilla.

Figure 2.13B,C. Axial and sagittal images clearly demonstrates the marked cosmetic deformation but also dentition problems and those related to sinus and nasal cavity obstruction (arrows). Also note that there is expansion and ground glass opacity in the base of left pterygoid plates (arrowheads), similar to the appearance in the maxilla.

DIFFERENTIAL DIAGNOSIS Rapid growth caused a concern that this may represent juvenile aggressive ossifying fibroma. Fibrous dysplasia rather than juvenile aggressive ossifying fibroma was considered far more likely once an additional focus of fibrous dysplasia involving the base of the pterygoid plates was identified.

Fibrous dysplastic bone may mimic reactive changes due to an adjacent meningioma or an intraosseous component of a meningioma. It may also be mistaken for an osteoblastic metastasis from solid tumors such as breast and prostate primaries and mixed osteoblastic and osteolytic changes seen with lymphoma or leukemia or mimic other matrix-producing bone lesions. Lack of adjacent soft tissue and/or dural changes usually make this differential straightforward.

Fibrous dysplasia is often so vascular that it might be mistaken for a slow-flow vascular malformation or other high vascular lesion unless the matrix is calcification is recognized.

DIAGNOSIS Fibrous dysplasia

DISCUSSION Fibrous dysplasia of the cranial and facial bones is often an isolated "monostotic" phenomenon, although it very often involves more than one contiguous part of the facial bones—for instance, being frontoethmoidal or sphenoethmoidal in its full extent. It can also be part of a more widespread polyostotic process and associated with endocrine problems as with Albright syndrome.

The craniofacial form of the disease is very common. It is often discovered incidentally on imaging studies done for unrelated complaints. The maxilla, ethmoid, sphenoid, mandible, and bones of the calvarium may be involved. Isolated areas in the sphenoid bone are often detected as bright areas in the base of the sphenoid bone on MRI as incidental findings. These may need to be differentiated from areas of fat in the skull base or zones of arrested sphenoid sinus aeration or a skull base transitional status in preparation for sphenoid sinus aeration. Whatever the case, such areas are almost always of low biologic activity and will be of no ultimate consequence to the patient. In multifocal or polyostotic (noncontiguous) disease, a syndromic association may be considered.

When clinical concerns related to fibrous dysplasia arise, they are most commonly related primarily to cosmesis. Functional problems do arise and include malocclusion, visual disturbances, and possibly compressive cranial neuropathy where the cranial nerves exit the skull. There may also be initial concerns about the lesion in question representing a more ominous condition.

Fibrous dysplasia may enter into a rapid growth phase during pregnancy and adolescence, as in this patient. In the latter instance, differentiation from juvenile active ossifying fibromas might be difficult, and that lesion must be brought into the differential consideration.

Question for Further Thought

1. How is this condition treated?

Reporting Responsibilities

In general, there is often little or no risk associated with these fibro-osseous lesions. Many times the craniofacial findings are incidental, as seen on studies done for other indications. When the imaging studies are done specifically for complaints related to the craniofacial skeleton, routine reporting almost always suffices. There might rarely be a complicating disease such as secondary mucocele or infections with possible intracranial complications that require verbal communication. Also, rarely the lesion will show an aggressive growth pattern suggestive of a superimposed sarcoma or a possible juvenile active ossifying fibroma variant; these findings also would be best communicated verbally to the referring health care provider.

What the Treating Physician Needs to Know

- Extent of disease and whether its pattern is consistent with a known or working clinical diagnosis
- If there are findings that specifically explain functional deficits
- If there are findings that might potentially cause a deficit with progression of the disease state
- Whether there is a complication of the underlying pathology such as acute or chronic infection, mucocele, or aggressive growth pattern that is potentially progressive and/or dangerous compared to the natural history of these usually benign conditions

Answer

1. Treatment is surgical and aimed at restoring cosmesis and preventing functional losses. Recent advances in craniofacial surgery and three-dimensional treatment planning have led to improved results in these patients.

LEARN MORE
See Chapters 91 and 40 in *Head and Neck Radiology* by Mancuso and Hanafee.

CLINICAL HISTORY *A 52-year-old male patient presented with facial pain, nasal obstructive symptoms, and a few episodes of nosebleeds. He also had many systemic symptoms including generalized malaise and right lower extremity radicular symptoms. CT and MR images are shown below:*

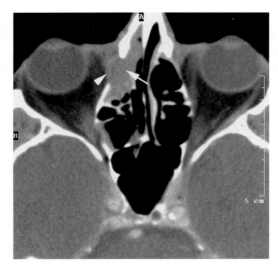

FIGURE 2.14A

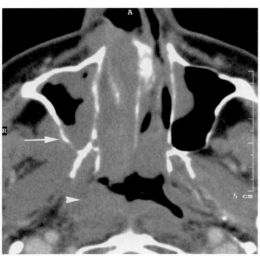

FIGURE 2.14B

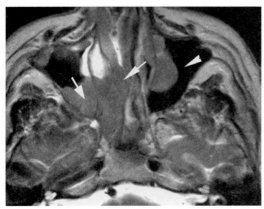

FIGURE 2.14C

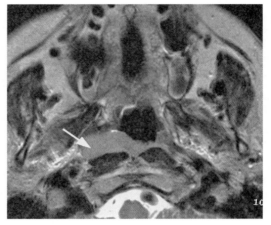

FIGURE 2.14D

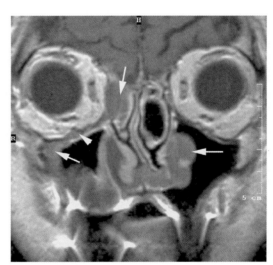

FIGURE 2.14E

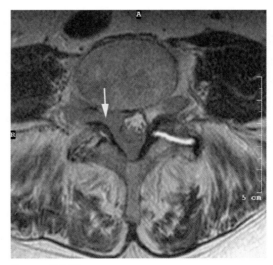

FIGURE 2.14F

FINDINGS

Figure 2.14A. CT shows a mass invading the anterior ethmoids from the anterior nasal cavity (arrow) with extension into the orbit (arrowhead) but no invasion of orbital fat.

Figure 2.14B. CT more inferiorly shows tumor throughout the nasal cavity but also invading through the posterior wall of the maxillary sinus (arrow) and a separate area of invasion in the nasopharynx (arrowhead).

Figure 2.14C. T2W image shows contiguous disease in the left nasal cavity and maxillary sinus (arrows) with a noncontiguous focus of disease in the left maxillary sinus (arrowhead).

Figure 2.14D. Another noncontiguous focus of disease seen on the CT study in (Fig. 2.14B) is confirmed in the nasopharynx (arrow).

Figure 2.14E. T1W CE image shows noncontiguous areas of disease in both maxillary sinuses and in the ethmoid sinus (arrows) as well as a suggestion of perineural spread along the right infraorbital neurovascular bundle (arrowhead).

Figure 2.14F. Additional invasion of the epidural space is seen, confirming the suspicion of systemic disease presenting as a sinonasal mass.

DIFFERENTIAL DIAGNOSIS Main differential diagnoses are Wegener's granulomatosis or sarcoidosis. Other differentials to consider include chronic fungal and other infections that cause skull base osteomyelitis and histiocytosis. These usually need to be excluded by some combination of clinical evaluation, imaging, and laboratory findings and ultimately tissue sampling.

DIAGNOSIS Sinonasal lymphoma

DISCUSSION Sinonasal lymphoma may affect the very young but more frequently occurs in middle-aged and older men. These are almost exclusively non-Hodgkin lymphoma, and most sinonasal presentation heralds stage IV disease requiring a systemic workup with imaging, laboratory studies, and often bone marrow biopsy. Children respond better to chemotherapy than adults. Relapse drops ultimate survival rates precipitously. Chemotherapy and radiotherapy are used in treating lymphoma, and the only role of surgery is to get an adequate tissue sample to accurately characterize this disease using modern pathologic evaluation including immunohistochemistry, tumor immunophenotyping, and molecular genetics.

The lymphomas are of B- or T-cell lineage with a broad range of biologic activity. B-cell lymphoma, T-cell lymphoma, and natural killer (NK)/T-cell lymphoma, depending on their immunophenotype, have different growth patterns, prognosis, and patterns of treatment failure and survival rates. The nasal cavity is the predominant site of sinonasal involvement in T-cell and NK/T-cell lymphoma. Sinus involvement without disease in the nasal cavity is common in B-cell lymphoma. NK/T-cell lymphoma is strongly associated with the Epstein-Barr virus.

The locoregional failure rates in these tumors are similar; however, distant failure is much more common in B-cell or NK/T-cell lymphoma than in T-cell lymphoma. T-cell lymphoma has the most favorable prognosis, and NK/T-cell has the worst.

Question for Further Thought

1. What are main imaging features of sinonasal lymphoma, and what are the implications of not recognizing this condition?

Reporting Responsibilities and What the Treating Physician Needs to Know

If the sinonasal mass is a new finding or this is the presentation of systemic disease, then direct verbal communication is recommended. Posttreatment surveillance can be reported routinely. Recognizing such disease at the time of initial presentation is often difficult but may be aided greatly by noncontiguous multifocal disease or atypical spread patterns. The report should also clearly describe the extent of disease in the sinonasal region and extension beyond the sinuses and the most suitable site for tissue sampling.

Answer

1. Sinonasal lymphoma and other similar systemic disease are recognized by how their spread patterns differ from other sinonasal cancers. The biggest clue is multifocal, noncontiguous disease with involvement of facial and/or Waldeyer's ring followed closely by a pattern that suggests a bone or bone marrow origin of the disease. A prominent perineural and/or perivascular component, especially combined with an unusual site of involvement, should raise the possibility of lymphoma. Skin and subcutaneous disease may be present.

   Most sinonasal cancers are of epithelial origin. The differences between those cancers and the sinonasal lymphoma and leukemia are most often substantial with regard to medical decision making, especially treatment options. However, failure to recognize the patterns of this disease can lead to unnecessarily morbid approaches to tissue sampling and even attempted unnecessary gross total excision.

   Modern pathologic evaluation including immunohistochemistry and tumor immunophenotyping only occasionally leaves the diagnosis in question once sufficient tissue has been obtained. When these cancers present as a solitary mass, their true nature is usually not apparent until the tissue is sampled.

LEARN MORE

See Chapters 92 and 27 in *Head and Neck Radiology* by Mancuso and Hanafee.

CASE 2.15

CLINICAL HISTORY A 55-year-old man presented to the emergency room with pain in his right shoulder after minimal trauma. He also gave history of progressive nasal obstruction of about 1 years duration. Multiple images are shown below:

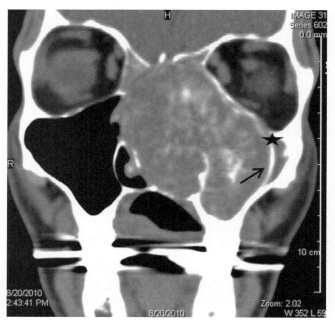

FIGURE 2.15A

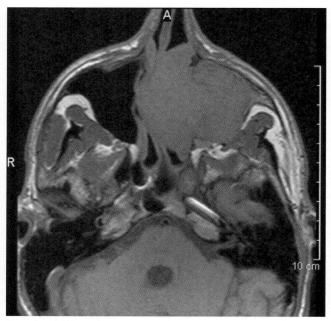

FIGURE 2.15C

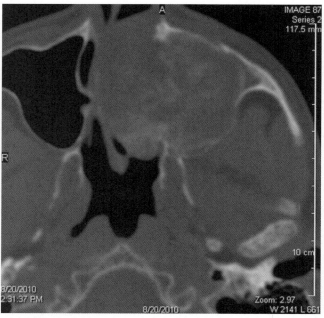

FIGURE 2.15B

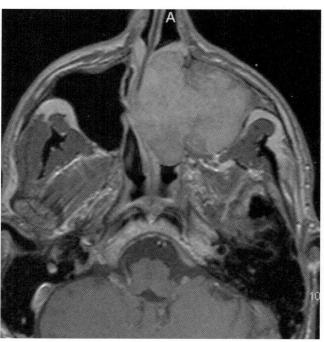

FIGURE 2.15D

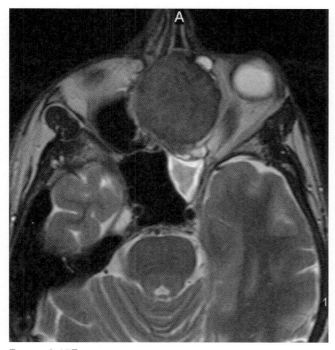

FIGURE 2.15E

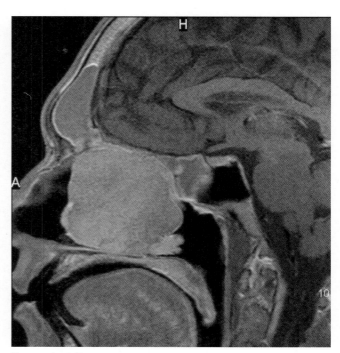

FIGURE 2.15G

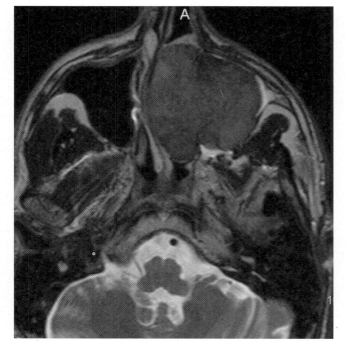

FIGURE 2.15F

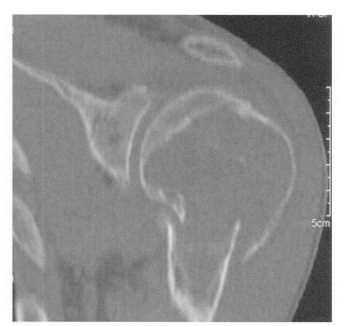

FIGURE 2.15H

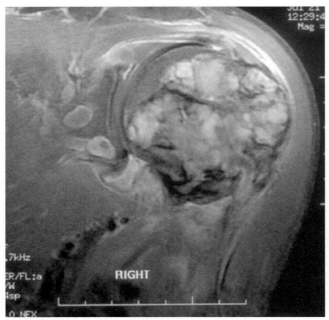

FIGURE **2.15I**

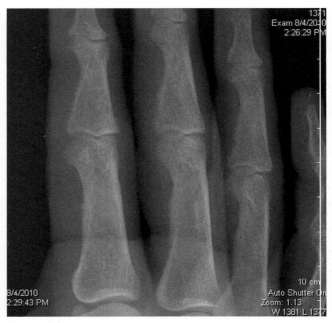

FIGURE **2.15J**

FINDINGS

Figure 2.15A,B. Coronal and axial CT images demonstrate a large mass in the nasal cavity centered on the left side extending superiorly from the cribriform plate to the hard palate inferiorly and anteriorly from the pyriform aperture to posterior choanae. There is extensive regressive remodeling of the medial wall of maxilla (black arrow) with a small residual left maxillary sinus (black star). Similar remodeling of the left orbital floor and medial wall is also noted. The mass shows heterogeneous calcified matrix.

Figure 2.15C,D. T1W and post gadolinium T1W images show the mass is isointense and mildly enhances.

Figure 2.15E,F. T2W images show that the mass is hypointense. Note that MR does not show the internal calcification/ossification like CT.

Figure 2.15G. Postcontrast T1W sagittal image shows the superior inferior extent of the mass with secondary obstruction to the left frontal and sphenoid sinus.

Figure 2.15H,I. Coronal reformatted CT of the right humerus shows a lytic lesion with pathologic fracture through the neck. Coronal proton density images show a heterogeneous mass lesion within the humeral head and neck.

Figure 2.15J. AP radiograph of the right hand shows subperiosteal resorption of the radial aspect of middle phalanges of the index and middle fingers.

DIFFERENTIAL DIAGNOSIS Generally, some sort of osteocartilaginous or fibro-osseous mass (i.e., ossifying fibroma, osteosarcoma, osteoblastoma, chondrosarcoma), olfactory neuroblastoma, extracranial meningioma (rare), giant cell granuloma, giant cell tumor, and metastasis

DIAGNOSIS Severe primary hyperparathyroidism with subperiosteal resorption, brown tumors in the sinonasal region and humerus (with pathologic fracture)

DISCUSSION In primary hyperparathyroidism, there is simply overproduction of parathormone (PTH). In secondary hyperparathyroidism due to renal failure, multiple mechanisms are at play including phosphate retention and diminished vitamin D transformation, both of which deplete calcium and lead to overproduction of PTH.

Brown tumors are focal osteolytic, sometimes aggressive-appearing lesions that primarily affect the mandible and maxilla. They are rare in the head and neck region. Multiple brown tumors can present as "cherubism."

Brown tumors are "expansile"-appearing lesions of bones with bony margins able to remain mineralized and/or show narrow margins of sharp or indistinct transition depending on the developmental cycle of the metabolic disorder. Soft tissue interfaces generally remain sharp but may be slightly indistinct as well. The extent of bony abnormality is best studied with CT.

The masses may appear solid or "multiloculated" (as in this patient the lesion in the humerus appears multiloculated) and enhancing internally on both CECT and CEMR. Brown tumors should not mineralize unless healing or if residual bone is being mistaken for tumor mineralization (as in this patient). Sometimes, fairly diffuse subtle mineralization in a trabecular-type pattern can be seen in the brown tumors as they begin healing.

The internal contents are usually isointense or hypointense to muscle on noncontrast T1W MR images unless they are hemorrhagic. Brown tumors tend to be between muscle and fat in signal intensity on non–fat-suppressed T2W images because of their fibrous tissue content unless truly cystic change, usually related to necrosis or hemorrhage, is present. Depending on the phases of evolution of hemorrhage, MR appearance may vary significantly. If actual fluid levels and an essentially entirely cystic nature are present, those findings suggest but are not specific for aneurysmal bone cyst since such regressive changes occur in traumatic bone cysts and brown tumors as well.

Question for Further Thought

1. How are brown tumors related to hyperparathyroidism treated treated?

Reporting Responsibilities

In general, there is often little or no acute functional risk associated with most metabolic diseases affecting the sinonasal region. Sometimes the craniofacial findings of metabolic disease are incidental as seen on CT and MRI studies done for other indications.

When the imaging studies are done specifically for complaints related to the craniofacial skeleton, routine reporting may be sufficient. There might rarely be a complicating condition, such a secondary mucocele, or infections with possible intracranial complications that might require verbal communication.

In this case, the nasal cavity obstruction was a known finding to the referring physician; the hyperparathyroidism was not known. The main responsibility here is to identify that the mass is likely of low biologic activity (low acuity but possibly high importance), remodeling the adjacent structures without invasion. Since it was atypical in appearance and could have been a sarcoma, a verbal contact was made. The presumptive diagnosis here was achieved by correlation with the shoulder and hand imaging (the latter suggested by radiology after the shoulder was made available to compare with the sinonasal imaging) and was confirmed with elevated PTH levels and tissue sampling of the nasal mass.

What the Treating Physician Needs to Know

- If a sinonasal mass has an atypical appearance for the more common epithelial pathology that arises in this region, what general category of disease might it represent? Is it more likely of mucosal, bone (bone marrow), or dental origin?
- If multifocal, could it be a systemic disease? If systemic, is it more likely neoplastic or metabolic?
- Would other imaging help in securing a diagnosis?
- Would other imaging help to find the most suitable site for tissue sampling—sinonasal or elsewhere?

Answer

1. The brown tumor in the nasal cavity can be surgically resected or debulked to relieve the nasal obstruction. However, the primary treatment is to identify the parathyroid adenoma and then surgically resect the lesion.

LEARN MORE

See Chapters 93 and 43 in *Head and Neck Radiology* by Mancuso and Hanafee.

CLINICAL HISTORY *A 6-month-old boy was referred to MRI because micropenis was noted on routine physical examination. Selected MRI images are shown below:*

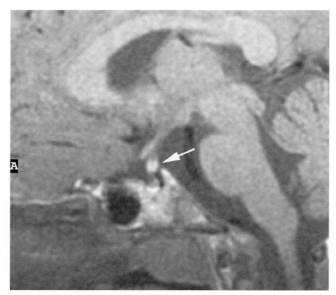

FIGURE **2.16A**

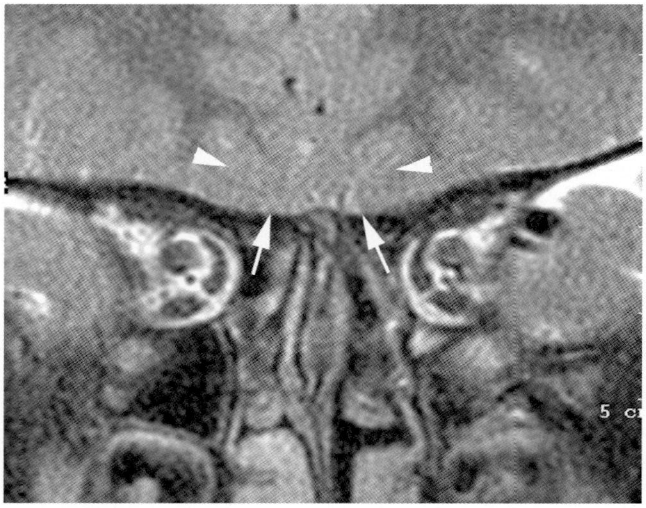

FIGURE **2.16C**

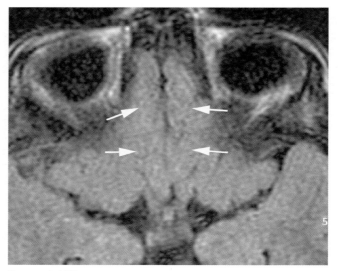

FIGURE **2.16B**

FINDINGS

Figure 2.16A. The anterior pituitary is difficult to identify, and the posterior pituitary (arrow) is ectopic.

Figure 2.16B. The olfactory sulcus is not developed (arrows).

Figure 2.16C. Coronal image confirmation of lack of olfactory sulcus development and imperceptible proximal olfactory tracts.

DIFFERENTIAL DIAGNOSIS None

DIAGNOSIS Kallmann syndrome

DISCUSSION Kallmann syndrome is a rare genetic condition associated with isolated hypogonadotropic hypogonadism and either anosmia or severe hyposmia. These patients have gonadotropin-releasing hormone (GnRH) deficiency. Hypothalamic-pituitary function is otherwise normal in most patients. In this patient, although the anterior pituitary gland was not clearly seen and the posterior pituitary gland was ectopic, the patient did not have any other hormone deficiency or diabetes insipidus.

Deficient hypothalamic GnRH secretion leads to marked abnormal gonadotropin secretion. This results in hypogonadism, infertility, and complete or incomplete puberty. The abnormal secretion of gonadotropin can be confirmed by patient response to pulsatile GnRH therapy.

Many genetic mutations have been described to be associated with Kallmann syndrome. The genes generally have been found to encode neural cell adhesion molecule, fibroblast growth factor receptor 1, or critical components of the prokineticin pathway. This disease is generally thought to be the result of abnormal neuronal migration during development.

A large proportion of patients with Kallmann syndrome have abnormal olfactory systems on MRI. These range from complete agenesis of olfactory bulbs and sulci to shallow olfactory sulci or medial orientation of the olfactory sulci. Although there are abnormalities of the olfactory system, most patients have a normal-appearing hypothalamus and pituitary gland. Idiopathic hypogonadotropic hypogonadism has only hormonal abnormalities without any imaging abnormality. Thus, imaging plays an important role in differentiating these conditions and other conditions of the hypothalamus and pituitary gland in patients who present with endocrine abnormalities.

Most patients may experience partial or no puberty. They rarely present at a very young age with micropenis, as did this patient. In general, the lack of gonadotropins leads to erectile dysfunction, decreased libido, decreased muscle strength, and diminished aggressiveness in men and amenorrhea and dyspareunia in women.

All patients with Kallmann syndrome have either anosmia or severe hyposmia. This condition may be associated with congenital heart disease or other neurologic manifestations such as color blindness, hearing deficit, and epilepsy.

Question for Further Thought

1. How is Kallman's syndrome treated?

Reporting Responsibilities

Getting the scan done with the right protocol is important; without the high-resolution T2W coronal images, it would be easy to miss this diagnosis. Any associated pituitary gland and hypothalamus abnormalities should be described. The report should also contain pertinent negative findings such as the absence of other congenital conditions like septo-optic dysplasia. No special communication is required.

What the Treating Physician Needs to Know

- If there is a structural cause for the olfactory dysfunction
- What is the site of origin?
- What is the likely diagnosis?
- Are there important associated findings?
- Degree of confidence of a negative study excluding significant causative pathology

Answer

1. If micropenis is identified early, it is treated with a short course of testosterone. Prolonged therapy is avoided to prevent virilization and bone maturation. However, it is still difficult to treat this condition. During adolescence, steroid hormone replacement is again begun mainly to increase libido, for erectile function, and to maintain muscle. These patients are prone to osteoporosis and need to be monitored and treated for the same. There is no treatment for anosmia.

LEARN MORE

See Chapter 94 in *Head and Neck Radiology* by Mancuso and Hanafee.

CASE 2.17

CLINICAL HISTORY *A 51-year-old female patient presented to the otolaryngology clinic with complaints of distressing left facial pain that has been gradually progressing for the last year and has become much worse in last 2 months. She had seen her primary care physician 6 months ago, but no imaging was performed. No other cranial neuropathy was detected on examination. CT with contrast was performed. Selected CT images are shown below:*

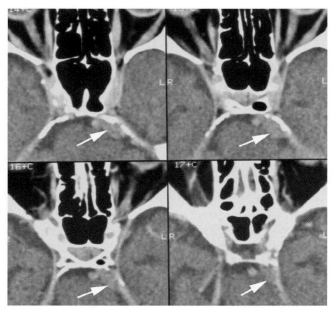

FIGURE 2.17

FINDINGS

Figure 2.17. The cause of the left fifth nerve symptoms as seen on this series of CT images is a dural-based mass projecting into the upper prepontine cistern (arrows). It slightly compresses the root entry zone of the trigeminal nerve.

DIFFERENTIAL DIAGNOSIS Schwannoma; dural and leptomeningeal pathologies including chronic inflammatory diseases as diverse as tuberculosis, sarcoidosis, and siderosis; and infiltrating malignancies such as lymphoma and leukemia and meningeal carcinomatosis

DIAGNOSIS Meningioma compressing the root entry zone of the left trigeminal nerve causing trigeminal neuralgia

DISCUSSION In this patient, it was important to determine clinically that symptoms are due to trigeminal neuralgia and not migraine or tension headache. This clinical determination is especially important when the pain is atypical for trigeminal neuralgia. Failure to identify the pain pattern as progressive, atypical facial pain can result in delay in requesting imaging, as in this patient. Progressive symptoms, especially when an atypical pattern for trigeminal neuralgia is present, require carefully constructed imaging protocols that cover the entire course of the trigeminal nerve and sometimes repeated imaging to search for a structural lesion when the initial, even carefully performed and interpreted, studies are negative.

Recognizing this condition is far easier when the pain involves only one or two divisions of the trigeminal nerve. Typical trigeminal neuralgia is almost unmistakable clinically. It will produce intermittent lancinating pain in any division of the trigeminal nerve, more commonly the second and third. There will often be a touch-sensitive triggering event such as shaving.

When more than one cranial nerve is affected, and possibly associated with other symptoms or neurologic deficits, localization may be much easier and a very "directed" and concise imaging evaluation is possible.

Sometimes, lesions outside the expected course of the nerves or involving end "organ" sites of sensory trigeminal nerve supply, such as sinus or dental disease, will be the source of symptoms. Therefore, imaging protocols are designed to not only image the trigeminal nerve but also all possible sources of such pain. It is critical to understand all of the neurologic deficits and complaints that might arise from the trigeminal nerve to enable effective imaging and interpretation of the images.

In this patient, since the meningioma was involved the nerve root entry zone and cisternal segment of trigeminal nerve, the patient had trigeminal nerve symptoms in all three divisions. If the meningioma was larger and extended more inferiorly, then sixth nerve involvement would be possible. If trigeminal neuralgia is associated with sensory and motor findings and perhaps other brainstem problems, then the lesion is usually located in the brainstem. Such lesions can range from intra-axial brainstem tumors to vascular disease to demyelination. If there is additional involvement of cranial nerves III, IV, and VI, the lesion is invariably located in the cavernous sinus region. More distal involvement is most commonly due to perineural tumor spread. Statistically, skin cancer is the most common etiology, followed by salivary gland neoplasms and lymphoma.

Question for Further Thought

1. How would you evaluate a patient with trigeminal neuralgia who has an obvious enhancing lesion in the cavernous sinus?

Reporting Responsibilities

In general, there is often little or no risk associated with the benign conditions; thus, no special communication is required. A likely cancer should be verbally communicated. It is important that the report contains a complete assessment of the extent of disease or tumor, including a statement of its relative significance to the diagnostic or therapeutic decision making at hand.

What the Treating Physician Needs to Know

- If there is a structural cause for the trigeminal neuropathy
- Is more than one nerve potentially involved?

- What is the likely diagnosis?
- If there is an alternative explanation for the symptoms or signs of the neuropathy affecting the end organ/endpoint of innervation
- Degree of confidence of a negative study excluding significant causative pathology

Answer

1. Clinically, cavernous sinus lesions present with associated neuropathy of cranial nerves III, IV, and VI in addition to trigeminal neuralgia. The differential diagnosis can range from aneurysms, neurogenic tumors, meningiomas, nasopharyngeal carcinoma (due to direct and/or perineural spread), lymphoma, metastatic disease, and other cancers that may be bloodborne or spread from adjacent bone. Less commonly, uncommon noninfectious inflammatory disease such as Tolosa-Hunt syndrome and sarcoidosis can present primarily as trigeminal neuralgia.

   A strong caveat here is that perineural spread of cancer may appear to be a primary process of this segment. The common error is to presume the enhancing cavernous sinus mass is a meningioma. When there is a mass in the cavernous sinus region, each branch of the trigeminal nerve should be traced to assure that the cavernous or paracavernous process is not a central expression of perineural spread of tumor from a more remote craniofacial site of origin.

> **LEARN MORE**
> See Chapters 95 and 31 in *Head and Neck Radiology* by Mancuso and Hanafee.

CLINICAL HISTORY *A 42-year-old male patient presents with fever and acute left jaw pain for the last 12 hours that has been progressive and now has swelling and induration of the floor of mouth and upper neck. CE maxillofacial CT was performed. Selected images, including reconstructions, are shown below:*

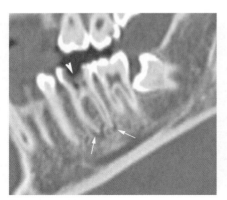
FIGURE **2.18A**

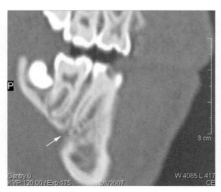
FIGURE **2.18B**

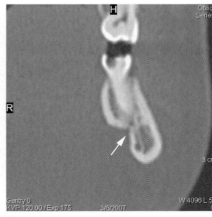
FIGURE **2.18C**

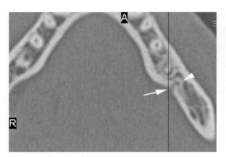
FIGURE **2.18D**

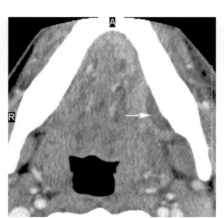
FIGURE **2.18E**

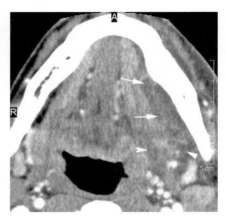
FIGURE **2.18F**

FINDINGS

Figure 2.18A. The gross endodontal disease (arrowhead) penetrates into the pulp cavity. There is secondary periapical change (arrowheads) related to the spread of disease through and possibly around the tooth.

Figure 2.18B. An oblique reformation shows the periapical disease penetrating the cortical surface of the mandible (arrow).

Figure 2.18C. The coronal reformation shows this tract of infectious disease penetrating inferiorly and medially (arrow).

Figure 2.18D. The axial view shows the defect in the lingual plate of the mandible (arrow) communicating with the periapical changes (arrowhead).

Figure 2.18E. A secondary subperiosteal abscess (arrow) resulted from this periapical infection. In this image, the abscess is fairly mature.

Figure 2.18F. A section somewhat lower shows spreading phlegmon beginning to organize into a submandibular space abscess (arrows) and less well organized more posteriorly (arrowheads). The more posterior disease is spreading into the parapharyngeal space and on its way to the deep neck.

DIFFERENTIAL DIAGNOSIS Sinus, skin, and major salivary gland inflammatory pathology may mimic the presentation of dental infection

DIAGNOSIS Endodontal disease with spreading abscess beyond the mandible

DISCUSSION Most head and neck abscesses outside of the orbit and temporal bone have the mandibular dentition as a source. Tooth-related infections that result in facial abscess are much less commonly related to the teeth of the maxillary alveolus.

Mandibular tooth infections arise from within the dental pulp, leading to periapical inflammatory disease, or from periodontal disease. Periapical inflammatory disease in teeth, depending on the virulence of the organisms involved and the host immune response, results in apical lucencies (rarefying osteitis), including periapical abscess, granuloma, and cyst. Usually, if left unattended or untreated, periapical inflammatory disease expands into the body of the mandible and produces subsequent complications. From there, the process can erode through the cortices into the subperiosteal layer and/or surrounding soft tissues resulting in osteomyelitis, cellulitis, or jaw trismus and eventually spreading into the floor of the mouth and fascial spaces as an abscess and sometimes the skin as a fistula.

These are mainly bacterial infections, both anaerobic and aerobic, although fungal disease is possible. Dental infections run a full range of relatively indolent processes to fulminate in necrotizing fasciitis.

Questions for Further Thought

1. What is the pathophysiology of this periapical dental abscesses?
2. How is a dental abscess treated?

Reporting Responsibilities

All cases where advance imaging is done for the suspicion of complications of an acute dental infection call for direct communication with the treatment team. This becomes a mandatory responsibility if there is any evidence to suggest a necrotizing infection or airway compromise or when maxillary tooth infections are seen, as they may also precipitate life-threatening situations such as cavernous sinus thrombosis.

The report should include the following information:

- Site (specific source) of origin and full extent of disease and whether the findings are consistent with the clinical diagnosis of dental infection
- Whether there are complications such as spreading abscess, osteomyelitis, orbital involvement, or vascular thrombosis
- If there is abscess, which spaces are involved?
- If there has been an attempt at prior drainage of the abscess, whether the drains have successfully drained each space involved
- Consider that a noninfectious inflammatory or other condition may be present if the pattern of disease suggests such an etiology.

What the Treating Physician Needs to Know

- Whether the findings are consistent with the clinical diagnosis of dental infection or if there is a more likely alternative

- Are there any complications, and does the situation constitute a medical urgency or emergency that might require urgent surgery?
- Origin and full extent of disease
- Are there findings that might influence surgical decision making?

Answers

1. Pyogenic dental infections that progress to the point where advanced imaging is indicated should be considered akin to an abscess or empyema, since it is essentially a collection of pus under pressure even when confined to the periapical region. It is this fundamental situation that creates the potential for the periapical or periodontal infection to spread beyond the maxilla and mandible. The pressure and local toxicity of the pyogenic material encourages bone resorption with eventual buccal or lingual cortical breakthrough and then subperiosteal accumulation of pus. Eventually, the pus will breach the periosteum and spread in adjacent and then more remote spaces. Since pressure is a driving force of these destructive and dissecting collections of pus, relieving this pressure by draining the causative dental abscess as soon as possible is the essential strategy aimed at the treatment and prevention of what can become life-threatening spread of the infection. This strategy usually begins and ends with extraction of the offending tooth but often requires more extensive drainage. The spread pattern is directed first by the point where the pus leaves its bony confines. Imaging provides the map for drainage procedure.

2. Empiric antibiotics are started after obtaining material for culture, targeting most common pathogens, including anaerobes, until the offending bacteria are confirmed. Specific antibiotic therapy is then the mainstay of therapy. Extensive abscesses, as in this case, would require an extensive open surgical procedure with debridement of infected, devitalized tissue and placement of drains. However, the mainstay of treatment is to eliminate the source of dental infection so that this does not recur. This is achieved by various endodontic microsurgical techniques. If the tooth cannot be saved due to extensive bone loss or resorptive changes, it is extracted.

> **LEARN MORE**
> See Chapters 97 and 13 in *Head and Neck Radiology* by Mancuso and Hanafee.

CLINICAL HISTORY *A 23-year-old male patient was brought to the emergency room by the emergency transport team. He was involved in motor vehicle collision. On examination, the left side of his head and face were bruised. He was in severe pain, was spitting out bloody saliva, and a crepitus was noted over the left mandible. Selected CT images are shown below:*

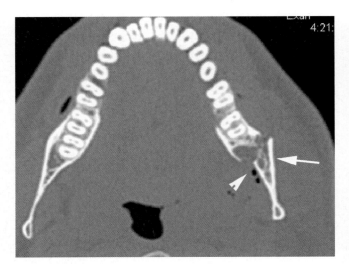

FIGURE 2.19A

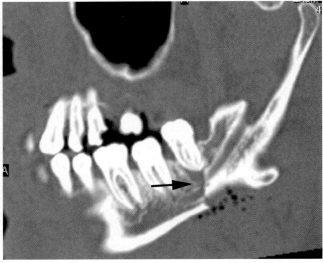

FIGURE 2.19D

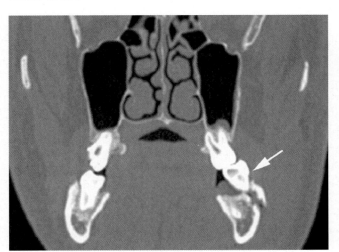

FIGURE 2.19B

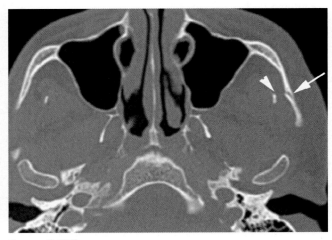

FIGURE 2.19E

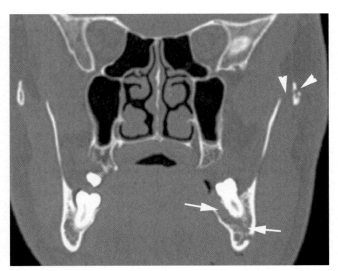

FIGURE 2.19C

FINDINGS

Figure 2.19A. There is lateral displacement of the ascending ramus (arrow) and a missing third molar as well as gas in the soft tissues (arrowhead).

Figure 2.19B. Coronal reformation shows the injured molar to actually be perched at the top of the fractured mandibular segment (arrow).

Figure 2.19C. Fracture extended forward to involve the root and root apex region of the adjacent second molar (arrows).

Figure 2.19D. Sagittal reformation shows the overall extent of the injury, including the interruption of the inferior alveolar canal (arrow). Both molars were extracted.

Figure 2.19E. There also was a fracture of the zygomatic arch (arrow) with possible impingement on the coronoid process (arrowhead).

DIFFERENTIAL DIAGNOSIS None

DIAGNOSIS Comminuted open fracture of the mandible with inferior alveolar nerve injury

DISCUSSION Motor vehicle crashes, fighting, and sports account for most mandibular fractures. Fractures most typically involve the body, ramus, and angle of the mandible. The ramus and coronoid process are relatively infrequent sites of injury.

Mandibular fractures can be classified as simple or communicated, open or closed, and additionally classified as "favorable" and "unfavorable" based on fracture orientation to the pulls of the muscles in the masticator space. An unfavorable fracture is one in which the natural pull of the involved muscles tends to displace the fracture, while a favorable fracture is one in which the involved muscles tend to reduce the fracture. Condylar fractures are described as extracapsular, intracapsular, or subcondylar as well as with regard to their degree of displacement.

In this patient, the fracture extended to third molar socket, thus communicating the fracture to the oral bacteria and risk of infection. Both molars were extracted. Interruption of the inferior alveolar nerve will result in numbness of this patient's chin and possible neuralgia later. The fractured zygomatic arch impinging on the coronoid process can result in temporalis tendon dysfunction.

Long-term complications of mandibular fractures may result in significant cosmetic deficits, mandibular dysfunction, and chronic pain. Nonunion, partial union, infection, construct failure, inadequate restoration of occlusion, and secondary temporomandibular (TMJ) dysfunction account for most of the complications. Injuries to the inferior alveolar nerve may also occur and produce neuralgia.

Question for Further Thought

1. How are mandibular fractures treated?

Reporting Responsibilities

All mandibular fractures are communicated directly to the health care provider—very urgently if there is any evidence of active bleeding, airway compromise, or associated cervical spine injury.

The report routinely should catalogue the following details:

- Whether or not there is bony injury.
- Basic fracture pattern should be identified if possible.
- Individual fractures should be described with respect to their complexity as nondisplaced, displaced, simple, or comminuted.
- With regard to dentition and occlusion, the report should contain details of displaced teeth, missing teeth (search for aspiration or swallowing), and potentially devitalized teeth with root fractures.

- Describe associated soft tissue injury, bleeding open wounds, and any other facial/hard palate fractures.

What the Treating Physician Needs to Know

- Is the mandible injured?
- Full extent of the injury and involved structures
- What complications might be anticipated based on the structures injured?
- Are there associated complications involving the mandible, TMJ, soft tissue structures, and/or airway?
- Is there a complicating infection?
- Are there any complications outside of those related to the mandible and remainder of the face?
- Are there findings that suggest a risk of delayed complications?
- Are foreign bodies noted or suspected based upon the mechanism of injury?

Answer

1. The choices for fixing the fractures are generally between open and closed procedures. Unstable fracture segments must be fixated to stable structures for surgical management to succeed. This objective can become quite challenging in patients with extensive mandibular fractures, poor bone stock, associated facial fractures, and/or significant comorbidities that might impair healing.

In combined mandibular and facial injuries, open reduction and internal fixation with miniplates and miniscrews is usually performed for best cosmetic and functional outcome. The mandible may then be managed opened or closed combined with the open facial procedure. Fracture fixation may be accomplished with miniplates, miniscrews, and compression plates or in rare cases with wire. External suspension-type procedures remain an option and often are combined with maxillomandibular fixation.

Treatment for a mandible fracture alone may be accomplished either through open or closed procedures. Closed reduction may be used for nondisplaced favorable fractures, grossly comminuted fractures, a severely atrophic mandible, pediatric fractures involving the teeth, coronoid fractures without zygomatic impingement, and selected condylar fractures. Open reduction is used if the occlusion cannot be restored with a closed procedure, for certain condylar fractures, those associated with complex facial injury, certain medically compromised patients, and nonunions and malunions.

Operated patients will often receive postoperative antibiotics in an attempt to reduce the potential for wound infections caused by intrinsic oral bacteria. Nonviable, loose, fractured, or possibly infected teeth will usually be removed.

LEARN MORE

See Chapter 98 in *Head and Neck Radiology* by Mancuso and Hanafee.

CLINICAL HISTORY *A 45-year-old black male presents to the dental clinic with left jaw swelling. He first noticed a slight swelling 1 year ago; since then, it has been gradually enlarging. He has no pain, and the deformity was the reason for seeking medical help. Selected CT images are shown below:*

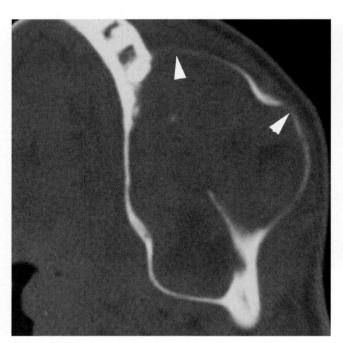

FIGURE **2.20A**

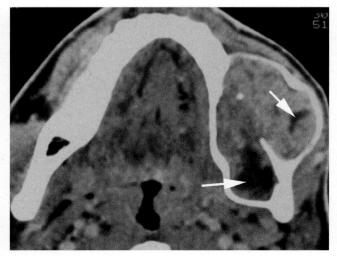

FIGURE **2.20B**

FINDINGS

Figure 2.20A. Bone windows from a CT study show a multilobulated mass with well-defined margins and some zones of almost dehiscent bone (arrowheads).

Figure 2.20B. Soft tissue view shows obviously solid and enhancing components of the mass and zones of cystic regressive changes (arrowheads). The mass, however, is contained within bone.

DIFFERENTIAL DIAGNOSIS Minor salivary gland tumor, plasmacytoma, fibro-osseous or chondroid bone tumors, giant cell granuloma or tumor, and a noninfectious inflammatory condition such as eosinophilic granuloma

DIAGNOSIS Ameloblastoma

DISCUSSION Ameloblastoma is a true neoplasm of odontogenic epithelium. These solid tumors arise from the enamel elements of the tooth and are locally aggressive but benign histologically, representing approximately 10% of all odontogenic tumors. They may originate from remnants of the dental lamina and dental organ. Ameloblastoma has been classified into solid/multicystic, desmoplastic, and unicystic subtypes.

The usual presentation is typically like this patient, with a relatively large multilocular mass but no pain. There is a predilection in males, more so in blacks between the ages of 20 and 50 years; 80% are found within the molar/ramus areas. Those discovered incidentally, usually by routine dental x-rays, may be small and unilocular.

An ameloblastoma will have a very thin cortical margin that is often focally dehiscent. It usually will bulge well beyond the limits of the mandible and will invade surrounding soft tissues. The tumor does not have a mineralizing matrix, although there is a fibrous variant that tends to be less locally aggressive.

Malignant forms of ameloblastoma are rare. The malignant carcinoma tends to create the most problems with regard to the local soft tissue extent, the main clinical problem being persistence or recurrence at the primary site. There is a relatively low risk of perineural and regional nodal disease in these rare cancers.

An ameloblastoma will have morphologic features on CT and MRI similar to any solid, benign epithelial neoplasm. However, unicystic and multicystic subtypes can look similar to other odontogenic cysts.

Question for Further Thought

1. How is this condition treated?

Reporting Responsibilities

In general, routine reporting suffices. Direct communication would be wise when an aggressive lesion is seen or when there is evidence of an excessively vascular mass or a vascular malformation that might pose a significant bleeding risk if biopsied. A pathologic fracture or proximate impending risk of one should also be reported immediately.

What the Treating Physician Needs to Know

- Whether the disease pattern is consistent with a known or working clinical or plain film diagnosis
- Full extent of disease—if it is solitary or multiple, the extent within soft tissues, the relationship to dentition and the inferior alveolar nerve (if mandibular)
- Whether the process is likely of high or low biologic activity
- If there are findings that suggest the lesion is a manifestation of a systemic or, rarely, a syndromic process
- Whether there is a complication of the underlying pathology such as pathologic fracture
- If there is a potential risk related to tissue sampling—fracture or excessive bleeding

Answer

1. These tumors are treated by gross total resection that must include a bony margin; thus, a segmental mandibular resection and reconstruction may be necessary. When there is soft tissue invasion, an adequate margin of normal tissue must be taken similar to the type of margin taken for a cancer operation. Most recurrences are in the soft tissue adjacent to the resection margin. Close imaging surveillance between 3- and 6-month intervals with CT and/or MRI is preferred until stability or regression of the soft tissue findings is clearly established.

LEARN MORE

See Chapters 99 and 21 in *Head and Neck Radiology* by Mancuso and Hanafee.

CLINICAL HISTORY *A 56-year-old woman presents to the dental clinic with left jaw pain of several months duration. Panoramic film demonstrated a lytic lesion. The patient was referred to CT for further evaluation. Selected images are shown below:*

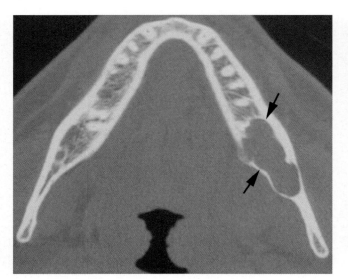

FIGURE **2.21A**

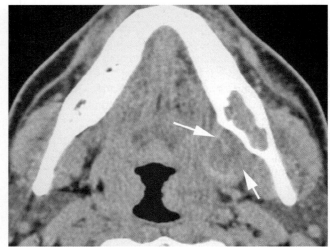

FIGURE **2.21B**

FINDINGS

Figure 2.21A. A fairly circumscribed mass is present in the region of the left retromolar trigone with a very narrow zone of transition. Normally, a dentigerous type of lesion would be considered most likely.

Figure 2.21B. However, there is also an obviously infiltrating mass in the adjacent peripharyngeal space (arrows). There also was a single 15-mm lymph node containing a focal metastasis in level 2 (not shown here). No mucosal mass was present.

DIFFERENTIAL DIAGNOSIS Submucosal SCCa, ameloblastoma, plasmacytoma, lymphoma, giant cell granuloma, or a noninfectious condition such as Langerhans cell histiocytosis is most likely given the appearance of the lesion. Imaging should help determine the next course of action, most typically tissue sampling. Sometimes, additional imaging or imaging-guided biopsy will be necessary before definitive therapy is planned. In this case, the metastatic node, practically speaking, limits the diagnosis to various malignant epithelial tumors.

DIAGNOSIS Mucoepidermoid carcinoma arising from minor salivary gland tissue beneath the mucosa of the retromolar trigone region

DISCUSSION Although most lesions of the mandible and maxilla are odontogenic in origin, a significant proportion are nonodontogenic in etiology. This differentiation aids in radiographic evaluation and subsequent medical decision making. Nonodontogenic cysts may be further divided into cystic and solid groups. Tumors and cysts of nonodontogenic origin may come from one of several cell lines that occupy and/or form the mandible and maxilla and their neurovascular constituents.

Various lesions come under this gamut. Nonepithelial lesions include cysts such as periapical inflammatory cyst, traumatic cyst, simple bone cyst, and Stafne defects. Epithelial cysts include nasopalatine duct cyst, nasolabial cyst, median palatal cyst, and median mandibular cyst. The osteocyte, osteoclast, chondrocyte, and fibrocyte cell lines may produce primary tumors of the mandible and maxilla. The mandible also has neurovascular constituents that may produce the full gamut of nerve sheath, neurogenic, and vasogenic lesions. Minor salivary glands also populate the mandible and maxilla, so any type of minor salivary gland epithelial tumor may arise. The marrow space of the mandible could give rise to lymphoma, leukemia, plasmacytoma, and Langerhans cell histiocytosis. Perineural tumor spread and metastases are also possible. Fibro-osseous lesions are a crossover group and can be of either odontogenic or nonodontogenic origin.

Differentiation of these wide varieties of conditions can often be challenging on imaging, as the above case illustrates that nonodontogenic masses can present with a wide range of morphologic aggressiveness and in some cases mimic odontogenic lesions. In reality, biopsy is the next step in most mandibular mass cases after imaging and a definitive way of arriving at accurate diagnosis.

Questions for Further Thought

1. What are two other common sites of high concentration of minor salivary gland in the oral cavity/oropharynx region?
2. How is a minor salivary gland cancer in this location treated?

Reporting Responsibilities

When the imaging studies are done specifically for complaints related to the jaws, routine reporting usually suffices. Direct communication is necessary when there might be a complicating disease such as a likely aggressive lesion that could represent a malignancy or evidence of an excessively vascular mass or a vascular malformation that might pose a significant bleeding risk if biopsied.

What the Treating Physician Needs to Know

- Whether the disease pattern is consistent with a known or working clinical or plain film diagnosis
- Full extent of disease—if it is it solitary or multiple, the extent within soft tissues, the relationship to dentition and inferior alveolar nerve (if mandibular)

- Whether the process is likely of high or low biologic activity
- If there are findings that suggest the lesion is a manifestation of a systemic or even syndromic process
- Whether there is a complication of the underlying pathology such as pathologic fracture
- If there is a potential risk related to tissue sampling—fracture or excessive bleeding

Answers

1. The soft palate and lining of the tongue base
2. Wide surgical resection with partial mandibular resection and reconstruction followed by radiation therapy would be the standard of care. Neck dissection may be required.

> **LEARN MORE**
> See Chapters 100 and 22 in *Head and Neck Radiology* by Mancuso and Hanafee.

CLINICAL HISTORY *A 34-year-old female patient presented to the dental clinic with pain in the right TMJ with clicking, progressive from the last 6 months. Selected MR images are shown below:*

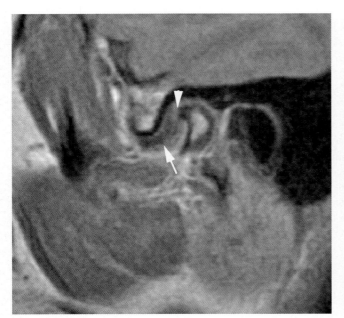

FIGURE **2.22A**

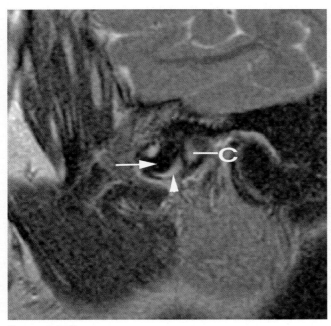

FIGURE **2.22B**

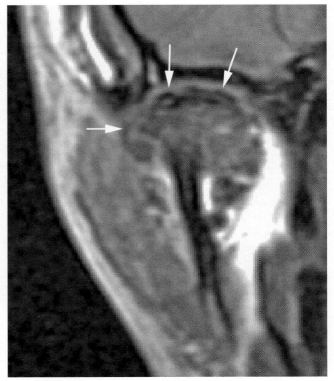

FIGURE **2.22C**

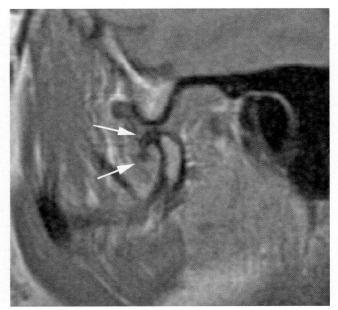

FIGURE **2.22D**

FINDINGS

Figure 2.22A. The articular disk (arrow) is well anterior to its expected position with respect to the condylar head (arrowhead).

Figure 2.22B. T2W image shows the articular disk anteriorly dislocated and somewhat more lateral than usual (arrow) relative to the condylar head (Fig. 2.22C), and there is an inferior joint space effusion (arrowhead).

Figure 2.22C. Coronal section shows the articular disk to be anteriorly dislocated and somewhat lobulated and dysmorphic with a component of lateral dislocation as well (arrows).

Figure 2.22D. Upon opening, the somewhat dysmorphic articular disk continued to be displaced anteriorly (arrows).

DIFFERENTIAL DIAGNOSIS None

DIAGNOSIS Anterior TMJ disk dislocation without reduction

DISCUSSION
Understanding the normal anatomy of the intra-articular disk is crucial to identify internal derangement of the TMJ. The intra-articular disk or meniscus separates the mandible and the glenoid fossa. It has an anterior and posterior band and a connecting central thin portion or zone. The disk is held in place mainly by medial and lateral capsular collateral ligaments and the medial and lateral capsular walls. The posterior band is connected to the joint capsule posteriorly by fibrovascular tissue called the *bilaminar zone*. The lateral pterygoid muscle has a connection to the medial aspect of the joint capsule.

The joint is capable, during opening, of rotation and anterior to posterior translation as well as medial to lateral gliding motions mediated with the muscles of the masticator space being the major contributors to this range of motions. In normal opening and closing, the intra-articular disk glides passively anteriorly and posteriorly on the articular surface of the condyle, between the condyle and the articular fossa.

MRI is the main imaging study used to evaluate internal derangements of the TMJ, replacing invasive arthroscopy of the joints. Standard MRI is most often performed only with sagittal opened and closed views.

Imaging findings mainly manifest as an abnormal position or abnormal morphology of the articular disk. Abnormal morphology may often be difficult to evaluate, particularly if there have been previous surgeries. It may manifest as just poor visualization of the normal disk anatomy or may show obvious fragmentation or fenestration. Morphologic abnormalities are much better judged by arthroscopy.

MRI is better at demonstrating an abnormal position of the disk, which may manifest as anterior dislocation with or without recapture upon opening, medial or lateral displacement seen more commonly in coronal images, and a "stuck" disk that fails to translate normally while the condylar head moves toward the articular tubercle.

The bilaminar zone may appear abnormally increased or decreased in signal intensity, suggesting edema or fibrosis, respectively.

Questions for Further Thought

1. If the condylar head is considered a clock face, between what hours is the posterior band bilaminar zone junction usually positioned?
2. How are TMJ internal derangements treated?

Reporting Responsibilities

TMJ internal derangements are generally reported routinely. Situations that require direct communication do arise, such as a periarticular mass affecting TMJ function that could be a malignancy or findings suggesting an infected joint.

What the Treating Physician Needs to Know

- Whether the findings explain TMJ symptoms and/or are consistent with the presumption of an internal derangement
- Full extent of disease, including the status of the articular surfaces, articular disk position and morphology in opened and closed positions, joint space, condylar marrow space, and periarticular soft tissues
- Whether there is an unexpected nonarticular finding that might be causing TMJ dysfunction

Answers

1. Between 11 and 1 o'clock.
2. This can be treated surgically with disk repair, repositioning, arthrocentesis, meniscectomy or meniscectomy combined with a construct made from tissue or artificial material, and condylotomy. More conservative care with physical therapy and splinting typically precedes surgery.

> LEARN MORE
> See Chapter 101 in *Head and Neck Radiology* by Mancuso and Hanafee.

CLINICAL HISTORY *A young adult female patient with autoimmune disease and bilateral TMJ pain and an abnormal mass presenting at the left external auditory canal near the tympanic ring. Selected MR images are shown below:*

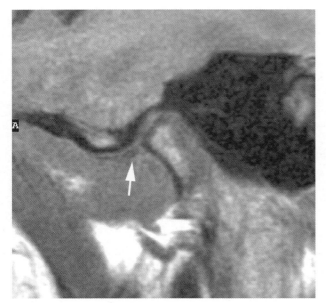

FIGURE **2.23A**

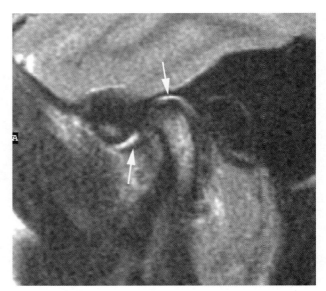

FIGURE **2.23C**

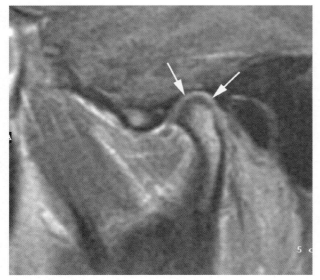

FIGURE **2.23B**

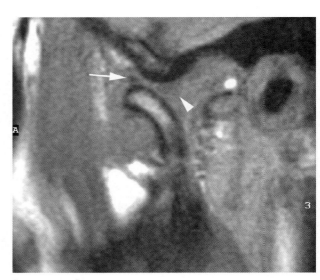

FIGURE **2.23D**

FINDINGS

Figure 2.23A. Noncontrast T1W image shows a dysmorphic, thin articular disk (arrow) that is anteriorly displaced.

Figure 2.23B. CE T1W image shows that the articular disk is difficult to identify and that there is enhancement of the synovium (arrows).

Figure 2.23C. T2W MR shows joint space effusion (arrow).

Figure 2.23D. In the open position, the noncontrast T1W image shows the anterior band (arrow) to be in relatively normal position and a dysmorphic posterior band

to be barely visible (arrowhead) but that the disk has recaptured.

Figure 2.23E. Axial T1W CE image shows the joint capsule (arrowheads) distended by enhancing synovium that has protruded into the external auditory canal near the tympanic ring (arrows), likely via the foramen of Huschke. The synovium appears to have herniated through the joint capsule.

Figure 2.23F. On the opposite side, the distended joint capsule is filled with enhancing synovium (arrow) and is slightly distended without synovial herniation as seen on the opposite side.

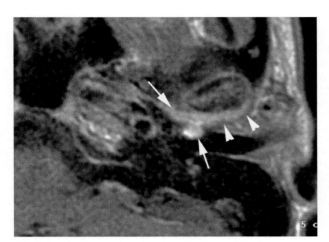

FIGURE **2.23E**

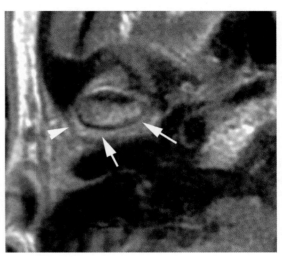

FIGURE **2.23F**

DIFFERENTIAL DIAGNOSIS None

DIAGNOSIS Anterior TMJ disk dislocation with reduction in a patient with bilateral autoimmune inflammatory synovitis worse on the left with the external auditory canal mass due to synovial herniation through the Huschke foramen

DISCUSSION Some of the unique features of TMJ pathology to be observed in head and neck problems are those related simply to it being a complex synovial joint. These observations are therefore similar to any that would be made in synovial joints that have meniscus elsewhere in the body. These critical points of analysis include erosion of the cortical and subchondral bone of both sides of the joint space, synovial changes, joint capsule distention, and the contents of the joint space and periarticular changes. Moreover, symptoms that might be attributed to ear "problems" fairly may really be of TMJ origin. In this case, the imaging was mainly done to sort out the origin of the submucosal mass in the external auditory canal.

Inflammatory TMJ conditions may be infectious, but the TMJ is more often involved in inflammatory arthropathy that is autoimmune, crystalline deposit related, and already manifested in other joints or due to isolated, acquired, noninfectious synovitis. Inflammatory arthropathies may eventually lead to fibrous and/or bony ankylosis; thus, the restricted opening in this setting typically will be studied with a progression from plain film studies to CT to MRI, the latter two studies usually without intravenous contrast depending on the complexity of medical decision making.

The rheumatoid and rheumatoid variant arthropathies that involve the TMJ will typically be present in the setting of known systemic autoimmune disease. Joint erosions, if present, may involve both articular surfaces, and the joint space may be narrowed or widened. These conditions, including rheumatoid arthritis and systemic lupus erythematosus, have been associated with condylar head resorption. MRI may show altered articular disk morphology, inflamed and thickened synovial lining, and joint effusions as in this case. The joint may eventually become ankylosed. Erosive osteoar-

thropathy can mimic autoimmune disease and more rare conditions such as pigmented villonodular synovitis (PVNS).

Questions for Further Thought
1. What other tissues can bulge through the Huschke foramen to produce an external auditory canal "mass"?
2. How are TMJ internal derangements treated?

Reporting Responsibilities
TMJ internal derangements are generally reported routinely. Situations that require direct communication do arise, such as a periarticular mass affecting TMJ function that could be a malignancy or findings suggesting an infected joint.

What the Treating Physician Needs to Know
- Whether the findings explain TMJ symptoms and/or are consistent with the presumption of an internal derangement
- Full extent of disease, including the status of the articular surfaces, articular disk position and morphology in opened and closed positions, joint space, condylar marrow space, and periarticular soft tissues
- Whether there is an unexpected nonarticular finding that might be causing TMJ dysfunction

Answers
1. Fat and the otherwise normal TMJ capsule
2. This can be treated surgically with disk repair, repositioning, arthrocentesis, meniscectomy or meniscectomy combined with a construct made from tissue or artificial material, and condylotomy. More conservative care with physical therapy and splinting typically precedes surgery.

LEARN MORE
See Chapters 102 and 20 in *Head and Neck Radiology* by Mancuso and Hanafee.

CLINICAL HISTORY *A patient with otalgia, mild trismus, and palpable left TMJ "fullness." Selected MR images are shown below:*

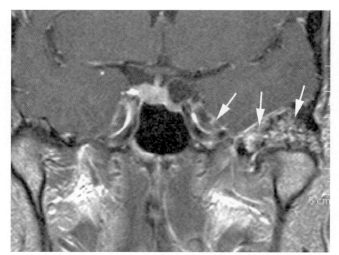

FIGURE **2.24A**

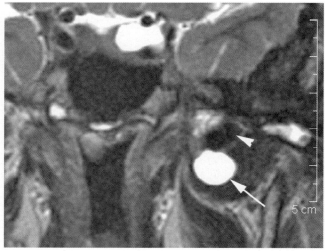

FIGURE **2.24C**

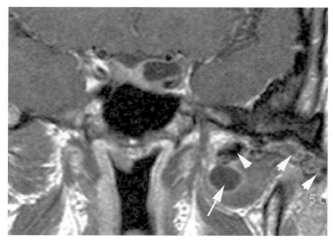

FIGURE **2.24B**

FINDINGS

Figure 2.24A. T1W CE image shows an enhancing nodular mass invading the bone of the condylar fossa and extending along the floor of the middle cranial fossa as far medial as the cavernous sinus lateral dura (arrows).

Figure 2.24B. T1W CE coronal image taken somewhat more posteriorly showing a mixed enhancing signal intensity pattern within the joint space with areas of diminished signal likely related to calcifications (arrowhead) and blood products and a fluid area possibly due to an area of prior hemorrhage and cyst formation (arrow).

Figure 2.24C. T2W coronal image for comparison with (Fig. 2.24B) shows the signal voids likely related to old blood products (arrowhead) and cyst formation possibly related to old hemorrhage (arrow).

DIFFERENTIAL DIAGNOSIS
Synovial osteochondromatosis (SOC)

DIAGNOSIS PVNS

DISCUSSION Most tumors or tumorlike conditions affecting the TMJ are extrinsic to the joint. These arise from the skin and subcutaneous soft tissues overlying the temporal bone and periauricular region and related lymph nodes, the parotid gland, parapharyngeal spaces, or masticator space, or they may be due to metastatic disease or a systemic malignancy such as lymphoma or plasma cell dyscrasia. Rarely, an actual TMJ-origin tumor or tumorlike condition will mimic one rising from one of these extrinsic sites, as in this case.

It is important to understand that tumors of structures surrounding the TMJ may present with TMJ pain or dysfunction; thus, images of the TMJ done with protocols dedicated to the evaluation of internal derangement must be searched for such extrinsic pathology. The corollary being that problems related to the ear clinically may actually be of TMJ origin and the joint must be carefully evaluated in patients with otalgia.

Benign or malignant tumors that arise primarily from the TMJ most often are of bony or marrow space origin. Aside from the fibro-osseous and osteochondral tumor origin, those other than metastases are uncommon.

Patients with the very uncommon benign and malignant tumors involving the TMJ often present with signs and symptoms identical with those of dental pathology disease, so these patients usually have had at least dental-type plain films, noncontrast CT, or cone beam volume CT by the time a tumor is confirmed by biopsy. A supplemental MRI may be useful, as was done in this case, in a patient who already had such prior imaging exams. MRI in these cases is usually focused on clarifying specific issues that may critically alter patient management, such as the extent of involvement beyond the TMJ.

One useful diagnostic approach to these conditions as seen on imaging is to first determine whether they arise intrinsic or extrinsic to the joint structures. Once that is established, a more specific odds determination can be reported with regard to the specific tissue or joint component of origin as well as the odds of it being benign or malignant.

The etiology of PVNS is unknown, with theories including metabolic lipid derangement, chronic recurrent nontraumatic inflammation, neoplasia, or a reaction to joint bleeding. PVNS results in a thickened synovium by a villous and/or nodular proliferation depending on the site of involvement. The nodular type occurs mainly in tendons and other or extra-articular soft tissues.

Microscopically, there are hemosiderin-laden giant cells and lipid-laden macrophages, fibroblasts, and other cellular elements. Hemosiderin also is found within periarticular tissues. The abnormal, hyperplastic synovium is hypervascular. These elements of the disease explain the thickened enhancing synovium and blood products seen on this MRI study both within the joint and in the periarticular soft tissues. PVNS invades local tissues and subchondral bone, the latter producing characteristic cysts. These findings explain the bone erosion and bone cysts seen on all imaging modalities and in particular on the MRI in this case.

SOC is perhaps the most reasonable alternative differential possibility in this case since a benign condition of the synovial membrane proliferates.

Question for Further Thought

1. What is the pathophysiology of SOC?

Reporting Responsibilities

There is only occasionally an immediate risk associated with these TMJ disorders, such as pathologic fracture, that requires direct communication. A TMJ mass may be found on studies done for routine dental or other indications. As these are unexpected findings, it is frequently wise to communicate directly with the referring provider depending on the perceived risk of a delayed or missed communication of that particular finding.

When the imaging studies are done specifically for complaints related to the TMJ, routine reporting may suffice since the pathology is often known to be present or highly suspected. The findings do frequently require direct communication since the discovered masses are not infrequently malignant or at least suspicious for malignancy.

What the Treating Physician Needs to Know

- Whether the findings explain TMJ symptoms and/or are consistent with the presumption of an internal derangement or whether there is an unexpected nonarticular finding that might be causing TMJ dysfunction
- Full extent of disease, including the status of the articular surfaces, articular disk position and morphology in opened and closed positions, joint space, condylar marrow space, and periarticular soft tissues

Answer

1. SOC is a benign condition in which the synovial membrane proliferates and undergoes metaplasia. The joint, bursa, or tendon sheath synovial lining proliferates and becomes nodular. The surface may fragment, and fragments collect in the joint space. The fragments may grow, sustained by synovial fluid, and calcify or ossify. The degree of calcification and fragment size varies. Fragments in the TMJ are typically a few millimeters. The disease progresses gradually with joint deterioration and secondary osteoarthritis, and it can be difficult to determine whether the findings are due to a primary degenerative process with multiple loose bodies or SOC. Malignant transformation is rare.

> LEARN MORE
> See Chapter 103 in *Head and Neck Radiology* by Mancuso and Hanafee.

Temporal Bone, Posterior Skull Base, Posterior Fossa, and Cranial Nerves VII–XII

CASE **3.1**

CLINICAL HISTORY *A 5-year-old boy with a malformed pinna and external auditory canal (EAC) atresia presenting with conductive hearing loss.*

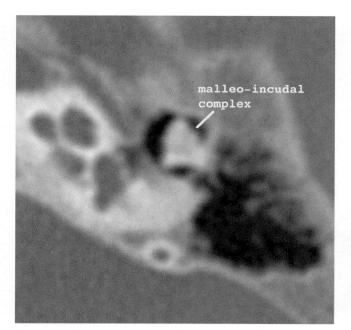

FIGURE **3.1A**

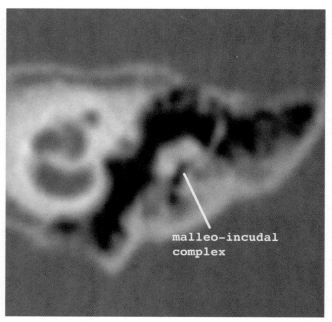

FIGURE **3.1C**

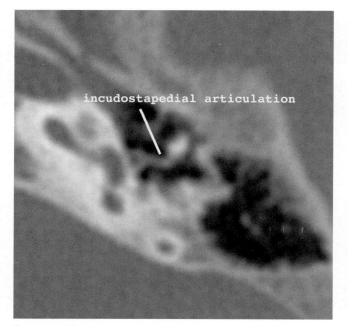

FIGURE **3.1B**

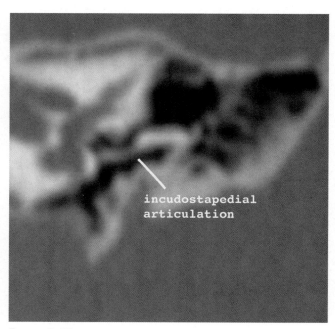

FIGURE **3.1D**

FINDINGS

Figure 3.1. In this patient with bony canal atresia figures A-D show, the malleus and incus are fused and incorporated in the atresia plate. The long process of incus is rotated and dysplastic, resulting in a dysplastic incudostapedial joint.

DIFFERENTIAL DIAGNOSIS Not applicable

DIAGNOSIS Aural atresia with fused and incorporated malleus and incus within the atresia plate with a dysplastic incudostapedial joint

DISCUSSION This patient had bilateral external and middle ear abnormalities. The left side had less severe developmental abnormalities and was the side of interest for reconstructive surgery. Audiometric evaluation should be performed as soon as possible after birth. Brainstem evoked response audiometry (BERA) or acoustic brainstem response (ABR) is used as objective measurement to evaluate the hearing threshold in babies. The involvement of the head and neck of the malleus, incudomalleal articulation, and the long process of the incus and the incudostapedial joint suggest involvement of both the first and second branchial arch development.

Imaging in aural atresia is typically delayed until surgical auricular reconstruction is planned, usually after 5 years of age. However, imaging can be performed earlier if the tympanic membrane cannot the visualized, especially to exclude congenital cholesteatoma. Computed tomography (CT) is used mainly because the critical information for medical and surgical decision making lies primarily in the bony anatomy. Magnetic resonance imaging (MRI) may be used in complex cases when there may be associated inner ear abnormalities and to evaluate anomalous brain development.

In this case, the stapes superstructure was intact and the oval window and the course of the facial nerve was normal— all findings that increase the chances of successful functional outcome after reconstruction surgery. A mesotympanum measuring less than 3 mm and a vertical height of an oval window less than 1 mm are generally considered inadequate for surgery. During development, contact between the stapes and the otic capsule is required to initiate development of the oval window and formation of the horizontal facial canal. Absence of the stapes leads to malpositioning of the facial nerve and absence of the oval window. If congenital or acquired cholesteatoma is suspected and the patient will not be treated operatively, it will be necessary to follow the changes with imaging yearly until the suspicious soft tissue changes have resolved or declared themselves to be progressive; in the latter case those changes may eventually require surgery. Noncontrast magnetic resonance (MR) could be used in such follow-up to avoid radiation in children.

Questions for Further Thought

1. What are most important factors for predicting successful reconstruction?
2. If reconstruction is not possible, what are the treatment options?
3. What is the ideal time for surgical intervention? Why?

Reporting Responsibilities and What the Treating Physician Needs to Know

- Is the bony EAC stenotic (≤4 mm) or atretic? If atretic, is there a fibrous or bony atretic plate, and if bony, how thick is the atretic bone?

- Size of the middle ear cleft, especially the mesotympanum (should be >3 mm in width)
- Status of the ossicles, especially the stapes, which is critical to the probable success of any attempted reconstruction
- Status of the oval window niche (vertical diameter <1 mm is considered a stenosis)
- Specific description of the entire course of the facial nerve to determine risk to the nerve during possible reconstructions to improve conductive hearing
- Status of the inner ear and internal auditory canal (IAC)
- Description of the pneumatization of the temporal bone
- Specific comment on presence or absence of congenital cholesteatoma
- Status of the sigmoid plate and roof of the mastoid
- Position of the carotid canal and jugular fossa and if there are any large anomalous vessels crossing the mastoid
- Whether the inner ear, brain, and cerebellopontine angle (CPA) appear normal.

Answers

1. The position of the facial nerve relative to the atretic plate, development of the middle ear space, and status of the stapes and oval window niche are some of the most critical features that go into planning the likelihood of operative success.

2. The bone-anchored hearing aid (BAHA) has become a valuable alternative to surgical reconstruction in terms of quality of outcome (hearing results, fewer complications) and cost-effectiveness. As a result, only patients with ideal middle ear and facial nerve anatomy are likely to be reconstructed in the future.

3. Surgical treatment is usually considered around the age of 5 to 6 years. At that time, accurate audiometric testing can be done and the pneumatization of the temporal bone is well advanced, facilitating surgical access. Moreover, it will provide the child with better hearing prior to starting school.

> **LEARN MORE**
>
> See Chapter 105 in *Head and Neck Radiology* by Mancuso and Hanafee.

CASE 3.2

CLINICAL HISTORY *A 2-year-old boy presented with delayed speech development. Audiometric evaluation demonstrated a profound sensorineural hearing loss (SNHL). CT and MRI of the right ear are shown below:*

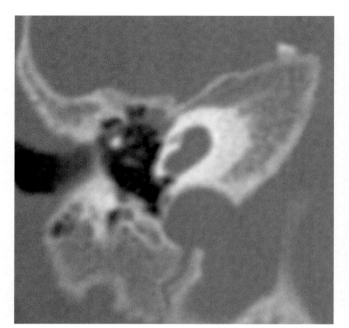

FIGURE 3.2A

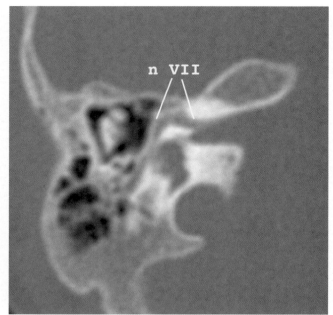

FIGURE 3.2C

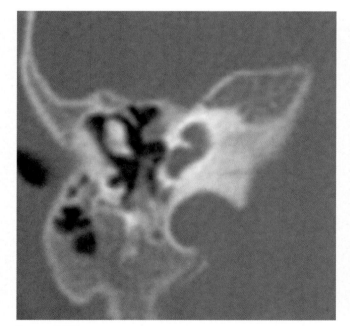

FIGURE 3.2B

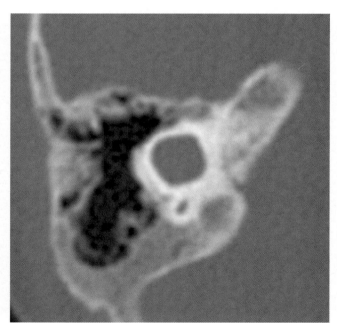

FIGURE 3.2D

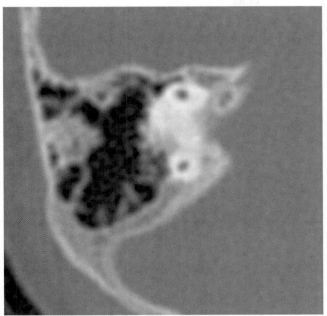

FIGURE 3.2E

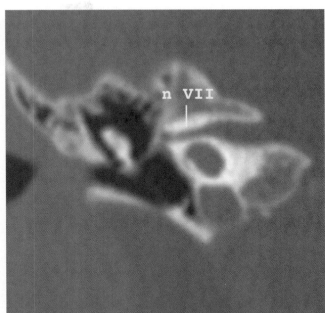

FIGURE 3.2G

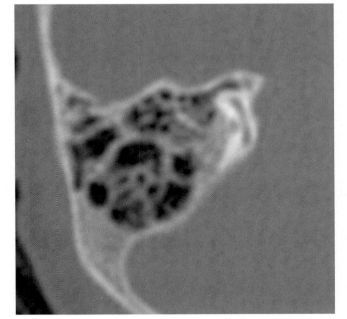

FIGURE 3.2F

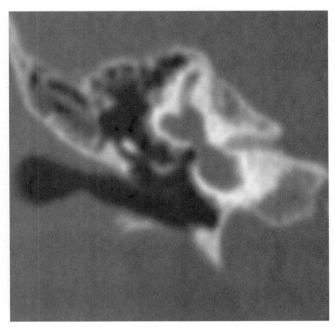

FIGURE 3.2H

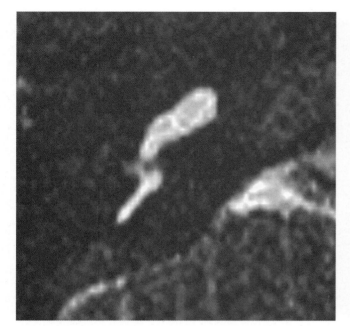

FIGURE **3.2I**

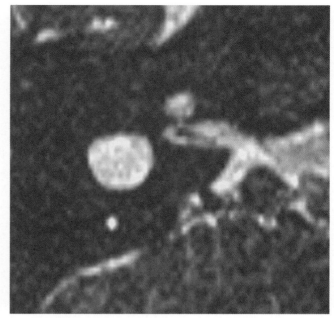

FIGURE **3.2K**

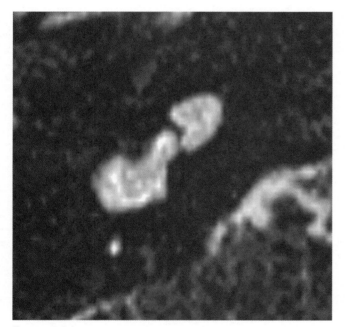

FIGURE **3.2J**

FINDINGS Axial (Fig. 3.2A–F) and coronal (Fig. 3.2G,H) CT images show a severely dysplastic cochlea. The basal turn is enlarged, and the second and apical turns are not formed. The lateral semicircular canal (SCC) is enlarged and incorporated into the vestibule, and the superior and posterior SCC are incompletely formed. There is no enlargement of the vestibular aqueduct. On axial high-resolution T2W MRI (Fig. 3.2I–K), no interscalar septum can be discerned within the malformed cochlea. It was not possible to determine whether a normal cochlear nerve was present.

RELEVANT EMBRYOLOGY The ectodermally derived inner ear begins as the otic pit before becoming the primitive otocyst. The otocyst first forms the saccule and utricle and then sends out three projections. The anterior projection develops into the cochlear duct, the lateral projection becomes the lateral SCC, and the posterosuperior projection becomes the superior and posterior SCCs. Cochlear development is complete at the 8th week of gestation. Formation of the saccule, endolymphatic duct, and utricle is completed within 11 weeks of gestation. The SCCs appear at the 6th week, and the superior SCC is completed by approximately 20 weeks, followed by the posterior SCC and finally the independently formed lateral SCC at about 22 weeks. The cochlear and vestibular aqueducts develop in conjunction with intracranial spaces, thereby completing the interconnection of the perilymphatic and endolymphatic spaces with the intracranial cerebrospinal fluid (CSF) spaces.

DIFFERENTIAL DIAGNOSIS Spectrum of findings and variations found when developmental arrest happens at 5 to 7 weeks (see the Relevant Embryology section above and the Discussion section below).

DIAGNOSIS Cystic cochleovestibular dysplasia (incomplete partitioning type II). This cochleovestibular anomaly is caused by developmental arrest presumably in about the sixth gestational week.

DISCUSSION This patient had bilateral inner ear abnormalities (only images from the right side were shown in Fig. 3.2).

Audiometric evaluation performed on the third day was abnormal. BERA was performed for objective measurement to evaluate the hearing threshold.

Involvement of the cochlea is consistent with developmental arrest before 8 weeks. Isolated involvement of the vestibule and SCCs happens when developmental arrest happens between 9 and 22 weeks. Generally, the later the arrest, the less severe is the abnormality.

Developmental arrest at 6 weeks would generally show at least partial cochlear development (generally the basal turn is formed, with fusion of the second and apical turns) compared to developmental arrest before 6 weeks, where there is either a large cystic structure without internal architecture (arrest at 4 weeks) or a cystic cavity with an anterior projection but without definite cochlear architecture (arrest at 5 weeks).

Other variations of developmental arrest at 6 weeks would include an abnormal course of the facial nerve with a long separate canal for the labyrinthine segment, absence of the round window, absence of the oval window, and concomitant malformation of the stapes and modiolar deficiency causing a wide connection between the cochlea and the IAC.

Questions for Further Thought

1. How is SNHL evaluated clinically?
2. What is the role of measurements in evaluation of inner ear abnormalities?
3. What are the imaging findings that make surgical intervention unsafe?

Reporting Responsibilities

For inner ear anomalies, the report is generally made routinely and must contain data with regard to the following issues:

CT and MRI

- IAC size
- Is the otic capsule normally mineralized?
- Is the cochlea normal (including the cochlear height, number of turns, status of the modiolus, and aperture of the cochlear nerve and cochlear aqueduct size)?
- Is the vestibular system normal (including the SCC size, shape, dehiscence, and size of the lateral SSC bony island, vestibular nerve canals, vestibular aqueduct, and sac region size/shape)?
- Are the round and oval windows normal?
- Specific description of the entire course of the facial nerve, which may be critical to recognizing a surgical hazard or associated anomalies
- Status of the external ear, middle ear, and mastoid in general and related major vascular structures

MR

- Status of cranial nerves VIII and VII—brainstem to end organ
- Status of the auditory cortex and any brain anomalies

What the Treating Physician Needs to Know

- Exact derangements of the sensorineural hearing pathway reported in a logical manner
- Whether there is an associated anomaly of the external or middle ear

- Whether there are any other associated abnormalities to suggest that this a syndromic situation
- Any potential for CSF leakage, perilymphatic fistula/gusher, or a potential route for meningitis
- Are there any alternative or additional findings that would explain the SNHL?
- Distorted anatomy that might create problems at surgery, including the status of the mastoid and middle ear roof, position of the facial nerve, major vessels, and any vessel that may travel an anomalous path through the temporal bone

Answers

1. Infants are routinely screened for hearing loss using otoacoustic emissions. This test may fail to identify children with abnormally developed or malfunctioning cochlear nerves and normally developed inner ears. The diagnosis of severe to profound hearing loss in early childhood is often made when the child misses normal speech development milestones. Audiometric evaluation should be done as soon as within 2 to 3 months after birth. Otoacoustic emissions reflect inner ear function. BERA or ABR is used as an objective measurement to evaluate hearing thresholds in babies, reflecting both cochlear and cochlear nerve function. With BERA, the structural integrity of the auditory pathway is measured. To confirm BERA findings, a behavioral audiogram can be done once the child is mature enough (at approximately 6 months).

2. Measurements of the cochlear and vestibular systems have contributed to the detection of cochlear and/or vestibular dysplasia. To increase sensitivity, measurements of the cochlear height on coronal images and of the lateral SCC bony island width should be performed. The height of a normal cochlea ranges from 4.4 to 5.9 mm. Cochlear hypoplasia (<4.4 mm) is associated with SNHL. A dimension of the bony island of the lateral SCC less than 2.6 mm is consistent with lateral SCC dysplasia. There is no consistent correlation between lateral SCC dysplasia and SNHL. Measurements above the range of normal for these structures may have no practical benefit in identifying inner ear dysplasias. Normal measurements do not exclude dysplasia; they are only another tool in a multifactor risk assessment for dysplasia.

3. CSF leaks occur on rare occasions in the setting of inner ear surgery, such as cochlear implant placement or stapedotomy, and inner ear dysplasia. The most clearly radiographically apparent anomaly associated with a perilymph (CSF) gusher (i.e., copious flow of CSF upon fenestrating the labyrinth) is a dilated IAC fundus with a deficient cochlear base. Distorted anatomy, including the status of the mastoid and middle ear roof, position of the facial nerve, major vessels, and any anomalous vessels, might create problems at surgery.

> LEARN MORE
>
> See Chapter 106 in *Head and Neck Radiology* by Mancuso and Hanafee.

CLINICAL HISTORY *A child with microtia.*

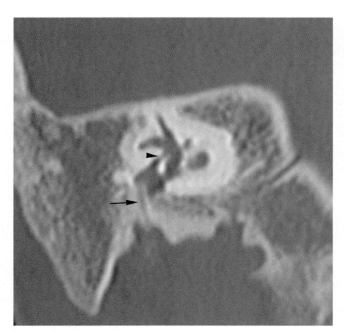

FIGURE **3.3A**

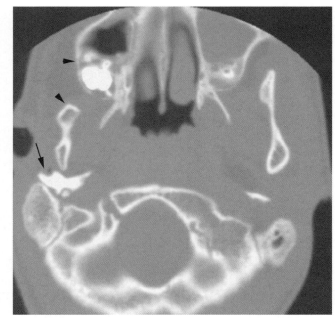

FIGURE **3.3C**

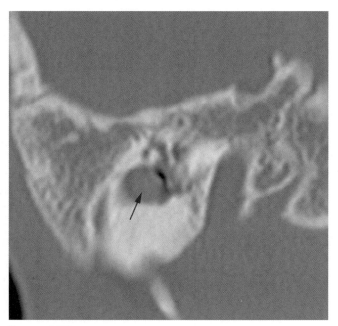

FIGURE **3.3B**

FINDINGS

Figure 3.3A. Coronal CT of the temporal bone showing aural atresia and middle ear "coarctation" with the facial nerve (arrow) descending through a thick atretic plate and markedly contracted oval window niche with no normal stapes (arrowhead).

Figure 3.3B. A coronal section more anteriorly shows an associated congenital cholesteatoma.

Figure 3.3C. Right side of the face microsomia manifest by a small maxilla and mandible (arrowheads). There is also a dysmorphic tympanic bone (arrow).

DIFFERENTIAL DIAGNOSIS Oculo-auriculo-vertebral spectrum (OAVS), most specifically hemifacial microsomia

DIAGNOSIS Goldenhar syndrome (GS)

DISCUSSION OAVS is a group of disorders that have unilateral or bilateral abnormalities of first and second branchial arches. These errors result in facial asymmetry and mandibular and/or maxillary hypoplasia.

OAVS includes hemifacial microsomia, GS, the first and second branchial arch syndrome, and facio-auriculo-vertebral syndrome.

Expressions of OAVS errors are generally associated with a spectrum of aural atresia and sometimes ocular abnormalities. GS has bilateral facial microsomia, vertebral anomalies, and epibulbar dermoid and sometimes abnormalities of the other organ systems. CT of the temporal bones in hemifacial microsomia and GS reveals unilateral or bilateral stenosis or atresia of the EAC, a small middle ear cavity, ossicular malformation, and atresia or stenosis of the oval window. Inner ear anomalies also sometimes occur in patients with GS.

Questions for Further Thought

1. What are the implications of the associated congenital cholesteatoma?
2. Give three reasons why conductive hearing cannot be restored.

Reporting Responsibilities

The written report of findings in anomalies of the temporal bone should reflect the developmental background of these anomalies. Such a report must include systematic documentation of the entire auditory pathway as seen on either CT or MRI, and a specific statement for each structure in this linkage should appear in every report. A reasonable approach to the general report format is to trace the sound, essentially vibrating air, from the outside to the brainstem and the facial nerve back out. For the purposes of discussion, the suggested report content in patients with syndromic hearing loss can be relatively conveniently divided into six basic categories:

- Those related to EAC atresia/middle ear anomalies
- Those related to possible inner ear anomalies
- Those that might impact cochlear implant candidates or those who are temporal bone surgical candidates for other reasons
- Anatomy of the facial nerve
- Visible and possibly related syndromic findings or clearly identifiable syndromes
- Suggestions for imaging or other clinical evaluation of organ systems that might express genetic defects

The reports can be sent routinely in almost all cases. If there might be a congenital cholesteatoma, it may be wise to discuss the implications of that verbally depending on the referral source to ensure adequate follow-up plans. Some syndromes have associations that require prompt intervention or investigation. Verbal communication is wise if such a circumstance is recognized.

What the Treating Physician Needs to Know

Reports must be logically constructed and comprehensive, anticipating all anatomic and pathologic findings that might lead to altered treatment plans.

Answers

1. Follow-up with imaging and likely eventual removal so that facial nerve function will not eventually be in jeopardy
2. Small volume of the middle ear cavity, no formed stapes, severely deformed oval window niche, and oval window region

> LEARN MORE
> See Chapter 107 in *Head and Neck Radiology* by Mancuso and Hanafee.

CASE 3.4

CLINICAL HISTORY *A 25-year-old female with history of dizziness, left-sided hearing loss, and pulse synchronous tinnitus. Physical examination revealed a pulsatile mass over the left promontory. CT and angiogram images are shown below:*

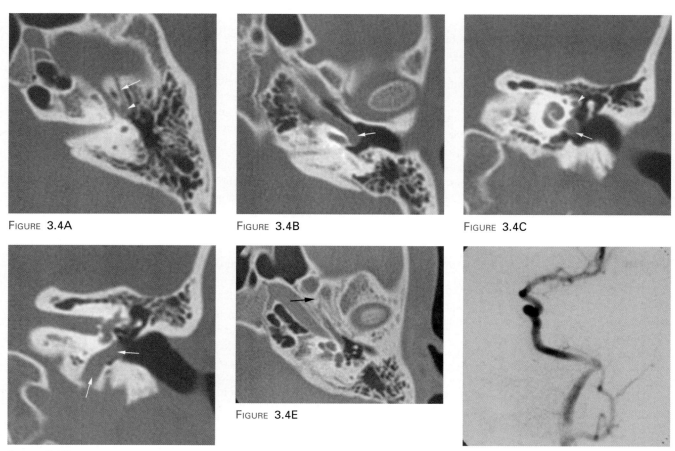

FIGURE 3.4A

FIGURE 3.4B

FIGURE 3.4C

FIGURE 3.4D

FIGURE 3.4E

FIGURE 3.4F

FINDINGS CT of a persistent stapedial artery (PSA) (arrow in Fig. 3.4A) as it joins the facial canal (arrowhead) with an aberrant carotid petrosal segment (arrows in Fig. 3.4B–D). Note how the facial canal is enlarged (arrowhead in Fig. 3.4C). The foramen spinosum is absent (arrow in Fig. 3.4E). Angiogram in (Fig. 3.4F) was unnecessary to confirm an anomalous course of the petrosal carotid segment.

DIFFERENTIAL DIAGNOSIS Glomus tumors, hemangioma of the mesotympanum, dural arteriovenous malformations, anomalous venous channels through and around temporal bone

DIAGNOSIS PSA in association with an aberrant internal carotid artery (ICA)

DISCUSSION When the stapedial artery persists into postnatal life, the middle meningeal artery typically arises from it. The foramen spinosum, which normally contains the middle meningeal artery, is absent. The PSA has a typical course. It arises from the petrous ICA, enters the anteromedial hypotympanum, and is contained in an osseous canal. The PSA crosses and is contained in Jacobsen's canal for a short segment. It leaves its osseous canal at the promontory and then courses dorsally and cephalad through the obturator foramen of the stapes and enters the facial canal through a dehiscence just behind the cochleariform process. The PSA travels anteriorly in the anterior facial canal and exits the canal just before the geniculate ganglion. It then travels anteriorly and cephalad in the extradural space of the middle cranial fossa.

The related embryology is complex and beyond the scope of this resource.

Question for Further Thought

1. What is importance of diagnosing a definitive cause of pulsatile tinnitus?

Reporting Responsibilities

Results can be communicated to the referring physician in a routine form, except when a biopsy is being contemplated or a surgical procedure is planned, in which case verbal communication would be wise to avoid inadvertent injury to the carotid artery.

What the Treating Physician Needs to Know

- Whether the vascular abnormality is a variant of normal or due to anomalous development or acquired disease
- If an anomaly, are their possibilities of associated abnormalities and/or syndromic associations?
- If acquired disease, what is the specific diagnosis, and are there any associated causative or complicating abnormalities?
- If a normal variant, does it likely relate to the patient's problem, or is it an inconsequential incidental finding?

Answer

1. Most cases of pulsatile tinnitus have no demonstrable structural cause. When no structural cause is found, it significantly allays the fears of the patient. The patient may need therapy and counseling to cope with this condition. When a structural etiology is found, such as paraganglioma, specific therapy such as radiation therapy or surgery is available to treat the underlying condition. When a structural cause such as ectopic carotid artery or PSA is found, the study is useful to prevent inadvertent biopsy. A vascular malformation may be treated with an endovascular approach and dural sinus thombosis may require medical management. This are a few examples of the conditions that may cause this symtoms and the diverse medical decision making that can result form such discovery.

> **LEARN MORE**
> See Chapter 108 in *Head and Neck Radiology* by Mancuso and Hanafee.

CASE 3.5

CLINICAL HISTORY *A 33-year-old white woman presented with pulsatile tinnitus for 1 month with complaints of some hearing difficulty in the left ear. The patient also complained of two episodes of loss of balance when she was listening to loud music while shopping for a home theatre system. On examination, there was mixed hearing loss and nystagmus with pressure on the EAC. CT temporal bone images are shown below:*

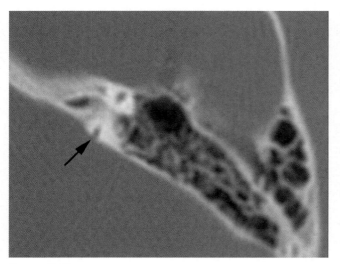

FIGURE 3.5A

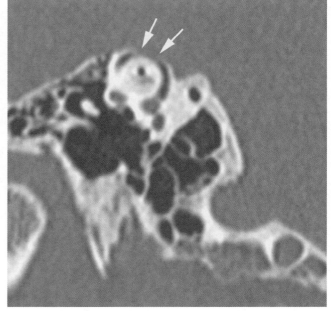

FIGURE 3.5B

FINDINGS

Figure 3.5A,B. CT images demonstrate a dehiscent SCC on the left side (arrows). In (Fig. 3.5A), an axial CT section shows a dehiscent SSCC. In (Fig. 3.5B), an oblique reformatted CT image shows dehiscence of the SSCC.

DIFFERENTIAL DIAGNOSIS None. This condition can be easily missed, especially if it is incidental and not specifically looked for as part of the routine analysis of temporal bone images.

DIAGNOSIS Superior SCC dehiscence

DISCUSSION A defect in the superior SCC can present with inner ear dysfunction. Dehiscence of the SCCs may be found at any age. Dehiscence of the superior (most commonly) and posterior canal later in life are felt to be acquired. Dehiscences are seen in children with similar forms of inner ear dysfunction. Most often, dysfunction will involve some degree of hearing loss—conductive, sensorineural, or mixed—as well as vestibular complaints. Pulsatile tinnitus has also been reported as a common presenting complaint. Classically, patients experience vestibular symptoms, mainly dizziness, in response to loud sounds or "Tullio's phenomenon or syndrome."

Dehiscence is also seen in a large proportion of patients without inner ear symptoms, which of course creates uncertainty about its causal relationship in patients with inner ear dysfunction.

Questions for Further Thought

1. What is the cause for hearing loss in this condition?
2. What treatment options are available for this condition?

Reporting Responsibilities

This condition is typically reported routinely unless it is associated with some erosive process that could possibly put the patient at risk for meningitis, such as chronic erosions into the mastoid by arachnoid granulations that might also cause dehiscence of the canal.

What the Treating Physician Needs to Know

- If a normal variant, does it likely relate to the patient's problem, or is it an inconsequential incidental finding?
- If an anomaly, are their possibilities of associated abnormalities and/or syndromic associations?
- If acquired disease, what is the specific diagnosis, and are there any associated causative or complicating abnormalities?

Answers

1. Hearing loss with the dehiscence has been attributed to a "third window" phenomenon in which the conduction of sound energy is diverted from the cochlea into the vestibular labyrinth. As a result, endolymph within the labyrinthine system continues to move in relation to sound or pressure, which causes an activation of the vestibular system.

2. Many patients with superior canal dehiscence have only mild to moderate symptoms. Treatment options should be considered on the basis of the character and severity of the patient's symptoms. For patients with primarily sound-induced symptoms, avoidance of loud noises may be sufficient to prevent the clinical manifestations. A tympanostomy tube can be beneficial for patients with symptoms arising mainly from pressure in the EAC.

Surgical repair of the dehiscence should be reserved for patients who are debilitated by their symptoms. Vestibular manifestations are usually the most troubling and are the ones for which surgical correction has been shown to be beneficial.

Resurfacing or plugging the dehiscence are two available surgical methods, generally by a middle cranial fossa approach and recently also via a transmastoid approach. Plugging or ablation has less incidence of recurrent symptoms after surgery. Surgery does not generally lead to improved hearing in adults.

LEARN MORE

See Chapter 109 in *Head and Neck Radiology* by Mancuso and Hanafee.

CLINICAL HISTORY *A 22-year-old male patient presented with progressively worsening acute onset of left ear pain, hearing loss, and fever for 3 days, with severe headache for the last 12 hours prior to admission. CT images of the temporal bone are shown below:*

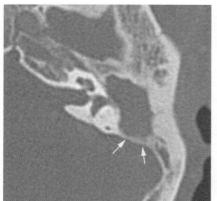

FIGURE **3.6A**

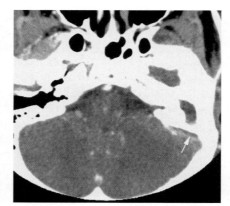

FIGURE **3.6B**

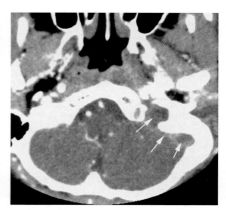

FIGURE **3.6C**

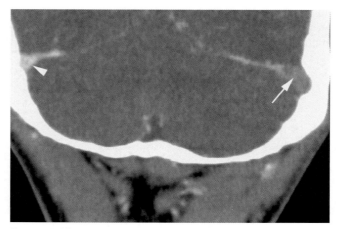

FIGURE **3.6D**

FINDINGS

Figure 3.6A. A CT image shows the remodeling of bone in the epitympanum and mastoid antrum and abnormal bone along the sigmoid plate.

Figure 3.6B. There is a small epidural abscess (arrow) along the sigmoid plate.

Figure 3.6C. Contrast-enhanced computed tomography (CECT) study shows thrombosis of the sigmoid sinus extending into the jugular bulb and thrombosis continuing into the neck.

Figure 3.6D. The junction of the transverse and sigmoid sinus shows minimal enhancement (arrow) compared to the opposite side (arrowhead). This could be due to enhancing thrombus with or without associated infection.

DIFFERENTIAL DIAGNOSIS Acute superimposed on chronic otomastoiditis, acute otomastoiditis in an immunocompromised patient. A more insidious onset and a less "toxic" patient with minimal tenderness and no clear evidence of sup-purative otitis media suggests acute otomastoiditis masked by incomplete treatment or an alternative diagnosis such as skull base osteomyelitis, petrous apicitis, eosinophilic granuloma, or tumor such as rhabdomyosarcoma or lymphoma.

DIAGNOSIS Acute coalescent otomastoiditis with intracranial extension causing a small epidural abscess and thrombosis of the sigmoid sinus and jugular vein

DISCUSSION Acute otomastoiditis is usually caused by an acute pyogenic bacterial infection of the mastoid air cells, most often seen as a complication of acute suppurative otitis media. Less frequently, acute otomastoiditis is seen secondary to chronic diseases of the middle ear, including cholesteatoma.

Untreated or undertreated and potentially masked, acute suppurative mastoiditis can lead to osteolytic changes in the walls of the mastoid air cells and cortex with spread beyond the tympanic cavity and mastoid; this is often referred to as coalescent mastoiditis (as in this case).

By the time mastoiditis comes to imaging, it may be in its coalescent state with the thin trabecular bone of the mastoid air cells and cortex appearing indistinct, either increased in density due to necrotic bone or frankly eroded. Similar thin bone separates the middle ear and mastoid from the middle cranial fossa, sigmoid sinus, and facial nerve. Suppuration may also spread through the oval or round window to the membranous labyrinth. Acute mastoiditis may also occur without evidence of middle ear disease if there is a mucosal block in the aditus ad antrum.

The pyogenic material under pressure may spread directly through the areas of inherent bony weakness to result in serious and potentially life-threatening complications. This sometimes predominantly thrombophlebitic spread pattern can lead to epidural and subdural abscess/empyema. Bland or infected venous thrombosis can involve most or all of the major dural sinuses; most typically, it is restricted to the ipsilateral sigmoid and transverse sinuses and jugular bulb. Jugular thrombophlebitis can continue well into the neck below the skull base. Imaging cannot differentiate a bland versus infected venous thrombosis. Infectious major arterial complications are rare. In this case, there was intracranial extension as epidural empyema as well as venous extension.

Venous disease can propagate into cortical veins and produce bland and/or infected cerebellar abscess and the particularly devastating infarct in the distribution of the vein of Labbé. Frank brain abscess may also occur as well as secondary leptomeningitis. Other routes of intracranial spread include a membranous labyrinthitis traveling via the cochlea and ducts and through preexisting surgical defects.

Less devastating but important spread through the mastoid to surrounding extracranial soft tissues can occur, resulting in cellulitis and/or abscess.

Questions for Further Thought

1. What is the pathophysiology for bone loss/decalcification in this condition? What are the usual sites of bone loss?
2. What are the indications for imaging, and what are the different imaging modalities available for this condition?

Reporting Responsibilities

Acute otomastoiditis is a clinical situation of relatively high acuity for proper diagnosis and triage. Direct verbal communication is necessary in most cases. The report should clearly state whether the findings are consistent with acute otomastoiditis and, if so, whether it is coalescent mastoiditis. It must also state whether there are extracranial or intracranial complications or a significant risk of intracranial complications based on the pattern of disease observed. A complete report generally should be structured in a way that assures the referring clinician that all pertinent observations about the extent of disease and possible complications have made. Such a structure should take into account the following:

- The primary site of disease origin and possible coalescent mastoiditis.
- Threat of early spread beyond the mastoid and middle ear.
- Intracranial spread, venous extension, inner ear extension, and related complications.
- Facial nerve complications.
- Spread into surrounding soft tissues.

What the Treating Physician Needs to Know

- Is the diagnosis of acute otomastoiditis correct?
- Is coalescent mastoiditis present?
- Are any intra- or extracranial complications of coalescent mastoiditis present?
- Is an alternative diagnosis more likely?

Answers

1. Prolonged infection results in mechanical compression of the bone by a swollen mucosal lining and retained secretions and creates hyperemia and localized acidosis. This leads to osteoclastic activity, decalcification, and bone resorption within the mastoid. This is the stage of coalescent mastoiditis. As the inflammatory process goes on, the osteoclastic resorption of bone proceeds in all directions and will cause regional complications. Trabecular bone of the mastoid air cells, Koerner's septum mastoid cortex, middle ear and mastoid roof (tegmen), sigmoid sinus plate, and facial nerve canaliculus are the usual sites of bone loss since bone in these regions is very thin.

2. Simple acute otitis media or otomastoiditis responsive to antibiotics is common in young children and adults and usually is not imaged. When no tympanic membrane perforation is found and no sample is available for culture/sensitivity, empiric antibiotic therapy may fail for the first time. In these cases and other cases presenting to the emergency room with low risk, noncontrast CT may be performed to confidently exclude coalescent mastoiditis. Coalescent mastoiditis is always treated surgically, even when the risk is low, and is best imaged with CECT. CECT not only allows evaluation of the early bone loss but also allows evaluation of other complications such as intracranial extension, venous involvement, and soft tissue extension. CECT should be done in a balanced arterial-venous phase to allow for the detection of both venous and arterial complications. MR should not be used for initial triage because of low sensitivity for bone loss. Other indications would include evaluation of causative pathology like nasopharyngeal mass and other complications like labyrinthitis and facial nerve involvement as well as assessment of the response to a trial of antibiotics. MR studies should include both MR venography and MR angiography. Diffusion-weighted images can be added for the assessment of potential areas of abscess, both intra- and extracranial. Fat-suppressed contrast-enhanced (CE) T1W images or a combination of pre- and postcontrast standard T1W images may be used.

> ### LEARN MORE
> See Chapters 110 and 15 in *Head and Neck Radiology* by Mancuso and Hanafee.

CASE 3.7

CLINICAL HISTORY *A 55-year-old homeless man presented to the emergency room with complaints of acute-onset left facial droop and dizziness. He had prior history of left eardrum perforation and chronic ear infection and was previously advised to have surgery; this advice was ignored. Selected CT images of the temporal bone are shown below:*

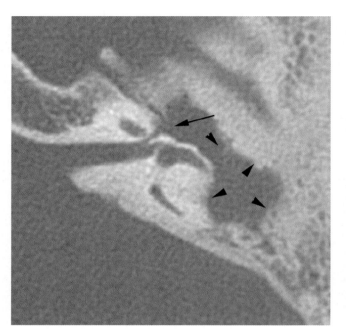

FIGURE 3.7A

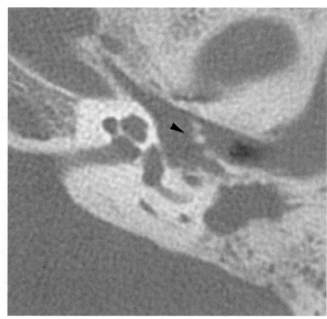

FIGURE 3.7C

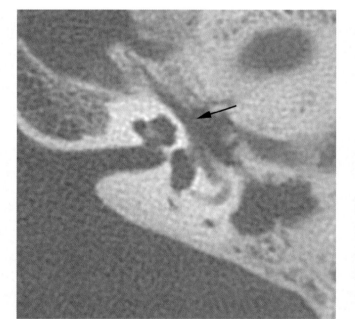

FIGURE 3.7B

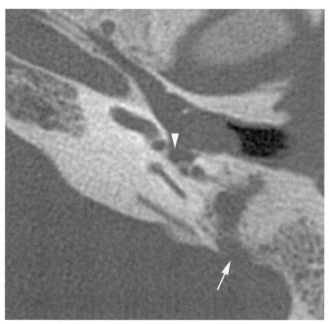

FIGURE 3.7D

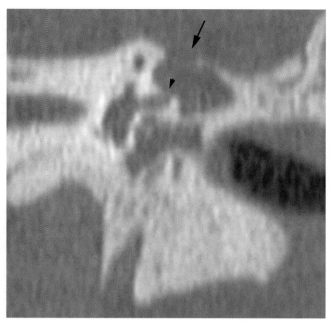

FIGURE 3.7E

FINDINGS

Figure 3.7A. Disease is spreading to the first genu of the facial nerve (arrow). It also widens the aditus ad antrum and erodes the mastoid antrum (arrowheads).

Figure 3.7B. Disease fills the mesotympanum (arrow), where it extends along the tympanic segment of the facial nerve. The ossicles are eroded.

Figure 3.7C. Disease material fills the mesotympanum, leaving only remnants of the malleus and incus (arrowhead). The stapes and incus bone process are completely eroded.

Figure 3.7D. Disease extends into the region of the descending facial nerve and into the lower aspect of the tympanic sinus and grows likely beneath periosteum along the descending facial canal (arrowhead). The disease has also eroded the central mastoid canal and the sigmoid plate (arrow).

Figure 3.7E. Coronal reformation shows erosion of the mastoid roof (arrow) and a lateral SCC fistula (arrowhead).

DIFFERENTIAL DIAGNOSIS None really—it is a clinical diagnosis.

DIAGNOSIS Extensive cholesteatoma with ossicular erosion and disruption, erosion of the facial nerve canal, and a lateral SCC fistula with erosion of the mastoid roof and sigmoid plate

DISCUSSION Acquired cholesteatoma often arises at the pars flaccida, the superior portion of the tympanic membrane, and extends into Prussak's space. Less commonly, the cholesteatoma arises from the pars tensa perforations and/or retention pockets of the tympanic membrane and extends into the facial recess and tympanic sinus; the latter sometimes is referred to as sinus cholesteatoma.

The clinical setting of chronic suppurative otitis media and physical findings including a perforated tympanic membrane and visible cholesteatoma usually make radiologic "diagnosis" of cholesteatoma a moot issue. Imaging is performed to establish the extent of disease; to detect any possible etiology such as a mass obstructing the eustachian tube, especially if the disease is unilateral; and to detect complications.

The pathophysiology of cholesteatoma is well established. Eustachian tube dysfunction associated with a retracted and/or perforated tympanic membrane leads to formation of retraction pockets, often in the pars flaccida portion. Squamous epithelium may grow through or within the areas of perforation or retraction pocket. The tympanic membrane collapses on the promontory, incus, and stapes, and this pocket deepens until exfoliated skin can no longer migrate laterally, which results in the trapped debris, along with body heat and moisture that promote growth of microorganisms. Secreted toxins stimulate a host inflammatory response including recruitment of white blood cells, formation of granulation tissue, and more rapid turnover of the squamous epithelium. Once formed, cholesteatoma can spread within the tympanic cavity and mastoid to points remote from the site of origin and can also "grow" beneath or along the periosteum. Thus, it might not be visible by inspection of the mucosa during surgery.

As an isolated finding, cholesteatoma is usually a round to lobulated, well-circumscribed mass most commonly originating in Prussak's space. The adjacent scutum is often eroded. The ossicles may be normal, displaced, demineralized, or eroded. The long process of the incus is most subject to erosion.

As in this patient, the disease can be more extensive with involvement of anterior genu and facial canal in the horizontal and descending segments and involvement of the membranous labyrinth with a vestibular fistula, most commonly at the lateral SCC with deafness and dizziness. The disease can extend intracranially through the tegmen or mastoid roof and cause meningitis and extra-axial abscess. Dural sinus thrombosis is possible with involvement of the sigmoid sinus. This can lead to hemorrhagic venous infarct, most commonly in the temporal lobe due to vein of Labbé thrombosis.

The role of imaging is to confirm cholesteatoma, describe its extent, and detect possible complications. CT remains the best modality for both primary and posttreatment surveillance imaging. MRI has a role in the preoperative evaluation in cases of cholesteatoma-caused complications, such as labyrinthitis and brain abscess.

Question for Further Thought

1. How will this patient be managed?

Reporting Responsibilities

Chronic suppurative otitis media and cholesteatoma are chronic clinical situations of relatively low acuity for proper diagnosis and triage. It only takes on high acuity when there is a suggestion of an acute superimposed and possibly complicated otomastoiditis, especially if intracranial or facial nerve complications are suggested clinically or by imaging. If the pattern of disease is consistent cholesteatoma, then the following guidelines should be incorporated in the diagnostic report. The structure of such a report may be as shown below:

- *For the main site of disease origin:* Status of mucosal sites in the middle ear and mastoid, including specific comments on the tympanic membrane and ring, Prussak's space, tympanic sinus, facial recess, round and oval window niche's, anterior epitympanic recess, protympanum, hypotympanum, mastoid antrum, central mastoid canal and related air cell tracts, roof of the middle ear, and roof of the mastoid. Also, status of bony checkpoints and structures, including the scutum, ossicles, Koerner's septum, central mastoid canal, walls of related air cell tracts and the sigmoid plate, bony integrity of the oval and round windows, and bone over the SCCs; the lateral SCC is most commonly affected.
- *For possible spread beyond the mastoid and middle ear:* Atatus of the roof of the middle ear and mastoid, perilabyrinthine air cell tracts
- *For facial nerve complications:* Evaluate the entire course of the bony canal nerve through the temporal bone, including the status of mucosal sites and mastoid air cells adjacent to the facial nerve canal
- *For spread to the inner ear:* Appearance of the oval window niche and bony integrity of the round window, oval window, cochlea, SCCs

- *For normal anatomic variations that might prove important at surgery:* Course and bony integrity of the facial nerve canal, position and bony integrity of the jugular bulb, presence on anomalous veins across the mastoid, course of the ICA, status of temporal bone air cell development, and adequacy of access along the usual path of atticotomy
- *For intracranial spread and related complications (in complicated disease only):* Patency of the sigmoid sinus, jugular bulb, vein of Labbé and other major dural venous sinuses, the appearance of the inferior surface of the temporal lobe and cerebellar hemispheres, and evidence of dural/leptomeningeal reactive changes or extra-axial collections or hydrocephalus

What the Treating Physician Needs to Know

- Imaging is usually more important to establish disease extent than to "make a diagnosis" of cholesteatoma.
- Soft tissue changes alone are nonspecific and cannot exclude chronic erosive middle ear disease.
- Noncontrast CT is the only study necessary in most cases.
- Imaging is limited in its ability to demonstrate minimal mucosal disease.
- Imaging reports should be precise and answer critical questions about extent of disease, including soft tissue changes, bony erosion, and anatomic variations, that might alter management.
- Imaging reports should delineate normal anatomic variants that might impact surgical planning.
- Acute complications of chronic disease might require CECT and contrast-enhanced magnetic resonance (CEMR).

Answer

1. This patient has extensive disease and has presented in too advanced a stage to salvage the ear function. The goal of treatment here would be to prevent intracranial complications, attempt to rescue the facial nerve, and to relieve the vestibular symptoms.

    The patient would be admitted and started on empiric parenteral antibiotics. Surgery would be performed, likely canal wall down mastoidectomy with removal of cholesteatoma as much as possible, especially around the anterior genu and remainder of the facial canal, sigmoid plates, and mastoid roof. Material would be sent to culture and more specific antibiotics instituted. Vestibular symptoms would be managed medically. The patient may eventually develop ossific labyrinthitis and completely lose all inner ear function. If the facial nerve function recovers and cholesteatoma does not recur and vestibular symptoms resolve, then this could be considered a desirable result for this advanced presentation. However, if facial nerve palsy persists and there is recurrent cholesteatoma, then a more radical surgery with more aggressive removal of cholesteatoma with obliteration of the middle ear and mastoid with bone chips and stripping of mucosa and occlusion of the eustachian tube may be required.

LEARN MORE
See Chapter 111 in *Head and Neck Radiology* by Mancuso and Hanafee.

CASE 3.8

CLINICAL HISTORY *A 38-year-old female patient presented with a severe left-sided headache for the last 3 days, with left facial pain and diplopia for the last 24 hours. On physical examination, a left sixth nerve palsy was noted. CT images are shown below:*

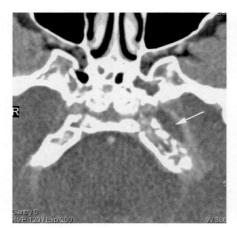

FIGURE **3.8A**

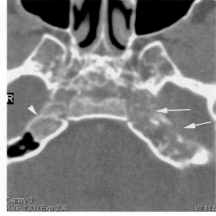

FIGURE **3.8B**

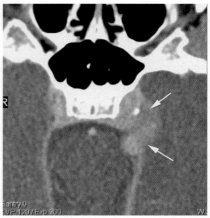

FIGURE **3.8C**

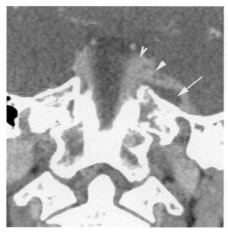

FIGURE **3.8D**

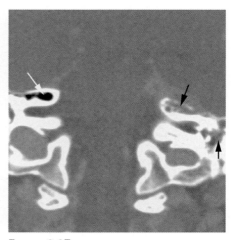

FIGURE **3.8E**

FINDINGS

Figure 3.8A. CECT study shows an epidural abscess along the petrous ridge (arrow).

Figure 3.8B. Bone detail images show erosion of the cortex of the petrous apex (arrows) compared to the normal cortical bone on the opposite side (arrowheads).

Figure 3.8C. There is extensive dural enhancement extending well beyond the area of obvious epidural abscess (arrows).

Figure 3.8D. Coronal sections show the epidural abscess (arrow) as well as the spreading dural phlegmon.

Figure 3.8E. The conduit for this disease was a tract of air cells seen on the normal side (white arrow) that allowed middle ear and mastoid disease to spread from the middle ear and mastoid to the petrous apex (black arrows).

RELEVANT ANATOMY The anatomy of interest is that of the petrous apex and mastoid air cell tract development as those air cells populate the petrous apex. Understanding the relationship of cranial nerves V and VI to the petroclival fissure region and the petrous segment of the carotid canal is also useful.

DIFFERENTIAL DIAGNOSIS Petrous apex cholesterol cyst, petrous mucocele

DIAGNOSIS Petrous apicitis with epidural abscess and dural phlegmon with involvement of the left fifth and sixth cranial nerves

DISCUSSION Petrous apex mucosal disease is an acquired inflammatory disease that arrives at that point usually along an air cell tract leading to the petrous apex. It is essentially the same disease that occurs in the middle ear and mastoid. The clinical presentation is due to the specific location and involvement of adjacent structures. Petrous apex mucosal disease may be limited to simple mucosal thickening with or without active inflammation, manifest by contrast enhancement. This mucosal change can more exuberant when due to bacterial or fungal infections causing localized bone erosion, such as that seen in coalescent mastoiditis; the process then is properly referred to as acute or subacute petrous apicitis and early osteomyelitis. This is a fairly serious disease process with life-threatening complications if left untreated. Such infectious petrous apicitis might progress to induce a nasopharyngeal abscess or dural phlegmon and then epidural or subdural empyema. The disease may propagate along veins to the dural sinuses and lead to substantial complications involving the brain and subarachnoid space. Cranial involvement is thought to result from direct spread of inflammation at the petrous apex. A petrous apex cholesterol cyst would demonstrate characteristic signal changes on MR, and a petrous mucocele would show regressive remodeling with expansion but without evidence of inflammation.

Questions for Further Thought

1. What is Gradenigo syndrome?
2. What are the treatment options?

Reporting Responsibilities

Simple mucosal disease is typically inconsequential and can be mentioned in the report. However, bone erosion with dural phlegmon, epidural abscess, and/or thrombophlebitis of dural sinuses should be urgently communicated verbally.

What the Treating Physician Needs to Know

- If the specific diagnosis of petrous apex infection can be confirmed and differentiated from minor air cell mucosal identification
- Extent of disease and extent of any related complications, including empyema, vascular occlusive and infectious complications, and those affecting the brain

- Relationship to surrounding anatomic structures best determined by a combination of CT and MRI
- Possible drainage pathways if CT is done
- Factors that might complicate a particular surgical approach such as high jugular bulb and variations in the mastoid
- If not a petrous apex infection, what is the most likely diagnosis?
- Likely need for and preferred imaging method of follow-up

Answers

1. The clinical triad of otorrhea, headache, and diplopia is known as Gradenigo syndrome. Diplopia is secondary to involvement of cranial nerve VI.

2. The etiology of infectious disease that is causing true petrous apicitis must be established and treated with appropriate antimicrobial therapy. Indications for surgery include drainable mucopyoceles of the petrous apex, a complicating empyema, and progressive cranial nerve deficits. The goal is to drain the lesion by exteriorizing it via the temporal bone. If labyrinthine function is poor, it is safest and easiest to use a direct translabyrinthine, usually transcochlear, approach. With intact labyrinthine function, the remaining transmastoid approaches are along the imaging demonstrated path of air cell development in that particular patient. CT with multiplanar and three-dimensional (3D) reconstruction plays a crucial role in surgical planning for the drainage pathway and its relationship to the carotid artery, jugular vein, and bony structures of the labyrinth.

> ### LEARN MORE
> See Chapters 112 and 13 in *Head and Neck Radiology* by Mancuso and Hanafee.

CASE 3.9

CLINICAL HISTORY *A 37-year-old male patient presented with chronic progressive headache for 2 years with recent onset of right ear fullness and diminished hearing. Physical examination showed serous effusion in the right middle ear with conductive hearing loss. Selected CT and MRI images are shown below:*

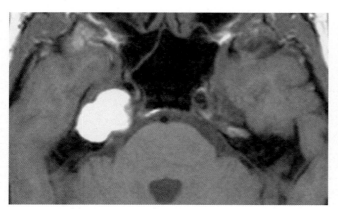

FIGURE **3.9A**

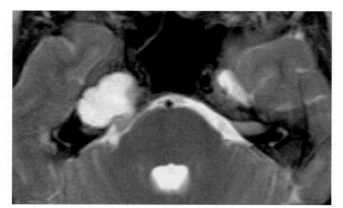

FIGURE **3.9B**

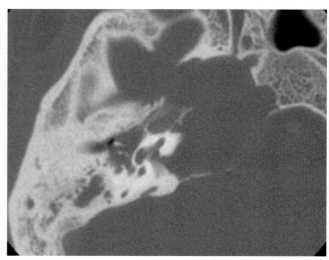

FIGURE **3.9C**

FINDINGS

Figure 3.9A–C. T1W noncontrast image (Fig. 3.9A) shows an expansile mass of the petrous apex of increased signal intensity equivalent to that of fat or brighter. T2W sequence (Fig. 3.9B) demonstrates the relatively watery nature of the mass but shows no evidence of blood products or internal heterogeneity of the mass. CT study (Fig. 3.9C) shows the evidence of relatively low biologic activity with chronic remodeling of the bone of the petrous apex, including much demineralization of the carotid canal.

Surgery revealed cholesterolosis. The opacification of the middle ear and mastoid visible on the MR study was due to the lesion occluding the bony eustachian tube.

RELEVANT ANATOMY The anatomy of interest is that of the petrous apex and mastoid air cell tract development as those air cells populate the petrous apex. It is also useful to understand the relationship of cranial nerves V and VI to the petroclival fissure region and the petrous segment of the carotid canal.

DIFFERENTIAL DIAGNOSIS Petrous apex mucocele or epidermoid

DIAGNOSIS Petrous apex cholesterol granuloma

DISCUSSION Cholesterol granuloma of the petrous apex is an acquired, sterile inflammatory reaction to blood breakdown products resulting from cyclical bleeding and accumulation of cholesterol crystals into a pneumatized petrous apex. Repeated hemorrhage into a pneumatized petrous apex results in accumulation of cholesterol and other end-stage blood products. The bleeding may be from inflamed mucosa and/or leakage from the vascularized skull base marrow space. Regressive remodeling of the surrounding bone occurs because the lesion is under constant pressure. The expansile mass may also compress cranial nerves V, VI, VII, and VIII and become adherent to major vessels, including the dural sinuses, carotid artery, and jugular vein. MRI provides essentially a definitive diagnosis of cholesterolosis when the signature signal intensities of the cyst and retained blood products changes are expressed on various pulse sequences as described previously. CT is excellent for determining whether bone is dehiscent—a factor that is sometimes used in determining timing and route of surgical intervention.

A mucocele occurs due to obstruction of an air cell tract leading to the petrous apex. Continued secretions from the mucosa will lead to expansion of the petrous apex without bleeding. Mucocele usually is low signal on T1W and high signal on T2W sequences without restricted diffusion unless complicated by infection. They can show smooth rim enhancement with contrast administration.

Epidermoid cysts are of ectodermal origin lined solely by stratified squamous epithelium and arise from inclusion of epithelial elements in abnormal location during embryogenesis. Epidermoid cysts are normally well-defined masses with a lobulated or irregularly nodular surface. The cyst is typically filled with waxy debris rich in cholesterol, resulting from constant sloughing of the keratin from the cyst wall. This cholesterol is, however, usually not "in solution"; thus, its potential to shorten T1 is most often not expressed. Epidermoid cysts follow CSF signal on T1W and T2W sequences, do not enhance with contrast, and demonstrate restricted diffusion on diffusion-weighted imaging. They are occasionally bright on T1W sequences.

All of the lesions just discussed appear similar on CT, with a smooth to lobulated expansile and typically low attenuation (although epidermoids are rarely high attenuation) mass, and MR is required to further differentiate them from other benign and malignant petrous apex lesions.

Questions for Further Thought

1. What is the role of CT in this condition?
2. When and how is this condition treated?

Reporting Responsibilities

This condition is chronic and can typically be reported routinely. If an alternative diagnosis such as chondrosarcoma is possible, direct verbal confirmation is wise. If an infectious complication might be present, direct communication is necessary. Dehiscence of bone raises the possibility of rupture, and the patient should be put in the hands of a neuro-otologist and/or neurosurgeon for appropriate timely disposition.

What the Treating Physician Needs to Know

• If the specific diagnosis of cholesterolosis or mucocele of the petrous apex can be confirmed; if not, what is the most likely diagnosis?

• Extent of bony dehiscence, relationship to surrounding anatomic structures, and possible drainage pathways if CT is done
• Factors that might complicate a particular surgical approach, such as a high jugular bulb variation in the mastoid
• Whether further follow-up is necessary; if surveillance is chosen, the preferred method(s) of such follow-up

Answers

1. CT alone cannot differentiate the different lesions in this region. CT is excellent for determining the extent of bony dehiscence and is indispensable for planning the operative approach. It may be preferable for surveillance when nonoperative watchful waiting is chosen as an alternative to drainage since progressive bony dehiscence may be a criterion that eventually forces a surgical option to reduce the risk of intracranial rupture. CT is also useful for postdrainage surveillance when recurrence is suspected since it can demonstrate whether the drainage tract has closed down more definitively than MRI.

2. If asymptomatic, the patient may be followed with imaging every 1 to 2 years to monitor the bony wall. Once that bone is demineralized, the risk of intracranial rupture becomes greater and aggressive intervention may be warranted. Indications for surgery include recurrent or progressive cranial nerve deficits and persistent headaches or otalgia and perceived risk of intracranial rupture. The surgical treatment is to drain the lesion by exteriorizing it via the temporal bone or sphenoid sinus. If labyrinthine function is poor, it is safest and easiest to use a direct translabyrinthine, transcochlear approach. With intact labyrinthine function, a transmastoid approach, basically along superior and infralabyrinthine tracts, is used. High-detail CT with 3D and multiplanar reconstruction, which are typically most informative along the long axis of the temporal bone, can help to establish whether these pathways are present and their relationship to adjacent vessels.

> LEARN MORE
> See Chapters 113 and 8 *Head and Neck Radiology* by Mancuso and Hanafee.

CLINICAL HISTORY *A 67-year-old male patient with uncontrolled diabetes presented with severe right ear pain, mild swelling, and mild ear discharge. CT images are shown below:*

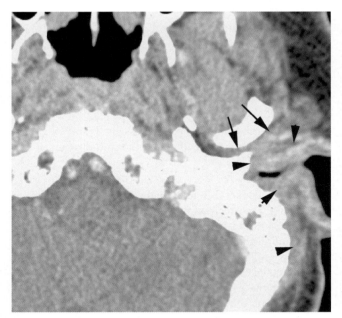

FIGURE **3.10A**

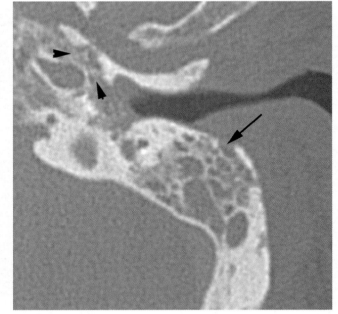

FIGURE **3.10C**

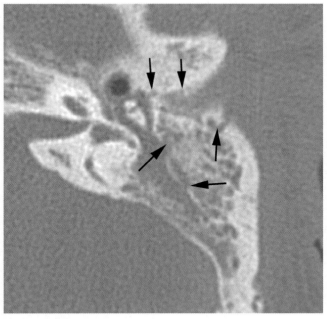

FIGURE **3.10B**

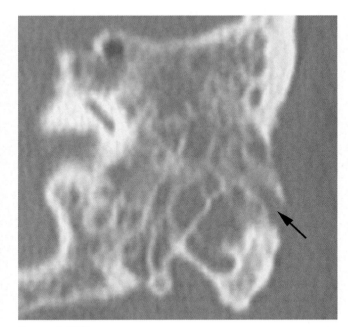

FIGURE **3.10D**

FINDINGS

Figure 3.10A. There is extensive soft tissue swelling of the external ear and along the mastoid (arrowheads) as well as along the posterior aspect of the temporomandibular joint (TMJ) (arrows).

Figure 3.10B. There is extensive bone erosion along the anterior wall of the EAC in addition to multiple areas of mastoid bone erosion.

Figure 3.10C. Bone erosion extends along the petrotympanic fissure in a fairly typical pattern (arrowheads), but it also involves the mastoid cortex in a less typical pattern.

Figure 3.10D. Coronal reformation shows the direct involvement of the mastoid laterally.

DIFFERENTIAL DIAGNOSIS Petrous apex infections, more generalized skull base osteomyelitis, relatively rare inflammatory conditions such as Wegener's granulomatosis and Langerhans histiocytosis

DIAGNOSIS Necrotizing (malignant) otitis externa (NOE)

DISCUSSION NOE is a spreading, necrotizing infection of the EAC soft tissue that can produce an osteomyelitis of the entire skull base. This sporadic condition occurs principally in elderly diabetic patients, usually caused by *Pseudomonas aeruginosa*. It may occur in other immunocompromised patients and less commonly with organisms like *Staphylococcus aureus*, *Proteus mirabilis*, and *Aspergillus*. NOE starts in the soft tissues and affects bone from the outside to the inside with a periosteal spreading pattern. The earliest finding is nonspecific soft tissue swelling within and around the EAC. The next stage shows bone demineralization at the petrotympanic fissure and then infiltration medially along the tympanic bone to its juncture with the petrous portion. Later-stage disease will spread along the periosteal surfaces of the mastoid and petrous portions of the temporal bone, usually following the eustachian tube, to the petrous apex and posterior skull base, frequently reaching the clivus. Frank subperiosteal or other abscess formation is rare and may suggest an etiology other the pseudomonas or a superimposed second bacterial infection with a more pyogenic organism. The intense cellulitis will involve the masticator and parapharyngeal spaces. This can result in a frank abscess in the parapharyngeal, retropharyngeal, and/or masticator space. Intracranial spread is a very late stage of the disease and is not commonly encountered since effective antipseudomonal antibiotics have been introduced.

CT is excellent for determining whether bone is eroded—a factor that is critical to establish the initial diagnosis and determine the extent of osteomyelitis. CT also shows the extent of soft tissue disease very well. Soft tissue changes, dural enhancement, and medullary changes of the bone are better shown and more obvious on MRI; however, MRI is not sensitive for bony changes.

The clinical setting and imaging can differentiate other conditions mentioned in the differential diagnosis from NOE.

Question for Further Thought

1. What treatment and surveillance options are available for this condition?

Reporting Responsibilities

If this is a previously undiagnosed infection, a positive study must be communicated verbally. Surveillance studies are reported routinely.

What the Treating Physician Needs to Know

- If the specific diagnosis of NOE can be confirmed and differentiated from other pathology.
- If not NOE infection, what is the most likely diagnosis?
- Imaging can be useful in confirming the effectiveness of antibiotic therapy.

Answer

1. NOE has been effectively treated with advanced-generation cephalosporins and fluoroquinolones for over two decades. Before the advent of those antimicrobial agents, the mortality of this disease approached 20% and the patients frequently underwent extremely morbid operative procedures as part of the treatment plan. Indications for surgery are not established but are performed generally for complications. This disease is best managed medically.

   Follow-up of treated NOE is clinical, with imaging surveillance predominantly relying on gallium SPECT imaging. CT and MRI can be useful initially to follow the soft tissue changes of NOE as a response to therapy, but bone changes lag behind, making them less useful for the definitive, long-term surveillance to ultimately determine that the disease has been cured. Bone/gallium or indium studies can be used to establish a baseline to monitor the effects of therapy. In general, antibiotic therapy will be continued well beyond the time when the radionuclide study normalizes to minimize the odds of recurrence.

> ### LEARN MORE
> See Chapters 114, 14, and 16 in *Head and Neck Radiology* by Mancuso and Hanafee.

CLINICAL HISTORY *A 70-year-old male patient presented with headache, fever, and right-sided facial pain. No history of diabetes. The patient was on steroids for chronic obstructive pulmonary disease.*

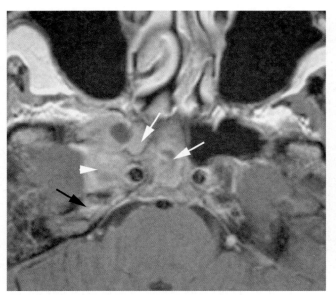

FIGURE 3.11A

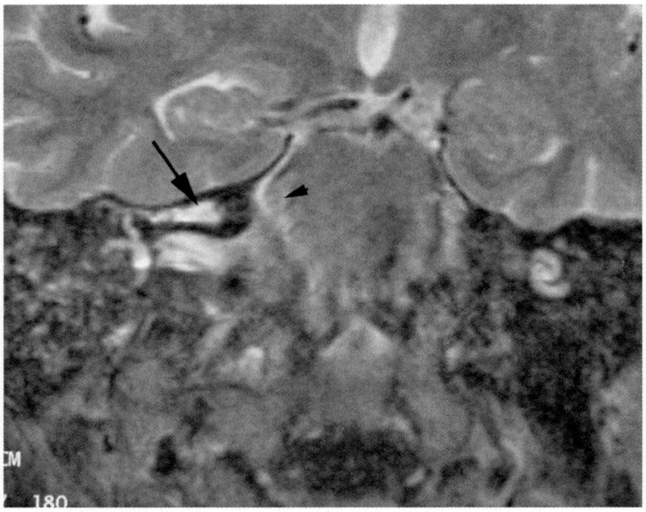

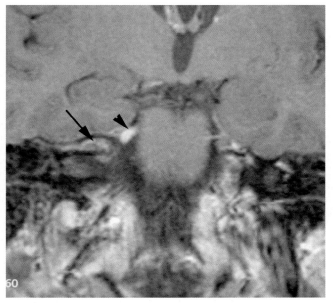

FIGURE 3.11C

FIGURE 3.11B

FINDINGS

Figure 3.11A. T1W CE image showing disease within the sphenoid sinus (white arrows) spreading to the adjacent cavernous sinus (arrowheads) and then secondarily to the petrous apex (black arrows).

Figure 3.11B. T1W coronal image showing that the disease has spread from the sphenoid bone into superior labyrinthine air cells (arrow). Also note inflammatory enhancement of the trigeminal nerve (arrowhead).

Figure 3.11C. T2W coronal image showing the inflammatory mucosal thickening in the petrous apex air cells (arrow) and edema at the root entry zone of the trigeminal nerve (arrowhead).

This was a biopsy-confirmed case of fungal skull base osteomyelitis with disease origin in the sphenoid sinus.

DIFFERENTIAL DIAGNOSIS Atypical presentation of NOE, primary and metastatic skull base malignancy or malignancy adjacent to the skull base such as nasopharyngeal carcinoma, rare inflammatory conditions such as Wegener's granulomatosis, other granulomatous diseases such as tuberculosis or sarcoidosis and Langerhans histiocytosis

DIAGNOSIS Fungal skull base osteomyelitis

DISCUSSION Skull base osteomyelitis other than that related to NOE is an uncommon disease. The portal of the infection might still be the middle ear or mastoid, but the disease is often bilateral and relatively symmetric, making some other source such as the nasopharynx, eustachian tube, or sphenoid sinus possible. Often, the site of original infection is not proven, and the specific organism might not be established. *S. aureus*, *Salmonella*, *P. mirabilis*, aspergillosis/mucormycosis, and actinomycosis are the causative conditions in most cases when the agent is identified. *Cryptococcus* and blastomycosis may also be causative agents. Patients are older and usually immunocompromised but not diabetic.

Skull base osteomyelitis may be a spreading, necrotizing infection of the soft tissues that affects bone secondarily, as seen in NOE. It may also be a primary osteomyelitis beginning in bone and spreading beyond its confines. The earliest findings may be nonspecific soft tissue swelling within the parapharyngeal spaces and nasopharynx, followed by bone demineralization. The site of bone destruction varies and usually is more extensive and bilateral at presentation. The pattern in some cases is very much like that seen in NOE, but the patients are not diabetic and the organism not predominantly *Pseudomonas*. Mastoid changes are often reactive to adjacent infection. Bone may demonstrate intensely sclerotic and a mixed sclerotic and lytic pattern. In later stages, there may be intense cellulitis that will involve the parapharyngeal and masticator spaces and may eventually lead to a frank abscess or at least soft tissue necrosis. Intracranial spread is typically limited to the dura and epidural space as phlegmon and/or abscess.

Question for Further Thought

1. What is the role of imaging in the diagnosis of and treatment for this condition?

Reporting Responsibilities

If this is a previously undiagnosed infection, a positive study must be communicated verbally since this is a potentially life-threatening disease.

What the Treating Physician Needs to Know

- If the specific diagnosis of skull base osteomyelitis can be confirmed and differentiated from NOE or other pathology
- If skull base osteomyelitis is confirmed, what is the extent of the disease?
- If not skull base osteomyelitis or NOE infection, what is the most likely diagnosis?
- Imaging can be useful in confirming the effectiveness of antimicrobial therapy.

Answer

1. Imaging plays a very important role in the diagnosis of and treatment for skull base osteomyelitis. CT is excellent for determining whether and how bone is eroded; these are factors critical to establishing the initial diagnosis and determining the extent of osteomyelitis. In skull base osteomyelitis from sinonasal mucormycosis, bony involvement occurs usually late in the disease due to the angioinvasion of the fungi. CT and MRI are excellent to show the extent of soft tissue disease, MR better than CT. MRI is also excellent for showing the extent of disease in the marrow space of the skull and extent of intracranial spread.

Radionuclide studies can be done with bone/gallium or indium studies. Radionuclide studies are used to establish a baseline suggestive of infectious disease and to monitor the effects of therapy. Nuclear medicine studies are better than CT and MRI for surveillance. Once the soft tissue abnormality resolves, the bony changes lag, making CT less useful to establish whether the disease has been ultimately cured. The antibiotic/antifungal therapy is continued for some time, usually about 6 weeks, after the gallium study returns to normal, to avoid the risk of recurrence.

LEARN MORE

See Chapters 115, 14, and 16 in *Head and Neck Radiology* by Mancuso and Hanafee.

CLINICAL HISTORY *A 5-year-old girl presented with swelling behind the left ear without fever or significant pain. She also had recently developed polydipsia and polyuria. CT and MRI are as shown below:*

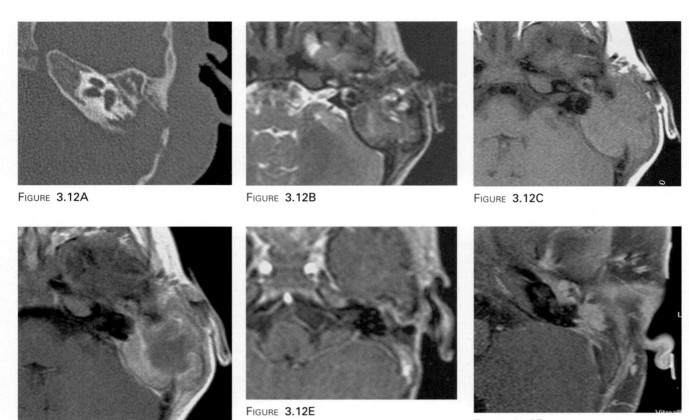

FIGURE **3.12A**

FIGURE **3.12B**

FIGURE **3.12C**

FIGURE **3.12D**

FIGURE **3.12E**

FIGURE **3.12F**

FINDINGS A lytic lesion of the temporal bone, mainly mastoid, with erosion of the sigmoid plate and lateral wall and a retroauricular soft tissue swelling, is present on CT (Fig. 3.12A). Corresponding MR images show a mass, a spectrum of signal intensity and heterogeneous enhancement pattern, extending into the middle ear and transcranially before treatment (Figs. 3.12B–D) and after treatment in (Figs. 3.12E and F).

DIFFERENTIAL DIAGNOSIS Rhabdomyosarcoma, chronic with superimposed acute or subacute suppurative mastoiditis, NOE, osteomyelitis from other infectious agents, Wegener's granulomatosis, metastasis, and posttransplant lymphoproliferative disorder (PTLD). The differential highly depends on the age and any associated or predisposing medical conditions of the patient. In this age group, the first two listed are the central, alternative considerations.

DIAGNOSIS Langerhans cell histiocytosis

DISCUSSION This patient had multiple other lesions in the calvarium, conductive hearing loss on the left side, and diabetes insipidus. Biopsy of one of the calvarial lesions showed Langerhans cell histiocytosis.

Langerhans cell histiocytosis is a disease of antigen–presenting cell or dendritic cells that are present in the epidermis basal layers, bronchial mucosa, thymic epithelium, and lymph nodes. Langerhans cell histiocytosis presents itself in three general clinical settings that may overlap. These include the following:

a. An acute, fulminating systemic disease in an infant or young child sometimes known as acute disseminated histiocytosis or Letterer-Siwe disease

b. A chronic, disseminated, multifocal systemic disease in young children and occasionally adults that can result in organ dysfunction, including diabetes insipidus, also known as the Hand-Schüller-Christian disease or syndrome

c. A solitary focus of eosinophilic granuloma that presents as a lytic lesion of bone.

The etiology of the disease is unknown. It is felt to be an aberrant immune response, probably to a viral antigen. The disease can present as nodal or extranodal. The focal extranodal form frequently involves the bones of the skull and face, especially the calvarium, temporal bone, and mandible, presenting with lytic lesions. The bone involvement seen in Langerhans cell histiocytosis may mimic that of metastatic disease, leukemia, and plasma cell dyscrasias and may even overlap with chronic osteomyelitis. The tissue within and outside the bone typically enhances considerably. Adjacent dura will enhance, and dural disease is most often a reflection of adjacent bone involvement.

Focal disease has a predilection for the temporal bone, especially the mastoid. As such, the presentation can mimic or be associated with chronic or subacute otomastoiditis, otitis externa, or a mastoid-region mass, as in the case above. However, if the sole presenting lesion involves the temporal bone, then it may delay diagnosis since it mimics otitis media.

Central nervous system involvement is usually due to leptomeningeal disease involving the hypothalamic-pituitary axis presenting with diabetes insipidus and anterior pituitary dysfunction.

Age at presentation, lack of fever, and other signs of septicemia are helpful to exclude infection. PTLD would have a prior history of transplantation, and cANCA would be positive in Wegener's granulomatosis. However, the definitive diagnosis is by biopsy.

Question for Further Thought

1. How is this condition treated?

Reporting Responsibilities

These cases typically mimic tumor or mastoiditis; thus, initial direct communication with the treating physicians is necessary to be certain of timely disposition to tissue sampling. Appropriate medical decision making then flows rapidly from that point. In the case of a complicating infection, the need for urgent communication is accelerated. The study can usually exclude infection as the primary diagnostic probability.

What the Treating Physician Needs to Know

- Imaging findings in focal noninfectious inflammatory diseases can mimic the appearance of malignant diseases and chronic infections.
- These diseases frequently enter the differential diagnosis when tissue sampling returns a "nonspecific inflammatory" result.

Answer

1. Solitary eosinophilic granuloma may be treated with curettage and/or low-dose radiotherapy if the mass threatens a vital structure or function. More disseminated forms of the disease are treated with steroids and other chemotherapeutic agents. In its most aggressive disseminated form, the prognosis can be poor. In this case, the patient improved on treatment as seen in Figures 3.12 E and F.

> ### LEARN MORE
> See Chapters 116 and 19 in *Head and Neck Radiology* by Mancuso and Hanafee.

CASE 3.13

CLINICAL HISTORY *A 35-year-old male patient was being treated for bacterial meningitis when he developed acute-onset tinnitus, hearing loss, vertigo with nausea, and a few bouts of vomiting. On examination, the patient had spontaneous nystagmus. Audiometry demonstrated profound bilateral SNHL. Pre- and postcontrast MRI was performed; images are shown below:*

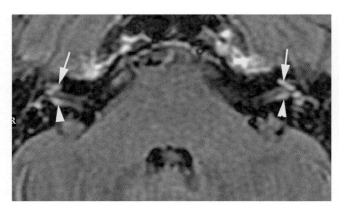

FIGURE **3.13A**

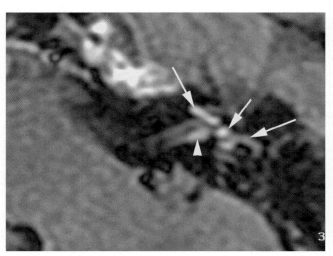

FIGURE **3.13B**

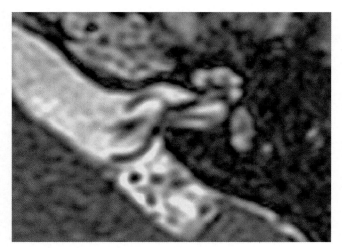

FIGURE **3.13C**

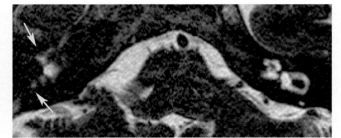

FIGURE **3.13D**

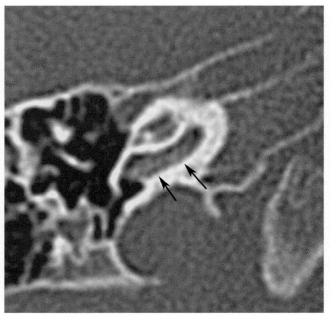

FIGURE **3.13E**

FINDINGS T1W CE images (Fig. 3.13A,B) show multifocal labyrinthine (arrows), meningeal, and perineural enhancement (arrowheads). The steady-state image in (Fig. 3.13C) shows little abnormality, likely reflecting the exudative nature of the labyrinthine disease. Figures 3.13 D (MRI) and E (CT) of another patient with the same disease process.

DIFFERENTIAL DIAGNOSIS Noninfectious inflammatory labyrinthitis due to vasculitis (neurovascular disease) or immune-mediated processes such as sarcoidosis, Wegener's granulomatosis, Langerhans histiocytosis, and autoimmune diseases

DIAGNOSIS Infectious meningitic labyrinthitis

DISCUSSION Acute suppurative (pyogenic) bacterial infections of the middle ear and mastoid can cause inner ear dysfunction due to involvement of the membranous labyrinth and/

or cochleovestibular nerve (CVN); this generally found to be associated meningitis and is a medical emergency at the time of the acute disease. Chronic infections such as skull base osteomyelitis, Lyme disease, and syphilis also may cause inner ear dysfunction due to labyrinthitis. The most common infectious condition causing labyrinthitis likely is viral neuritis, which typically is a presumptive diagnosis confirmed clinically by its response to therapy and/or associated clinical findings. Bacterial meningitis is the most common cause of postnatally acquired SNHL and has been reported to cause permanent hearing loss in 10% to 14% of those affected. Younger children and young adults are at more risk for labyrinthine dysfunction secondary to acute or chronic otomastoiditis.

An offending infectious agent itself may enter the labyrinth along the CVN via the round or oval window or from the CSF via the cochlear aqueduct or IAC. Bacterial endotoxins and the host response (inflammatory mediators) may involve the labyrinth without direct invasion of the bacteria; this is referred to as serous/eosinophilic labyrinthitis. Infectious disease of the labyrinth may also be bloodborne due to meningovascular disease. On rare occasions, this may be iatrogenic following stapedectomy.

The portal of entry in this patient was possibly from meningitic spread via the cochlear aperture, reflected by the enhancement in the IAC.

MRI should be done first since it most confidently excludes causative pathology of the labyrinth as well as all segments (i.e., brainstem, cisternal, exit canal/foramen, extracranial) of the CVN. MRI is also more sensitive than CT for excluding intra-axial pathology that presents in a manner identical with labyrinthitis. CT may be necessary to most confidently exclude conditions of the middle ear and mastoid as sites of a primary inflammatory process or CSF leakage—inner ear anatomic variants that might predispose to infection of the labyrinth. MR is sensitive for enhancement and CT for bone erosion. A negative MRI never *excludes* meningitis or labyrinthitis.

It is difficult to differentiate noninfectious causes from infectious labyrinthitis by imaging alone since imaging findings are similar. Other imaging findings, clinical findings, laboratory findings, and history are helpful, for instance, in a patient developing labyrinthitis who has known vasculitis.

Medical treatment relies on identification of the infectious agent and specific antimicrobial agent treatment. Anti-inflammatory or immunosuppressive therapy may be indicated in noninfectious diseases. If acute otomastoiditis is considered the cause, the mastoid and middle ear may need to be decompressed.

Question for Further Thought

1. What are the complications of this condition? What is the best modality to detect these changes?

Reporting Responsibilities

Bacterial infectious meningitis is a medical emergency, so direct rapid communication of the findings is essential. If the meningitis is recurrent, a portal of entry via the tempo-

ral bone should be sought. The clinicians should understand that a negative imaging study never excludes meningitis, and that should be so stated in the report.

What the Treating Physician Needs to Know

- Whether a structural lesion involving the labyrinth, CVN, CPA dura, or leptomeninges is producing the patient's symptoms.
- Is the membranous labyrinth involved? If so, what is the precise extent of disease?
- If a nerve lesion is also present, what segments of the CVN are involved?
- Are there findings that suggest a specific causative condition?
- If the lesion is enhancing, is it likely to be inflammatory or infectious?
- Are there any findings that suggest a condition, inflammatory or otherwise, that may require urgent or emergent intervention?
- If there is no structural lesion, is there a clue to an alternative diagnosis, and is there any other imaging that might prove useful in medical decision making?

Answer

1. Labyrinthitis leads to irreparable inflammation of the membranous labyrinth. The delayed effect of such inner ear infection is often a chronic, fibro-osseous obliterative labyrinthitis. This condition replaces the normal fluid and membranes of the labyrinth with fibrosis and later with new bone with damage to nerve cells and the organ of Corti.

   CT may not reflect a purely fibrous replacement of the labyrinth or a labyrinth that is filled with an exudate or blood. Obliteration by calcification or new bone is well seen with CT (Fig. 3.13D shows CT and MR images in a different patient with streptococcus infection with fibro-osseous obliterative labyrinthitis.) Advanced fibro-osseous obliteration is most commonly seen in patients with long-standing SNHL.

   Loss of normal bright fluid signal on steady-state MR images within the labyrinth serves as evidence of fibrous replacement or fibro-osseous obliteration of the labyrinth. Therefore, steady-state MRI is a must for inner ear evaluation and more sensitive than CT in the early stage of disease.

   Profound hearing loss due to labyrinthitis is considered an indication for cochlear implantation. Obliteration due to ossification will complicate surgery and may prevent complete insertion of the cochlear implant. Because of the possible rapid progression of fibro-osseous changes, swift action becomes necessary. In cases of extensive obliteration, out of reach for surgical removal, a double array implant may be used.

> LEARN MORE
>
> See Chapters 117 and 13 in *Head and Neck Radiology* by Mancuso and Hanafee.

CASE 3.14

CLINICAL HISTORY *A 35-year-old male farmer presented with history of gradual-onset hearing loss for the last 5 years that has progressively worsened, more on the right than left side. He recently started having intermittent tinnitus. The patient's older brother also had similar complaints and was surgically treated. On examination, the patient had mixed hearing loss and demonstrated pink discoloration of the promontory. CT images from the right side are shown below:*

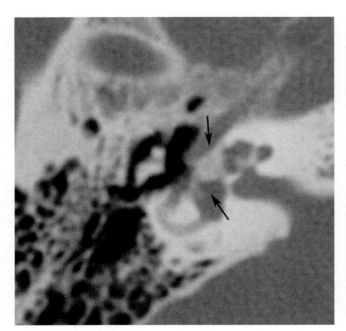

FIGURE 3.14A

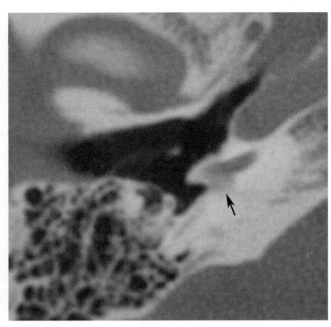

FIGURE 3.14C

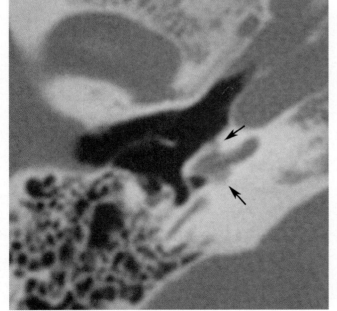

FIGURE 3.14B

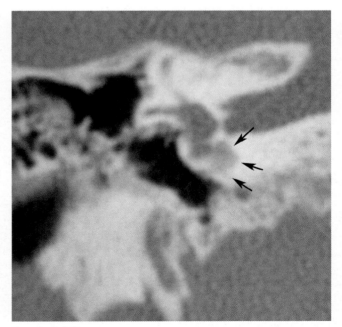

FIGURE 3.14D

FINDINGS

Figure 3.14A–D. Focal areas of demineralization at the fissula ante fenestram with associated bony proliferation changes encroach the oval window and also involve the round window (arrows).

DIFFERENTIAL DIAGNOSIS Paget disease, osteogenesis imperfecta

DIAGNOSIS Otosclerosis

DISCUSSION Otosclerosis is a disease unique to the otic capsule of humans. The disease is seen mainly in the white population, uncommon in blacks, and exceptional in the Asian population. The otic capsule is normally inert with minimal bone turnover. Otosclerosis increases bone turnover. It typically begins in the region of the fissula ante fenestram as a focus of osteolysis. The repair bone that follows the osteolysis is laid down in a degraded bony endosteal matrix, resulting in the altered bone density and intensity and is accompanied by increased vascularity. This process in the oval window may spread across the annular ligament to immobilize the stapes. Extension over the inner ear is accompanied by collateral damage to the membranous labyrinth that manifests as SNHL, tinnitus, and vertigo.

CT is usually performed first since it is quite sensitive in detecting the bony changes and also in evaluating other causes of conductive hearing loss. MRI will be extremely insensitive except to very advanced bony changes; even when advanced, the changes may go unnoticed depending on the study quality and disease activity. When this disease is detected on MRI, it is usually due to observing abnormal enhancement of the otic capsule.

Paget disease is rare and virtually never limited to the otic capsule when seen in the temporal bone; it may also involve multiple other bones. Features of osteogenesis imperfecta such as blue sclera and young age help to differentiate from otosclerosis, although tarda or less expressed varieties of that disease should be considered in the adult population.

Questions for Further Thought

1. How is this condition evaluated clinically, and what role does imaging play?
2. What treatment options are available for this condition?

Reporting Responsibilities

This is typically a chronic disease requiring only routine reporting.

What the Treating Physician Needs to Know

- Whether there is evidence of otosclerosis.
- If surgery is considered, whether there is evidence of obliterative otosclerosis at the oval or round window. In the case of cochlear implantation, whether there are anatomic distortions including scala tympani involvement and otosclerotic foci between the cochlea and the labyrinthine segment of the facial nerve.
- If there is no otosclerosis, is there a clue to an alternative diagnosis (like enlarged vestibular aqueduct, potential stapes gusher, SSC dehiscence, or tympanosclerosis)?
- In the case of posttreatment imaging findings, the position of stapes prosthesis and ossicular continuity should be noted.

Answers

1. These patients will generally present with progressive conductive or mixed hearing loss. Tinnitus or dizziness may accompany the hearing loss. It may present as pulse synchronous with a reddish retrotympanic mass versus nonpulsatile tinnitus. This discoloration of the promontory is pathognomonic for otosclerosis and is called the *Schwartze sign*. Audiometry will often suggest this as a primary working diagnosis due to the low frequency loss, especially when no other cause of a conductive loss is apparent. The stapedial reflex is usually absent when conductive hearing loss is found. Imaging is done only if there is a doubt about the clinical diagnosis and in cases of fluctuating hearing loss.

2. Fluoride has been found to be of value in treatment for otosclerosis. Fluoride ions replace the hydroxyl group in hydroxyapatite to form a fluorapatite complex that is resistant to osteoclastic degradation. Oral intake has been shown to stabilize hearing loss, both conductive and sensorineural. Hearing aids will commonly be used before proceeding to surgery. Surgical treatment is primarily by stapedectomy, which consists of removal of the stapes superstructure and drilling a small hole into the footplate, through which a prosthesis is inserted. If the result is unsatisfactory, and in very advanced cases with profound deafness, cochlear implantation can be considered. This surgery can be challenging because of anatomic distortions and obliteration of the basal turn with higher risk of partial insertions or misplacement of the electrode array.

LEARN MORE
See Chapters 118 and 43 in *Head and Neck Radiology* by Mancuso and Hanafee.

CLINICAL HISTORY *A young adult with a temporal bone region mass and progressive, mild otalgia.*

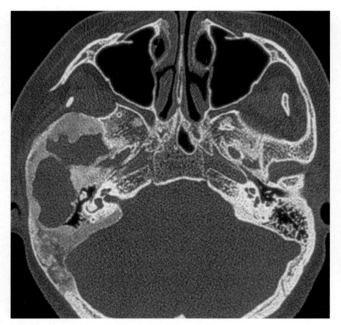

FIGURE 3.15A

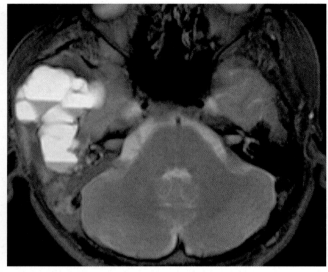

FIGURE 3.15C

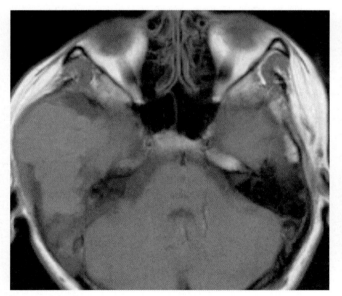

FIGURE 3.15B

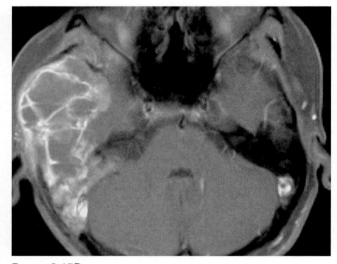

FIGURE 3.15D

FINDINGS CT (Fig. 3.15A) shows an expanded appearance of the temporal bone with predominant ground-glass appearance and cyst formation in multiple parts of the temporal bone. Some components have relatively low signal intensity compared to brain on T1W (Fig. 3.15B) and T2W images (Fig. 3.15C), the latter sequence also showing multiple cystic spaces with fluid–fluid levels with significant enhancement on the postcontrast T1W image (Fig. 3.15D).

DIFFERENTIAL DIAGNOSIS Paget disease, sarcoma

DIAGNOSIS Fibrous dysplasia with an aneurysmal bone cyst

DISCUSSION The conditions that primarily effect bones throughout the body can express themselves in isolated form in the temporal bone. More commonly, the temporal bone expression is part of a bony condition that involves more than one segment of the skull base and/or facial bones. The temporal bone involvement may also be part of a systemic process. These processes may be generally categorized as developmental/dysplastic, metabolic/dystrophic, and reactive. Patients may present with various complaints, physical findings, and functional deficits that are common in many other temporal bone pathologic conditions. The complaints in this patient are fairly typical.

Temporal bone involvement in fibrous dysplasia is less common than that of the facial bones but by no means is unusual. An exophytic growth of dysplastic bone will typically cause it to present as a mass in the mastoid region. Pain, especially when progressive, is usually a sign of a complicating factor. There is very small risk of transformation rate to a sarcoma or aneurysmal bone cyst formation; the latter is present in this case.

Partial surgical removal can be performed to improve function such as a conductive hearing loss or cosmesis.

Question for Further Thought

1. What other type of complaints or complications may be seen with temporal bone fibrous dysplasia?

Reporting Responsibilities

In general, there is often little or no immediate risk associated with such conditions. Sometimes the temporal bone findings are incidental and seen on studies done for other indications. When the imaging studies are done specifically for complaints related to the temporal bone, routine reporting usually suffices. There might be a complicating disease such a secondary acute otitis media with possible intracranial complications that might require verbal communication.

What the Treating Physician Needs to Know

- Extent of disease and whether its pattern is consistent with a known or working clinical diagnosis
- If there are findings that specifically explain functional deficits
- If there are findings that might potentially cause a deficit with progression of the disease state
- If there are findings that may reduce the likelihood of successful surgical intervention
- Whether there is a complication of the underlying pathology such as acute or chronic otitis media or cholesteatoma that is potentially progressive

Answer

1. Fibrous dysplasia is associated with SNHL and/or vertigo when it involves the otic capsule and a compressive seventh nerve palsy when it involves the facial canal. Conductive hearing loss may be due to EAC stenosis or middle ear obstructive changes that may progress to chronic otitis media and cholesteatoma.

> **LEARN MORE**
> See Chapters 119 and 40 in *Head and Neck Radiology* by Mancuso and Hanafee.

CASE 3.16

CLINICAL HISTORY *A 21-year-old male patient presented to the emergency room following assault to the right side of the head with a baseball bat. He was conscious and complained of pain and decreased hearing in the right ear. On examination, he had right facial droop. CT of the head demonstrated contusions to the right temporal lobe. Temporal bone CT was also performed; two selected images are shown below:*

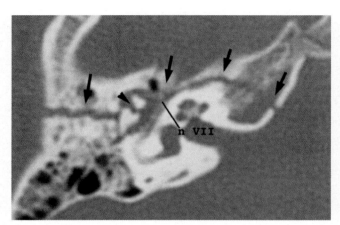

FIGURE **3.16A**

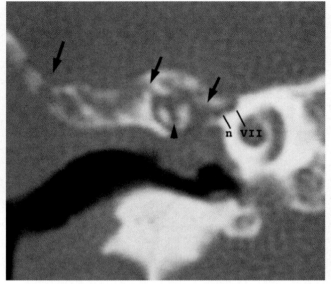

FIGURE **3.16B**

FINDINGS

Figure 3.16A,B. The patient had facial nerve paralysis immediately after the trauma. A fracture (arrows) through the roof of the EAC and extending to the petrous apex involves the anterior genu of the facial nerve (cranial nerve VII). There also is malleoincudal disruption (arrowheads).

DIFFERENTIAL DIAGNOSIS None

DIAGNOSIS Temporal bone fracture with facial nerve injury and ossicular disruption

DISCUSSION Trauma to the temporal bone is most commonly due to blunt-force skull injuries as a result of motor vehicle accidents, falls, assaults, and sports injuries. Penetrating trauma is much less common.

The facial nerve may be involved by fractures either within the IAC or in its more peripheral portion from the geniculate ganglion to the stylomastoid foramen. Facial nerve injury can be caused by transection, intraneural hematoma or edema, and/or bony impingement of the nerve. An accurate determination of the level of fracture and any fragments within the canal may play a central role in patient management. Disruptions at the anterior genu or posterior genu are among the most common locations of injuries and also constitute two areas where it may prove most difficult to detect

a fracture. The labyrinthine segment of the facial nerve is the narrowest and tightest part of the facial canal; it is here that edema within the facial nerve is most likely to result in a compressive neuropathy; thus, surgical decompression must include this portion of the canal even though it may not be obviously disrupted.

Ossicular disruptions will appear as separations of the head of the malleus and body of the incus and displacement of these larger ossicles in the epitympanic recess. Fractures of the stapes crura may mainly manifest as incudostapedial joint disruption.

Questions for Further Thought

1. How would this patient be treated?
2. Describe briefly the other injuries to temporal bone and their clinical management.

Reporting Responsibilities

Posterior fossa extra-axial hematoma, obvious injury to the facial nerve canal, and fractures across the carotid canal should be reported urgently and communicated verbally. Other injuries can be reported promptly but require no verbal communication except when there is risk of meningitis.

What the Treating Physician Needs to Know

- Is there a posterior fossa extra-axial hematoma or large intra-axial hematoma?

- Is there injury to the facial canal?
- Is there injury to the carotid canal and ICA?
- Is there extensive pneumocephalus or a distracted mastoid or middle ear fracture?
- Is there potential communication between the middle ear and mastoid and CSF spaces?
- Is there ossicular disruption?
- Is there a fracture through the inner ear?
- Is there a fracture involving the TMJ?

Answers

1. This patient can be treated watchfully with steroids and nerve function monitoring. If function does not improve, surgical decompression can be performed. This patient was treated with a limited labyrinthine segment decompression. In the same setting, ossicular reconstruction was performed. Patient recovered both the nerve function as well as hearing.

2. Other injuries and their clinical management are briefly detailed below:
   - Fractures across the transverse and sigmoid sinus raise the risk of extra-axial posterior fossa hematoma; an extracranial posterior fossa hematoma is a medical emergency. Many patients with such injury die at the scene of the accident.
   - Dissections or related pseudoaneurysms of the petrous segment of the ICA are uncommon injuries and can secondarily lead to thromboembolic phenomena.
   - The CSF spaces may communicate with the middle ear via fractures through the tegmen tympani, the footplate of the stapes and oval window, or disruptions around the round window. CSF otorrhea and herniation of meninges and the temporal lobe into the middle ear cavity is possible after trauma. Tears of the dura or loss of cortical integrity heal quite slowly, if at all. The meninges are able to pulsate and project into the middle ear cavity, thus creating a mass that interferes with conductive hearing. If CSF otorrhea is present, it will test positive for beta-2 transferrin. Even a tiny pneumocephalus suggests a dural tear. If CSF leak does not stop within a week with medical treatment, the potential for meningitis increases, and these are usually fixed surgically. MRI is more useful than CT in detecting meningoencephaloceles that may occur through these defects, which usually present later, mostly as conductive hearing loss or meningitis.
   - Fracture through inner ear structures could lead to SNHL and vestibular symptoms. Hearing loss may require the need hearing aids and rehabilitative therapy. Vestibular symptoms have a good prognosis for full recovery with vestibular rehabilitation techniques.
   - Fractures may also disrupt the bony eustachian tube and cause long-term chronic eustachian tube dysfunction and secondary chronic otitis media.

LEARN MORE

See Chapter 120 in *Head and Neck Radiology* by Mancuso and Hanafee.

CLINICAL HISTORY   *A 28-year-old male patient presented with gradual difficulty in hearing from the left ear. On examination, there was narrowing of both EACs. Additional history revealed that the patient often swims and surfs in cold water. CT images are shown below:*

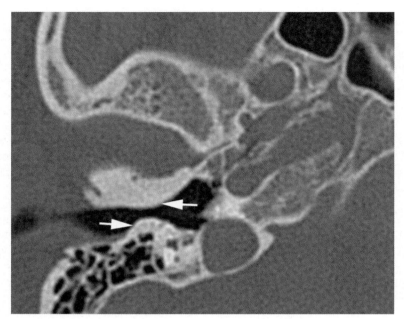

FIGURE 3.17A

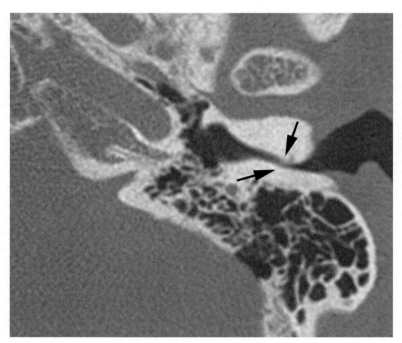

FIGURE 3.17B

FINDINGS

Figure 3.17A,B. Marked bone thickening of both EACs, the left more than the right. Bone thickening is circumferential and on the left side nearly occludes the canal.

DIFFERENTIAL DIAGNOSIS A wide range of differentials can be considered from the history and examination; however, with imaging, it is diagnostic of reactive exostosis of the EAC due to prolonged cold water exposure.

DIAGNOSIS "Surfer's ears" (reactive osteitis)

DISCUSSION This patient started cold water surfing almost 10 years ago. The marked narrowing of the left EAC caused partial conductive hearing loss. The pathophysiology of this condition is not well understood. It has been observed that cold water surfing (and diving) has much high propensity to develop this condition than warm water sports such as surfing. The bony exostosis can involve the canal completely or partially. Predominant involvement of the outer portion of the canal can lead to accumulation of water, debris, and cerumen, leading to higher chances of secondary infection and earlier onset of conductive hearing loss. Infections are harder to treat since the deeper canal cannot be completely cleaned. The patient may also present with otalgia, although most patients are asymptomatic until they develop infection or significant hearing loss.

Focal osteoma of the EAC appears similar to pedunculated osteomas elsewhere and are not related to cold water surfing.

Question for Further Thought

1. How is this condition treated?

Reporting Responsibilities and What the Treating Physician Needs to Know

- Imaging explanation of the reasons for EAC narrowing, including the most possible cause, based on the tissue characteristics
- Additional information regarding complications and status of the tympanic membrane and middle and inner ear
- Whether a biopsy can be safely performed by the clinician

Answer

1. Definitive treatment is by surgery that involves removing the excess bone by chipping and drilling. If the canal immediately adjacent to the tympanic membrane is affected, a mastoid approach is used to prevent tympanic membrane injury.

   The best treatment is prevention by using ear plugs that avoid the contact of cold water and air to the EAC.

LEARN MORE
See Chapters 121 and 38 in *Head and Neck Radiology* by Mancuso and Hanafee.

CASE 3.18

CLINICAL HISTORY *A 68-year-old male patient presented with a lesion in the right ear canal for the last 18 months that has been slowly growing. He did not seek medical attention since there was no pain. For the last few months, he has noticed minimal bleeding, discharge, and itching. He has also noticed decreased hearing on the right side and has pain while chewing. Selected CT and MR images are shown below:*

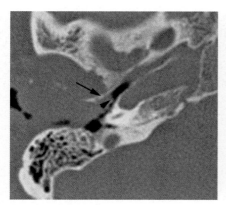

FIGURE **3.18A**

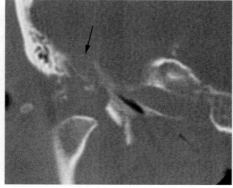

FIGURE **3.18B**

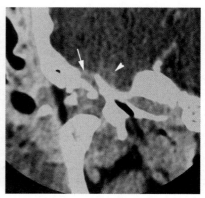

FIGURE **3.18C**

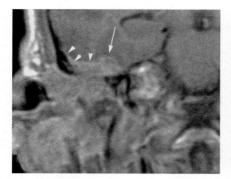

FIGURE **3.18D**

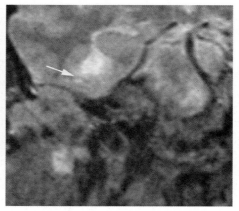

FIGURE **3.18E**

FINDINGS

Figure 3.18A. There is destruction of the EAC and tumor extending along the bone of the hypotympanum (arrow) with tumor growing toward the bony eustachian tube (arrowhead).

Figure 3.18B. There is destruction of bone between the glenoid fossa and the floor of the middle cranial fossa (arrow).

Figure 3.18C. CECT viewed at brain windows shows intracranial spread with an apparently sharp dural interface at one point (arrow) and possible brain invasion (arrowhead) at another. The relationship of tumor to brain and dura is uncertain.

Figure 3.18D. T1W coronal image with contrast shows reactive dural changes (arrowheads) along most of the intracranial invasion interface; however, there is also evidence of leptomeningeal enhancement (arrow).

Figure 3.18E. T2W coronal image shows evidence of brain edema. Surgery confirmed early brain invasion.

DIFFERENTIAL DIAGNOSIS The differential diagnosis of EAC cancer includes inflammatory otitis externa, especially necrotizing (malignant) otitis externa, chronic bacterial or fungal skull base osteomyelitis, and pyogenic infections. Chronic granulation tissue can mimic tumor and erode bone, as can EAC cholesteatoma or keratosis obturans. A foreign body reaction can also produce such findings. External canal osteoma can mimic a submucosal cancer. Benign tumors occur but are rare. In the pediatric age range, rhabdomyosarcoma becomes a primary consideration.

DIAGNOSIS Advanced squamous cell carcinoma (SCCa) of the ear with intracranial invasion and extension into the TMJ

DISCUSSION SCCa of the EAC can arise from any location along the canal and may be associated with chronic otorrhea. Growth is initially contained by the bony/cartilaginous walls and the tympanic membrane; thus, the cancer fills up the EAC and attaches to underlying perichondrium or periosteum. Tumor then invades the cartilage and/or bone and grows through the tympanic membrane to the middle ear and mastoid.

Once the middle ear is involved, the tumor can involve the eustachian tube, carotid artery, jugular fossa, and sigmoid sinus plate.

Tumor may spread intracranially through the roof of the middle ear and mastoid. MRI is more sensitive than CT for evaluation of intracranial extension. After bone destruction, the adjacent dura is involved, followed by pia-arachnoid and then brain invasion. Brain invasion is a strong indicator of poor prognosis. Cortical vein and dural sinus occlusion can cause venous congestion and infarction in the brain that might mimic signs of early brain invasion.

Anterior inferior growth eventually involves the TMJ, masticator space, parotid gland, and parapharyngeal space. Parotid involvement is facilitated by the insertion of the parotid capsule on the cartilage portion of the EAC.

SCCa has a 15% to 20% incidence of nodal involvement at the time of presentation. CT is preferred for nodal staging. Regional lymph node spread is to the parotid nodes and levels 2 through 5 predominantly.

Imaging appearance of other conditions mentioned in differential diagnosis can appear similar, especially chronic bacterial and fungal osteomyelitis with associated granulation tissue.

Questions for Further Thought

1. What nerves are at risk for perineural tumor spread?
2. How is this condition treated?

Reporting Responsibilities

EAC cancers are usually chronic problems. A rare secondary infection or brain complication that might progress would require more urgent communication. Reports must contain information about the full extent of tumor. If there appears to be a disparity between the pattern of disease seen on imaging and the working diagnosis, a plan to resolve those differences such as imaging-directed biopsy should be offered.

What the Treating Physician Needs to Know

- Is the suspected or histologically confirmed clinical diagnosis keeping with the imaging findings?
- Precise extent of bone involvement in particular medial boundaries
- Extent of involvement of surrounding structures and spaces
- Presence and extent of perineural and perivascular spread
- Is there evidence of meningeal or brain involvement?
- Is there evidence of disseminated pia-arachnoid disease?
- Are other major vascular structures at risk or involved?
- Is there regional lymph node disease (parotid, levels 2 through 5, occipital, mastoid, retropharyngeal)?
- Is there systemic or distant disease?

Answers

1. Perineural spread along the facial nerve and auriculotemporal branch of the mandibular nerve to the V3 trunk is possible in all cancers in this region. Facial nerve involvement may spread to the greater petrosal nerve. The auriculotemporal nerve is at risk when the upper parotid gland and perimandibular region is invaded; this can lead to V3 and more proximal perineural spread along this trigeminal nerve connection.

2. Surgery and radiation therapy are the primary means of treatment for cure. They are often combined. Surgery is usually done first. The common surgical approaches are temporal bone resections that include sleeve resection, lateral temporal bone resection, subtotal temporal bone resection, and total temporal bone resection depending on the extent of tumor involvement. Postoperative radiation is usually indicated for more advanced lesions and pathologic perineural invasion or close surgical margins. Radiation may also be used as a palliative therapy. Radiotherapy by itself generally is not considered curative in bone invasion.

> ### LEARN MORE
> See Chapters 122 and 24 in *Head and Neck Radiology* by Mancuso and Hanafee.

CLINICAL HISTORY *A 48-year-old female presented with pulsatile tinnitus for the last 2 weeks. On examination, a bluish-red mass could be visualized behind the tympanic membrane. CT images are shown below:*

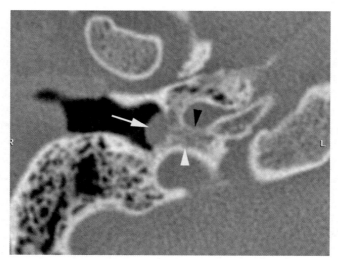

FIGURE **3.19A**

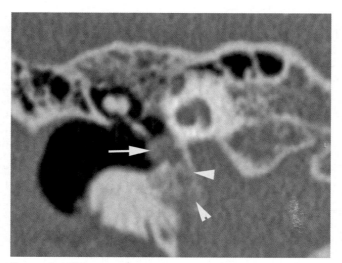

FIGURE **3.19B**

FINDINGS CT (Fig. 3.19A,B) shows a well-defined soft tissue mass in the hypotympanum (arrows) with aggressive-appearing bone erosion between the jugular fossa and carotid canal (arrowheads). The inner cortex of the jugular foramen and carotid canal are intact but undermined by tumor along their outer cortical margins.

DIFFERENTIAL DIAGNOSIS Aberrant carotid artery and high jugular bulb may be considered on the basis of the clinical evaluation. Following imaging, a nerve sheath tumor and occasionally an intraosseous or transcranial meningioma or a rare hemangioma might enter the differential.

DIAGNOSIS Paraganglioma of the jugulotympanic type

DISCUSSION The paraganglia cells of neural crest origin give rise to usually sporadically occurring paragangliomas. Depending on the site of tumor, they are named differently. They can be multicentric and associated with familial disease and multiple endocrine neoplasia (MEN) syndromes.

In this patient, the mass has a hypotympanum/promontory component as well as extension into the tympanic canaliculus (between the jugular fossa and carotid canal). This location indicates that the paraganglioma arose along Jacobson's nerve, a branch of the glossopharyngeal nerve. These are benign tumors but virtually always show an indistinct aggressive-appearing erosive pattern along their interface with bone, as is clearly seen in this patient in Figure 3.19B. If this mass presents more posteriorly adjacent to the descending facial canal, then it is arising from the paraganglia along Arnold's nerve in the mastoid (or inferior tympanic) canaliculus, a branch of the vagus nerve. Imaging is central to diagnosis and clinical decision making in a patient with a paraganglioma. Noncontrast CT can clearly differentiate between glomus tumors and other conditions such as a high jugular bulb and an aberrant carotid artery, which could also present with pulse synchronous tinnitus. MRI is less sensitive for initial diagnosis since bony changes are best seen on CT. MRI better demonstrates the enhancement and flow voids and can be used in follow-up after radiation therapy. Additional lesions should be searched for in other known sites when one paraganglioma is diagnosed; this is most efficiently accomplished by CT angiography with selected images also postprocessed for temporal bone detail on each side individually.

Patients such as the one shown in Figure 3.19 sometimes are mistaken as having tumors limited to the middle ear cavity resulting in partial resection. Patient symptoms then remain unrelieved or recur soon after surgery, necessitating repeated treatment.

Questions for Further Thought

1. What is the Fisch and Mattox classification for paragangliomas?
2. What are the treatment options for this patient?

Reporting Responsibilities

Paragangliomas are generally tumors that do not require direct communication, but if there is a known planned surgical biopsy of a middle ear or posterior fossa mass, this should likely be averted. Discovery of a mass in the head and neck region that would pose a significant hemorrhagic risk at biopsy should be discussed with the referring provider directly at the time of initial diagnostic concern for such a lesion.

What the Treating Physician Needs to Know

- Most likely alternative diagnosis if not a paraganglioma
- If the diagnosis remains in question, what additional studies or other means of confirmation are appropriate as a next step?
- If a paraganglioma, its full extent since it has the potential to alter the approach to treatment

- Particularly, the precise relationship of the tumor to the carotid canal and jugular fossa, if tumor extends beyond the middle ear cavity
- Whether the tumor is confined to the middle ear or has spread to or from there along the inferior tympanic and/or caroticotympanic canaliculi and adjacent infralabyrinthine bone between the jugular fossa and carotid canal

Answers

1. An excellent classification system for temporal bone–origin paragangliomas was developed by Fisch and Mattox. It sets a reasonable framework to decide whether surgical treatment is an equal or more reasonable choice than radiation therapy.
   - Class A glomus tympanicum tumors are limited to the middle ear.
   - Class B jugulotympanic tumors arise in paraganglia of the inferior tympanic and caroticotympanic canaliculi and invade the middle ear and mastoid, eroding the bone within and inferior to the hypotympanum but sparing the jugular bulb.
   - Class C glomus jugulare tumors arise from the jugular bulb and invade the surrounding bone. The extent of tumor relative to the carotid canal and artery is used to separate class C tumors into four subgroups.
   - Class D glomus jugulare tumors have spread intracranially, and this group is further subdivided by the size of the tumor and dural extent.

2. This patient could be treated with surgery or radiation therapy. A mastoidectomy and removal of the inferior bony tympanic ring will provide the added exposure necessary for the complete resection of this small class B tumor. The ossicular chain may be reconstructed if necessary. This patient opted for radiation therapy and received 4,500 cGy given in 25 fractions over 5 weeks. The pulsatile tinnitus symptoms resolved. Subsequent follow-up has shown minimal decrease in size.

> ## LEARN MORE
> See Chapters 123 and 33 in *Head and Neck Radiology* by Mancuso and Hanafee.

CASE 3.20

CLINICAL HISTORY *A 45-year-old female presented with diplopia and mild right facial pain. On examination, right sixth nerve palsy was noted. MR images are shown below:*

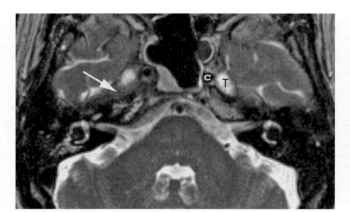

FIGURE **3.20A**

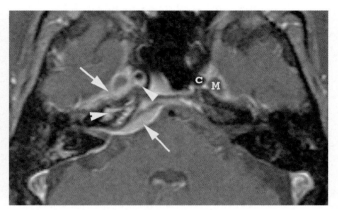

FIGURE **3.20C**

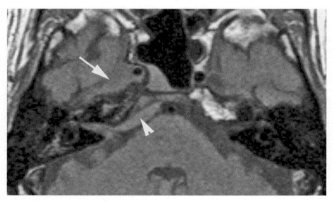

FIGURE **3.20B**

FINDINGS A dural mass (arrows), isointense to brain tissue on a T2W image (Fig. 3.20A) and T1 (Fig. 3.20B) with homogeneous intense enhancement (Fig. 3.20C) is seen along the anterior and posterior dural surfaces of the petrous apex and the clivus. The changes in the petrous apex air cells are due likely to reactive mucosal disease based on the high signal intensity in (Fig. 3.20A) and inflammatory changes in the right mastoid. However, there is limited intraosseous spread in the petrous apex and extension to the trigeminal cistern (*T*), encroachment and narrowing of the cavernous carotid artery. Within the IAC and along the clivus there is a dural tail due to either tumor or reactive changes.

DIFFERENTIAL DIAGNOSIS Sarcoidosis or other granulomatous pachymeningeal disease, lymphoma and metastases based on the appearance on imaging

DIAGNOSIS Meningioma of the petrous apex with intraosseous extension

DISCUSSION Petroclival meningiomas arise from the arachnoid villi of the clivus or the mesial petrous apex. Menin-giomas may be largely intraosseous; however, most grow in an exophytic manner along the dural surfaces. In this patient, the predominant component is en plaque with small intraosseous extension.

The sixth nerve palsy is secondary to involvement of Dorello's canal along the upper clivus. The facial pain is due to extension of the meningioma into the trigeminal cistern. Depending on the extent of the lesion and involvement of adjacent structures, a patient may present with other symptoms such as conductive hearing loss either due to eustachian tube obstruction or direct extension into middle ear and involvement of ossicles or sensorineural loss or vestibular symptoms due to involvement of the CVN. Facial nerve involvement can cause facial weakness.

MRI essentially provides a definitive diagnosis when typical morphologic features and growth pattern of the mass are expressed on various pulse sequences. Conditions such as lymphoma, PTLD, and Castleman disease and granulomatous pachymeningeal diseases such as Wegener's granulomatosis and sarcoidosis are usually not focally restricted to the petrous apex, but when they present in that manner, those conditions clearly become differential considerations when there is this type of infiltrating and dural-based morphology.

Questions for Further Thought

1. What is a predisposing condition for meningiomas?
2. What two infectious processes might be included in the differential diagnosis of this case given the right clinical circumstances?

Reporting Responsibilities

While a meningioma requires no special reporting, the other conditions in this differential diagnosis may lead to progressive neurologic deficits and might include a malignant neoplasm; therefore, direct communication is always wise at the time of initial discovery.

What the Treating Physician Needs to Know

- If the specific diagnosis of benign tumor or slow-flow vascular malformation of the petrous apex can be confirmed or if there are other reasonable differential considerations that require further workup such as CSF sampling and/or laboratory testing (e.g., cANCA)
- If not a benign tumor of the petrous apex, what is the most likely diagnosis?

- If a benign tumor, the full extent of disease both within bone, intracranial and extracranial
- Specific anatomic relationship to surrounding anatomic structures
- Best surgical approach based on the extent of disease
- Factors that might complicate a particular surgical approach, such as a high jugular bulb and variations in the mastoid

Answers

1. These are mainly sporadic tumors usually with no known predisposing conditions. Patients with neurofibromatosis type 1 (NF1), neurofibromatosis type 2 (NF2), and mosaics of those conditions are more likely than the general population to have a meningioma.
2. Skull base osteomyelitis and petrous apicitis

> **LEARN MORE**
>
> See Chapters 124 and 31 in *Head and Neck Radiology* by Mancuso and Hanafee.

CASE 3.21

CLINICAL HISTORY *A 53-year-old male patient presented with left facial and retro-orbital pain for the last 6 months that has progressively worsened, with poor control of pain by over-the-counter pain medicines. He also had intermittent diplopia that became constant 5 days before presentation. Physical examination revealed a left sixth nerve palsy and mild facial nerve palsy. CT and MR images are shown below:*

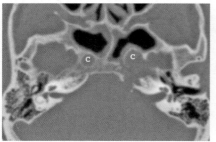

FIGURE **3.21A**

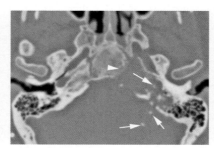

FIGURE **3.21B**

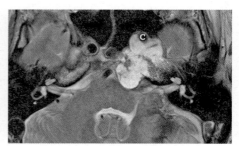

FIGURE **3.21C**

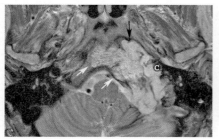

FIGURE **3.21D**

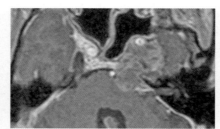

FIGURE **3.21E**

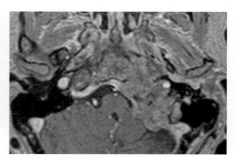

FIGURE **3.21F**

FINDINGS

Figure 3.21A,B. CT shows a mass eroding the bone at the left petroclival junction and carotid canal (*C*) with internal chondroid matrix calcifications (arrows in Fig. 3.21B). The margin at the clivus is fairly sharp with a narrow zone of transition suggesting low-grade behavior.

Figure 3.21C–F. MRI allows for better delineation of the extent of the mass, which involves the prevertebral space (black arrow), clivus (white arrow), and posterior fossa and displaces the carotid artery (*C*) anteriorly. The MR images confirm sharp bony margins with narrow zones of transition. T2W images show the predominantly CSF equivalent signal intensity within the mass corresponding to variably mineralized chondroid matrix (Fig. 3.21C,D). Postcontrast heterogeneous somewhat "solid"-appearing enhancement is seen (Fig. 3.21E,F).

DIFFERENTIAL DIAGNOSIS Clinically, most possible petrous apex lesions are in the differential. By imaging, cholesterolosis, mucocele and epidermoid cyst, unusually prominent arachnoid granulations, and the few benign (meningioma and nerve sheath and paraganglioma) and malignant neoplasms (chordoma, a rare metastasis and spread of nasopharyngeal carcinoma) may be considered.

DIAGNOSIS Chondrosarcoma of the petrous apex

DISCUSSION Chondrosarcomas arise close to or within the petroclival fissure from persistent embryologic cartilage rests near the petroclival synchondrosis. They extend predominantly lateral to the petrous apex and to a lesser extent medially to involve the basisphenoid/upper clivus. When the extent is predominantly medial, the spread pattern mimics that of a chordoma. There is potential to involve cranial nerves III through XII, other adjacent structures like dura, cavernous sinus, carotid artery, jugular vein, and eventually the bony labyrinth depending on the size and extent of the lesion.

A chondroid matrix, T2 signal intensity predominantly equivalent to CSF in a bone destructive lesion in the petrous apex is highly suggestive of a chondrosarcoma. Mild to moderate enhancement suggests a higher-grade lesion.

The combination of MRI and CT easily differentiates petrous apex cholesterolosis and mucocele from an epidermoid cyst, arachnoid granulations, the few benign (meningioma and nerve sheath tumors) and malignant neoplasms, and the relatively uncommon inflammatory pathologies that can involve the petrous apex. Chordoma is usually more medial in location, centered in the clivus, and has large components that appear markedly hyperintense to CSF on T2W images and relatively low density approaching that of fluid on CT. There may be stippled calcification that can be sometimes confused with matrix calcification of chondrosarcoma. Chordoma enhances less than chondrosarcoma.

Question for Further Thought

1. What treatment options are available for this patient?

Reporting Responsibilities

Chondrosarcomas are generally slowly progressive conditions; therefore, if a diagnosis of a petrous apex chondrosarcoma is made, no special communication usually is required. In the unusual instance that there is a complicating obstructive hydrocephalus or otherwise threatening mass effect, this should be communicated verbally. If an alternative etiology is discovered such as an aneurysm or dissection of the carotid artery that might have thromboembolic implications, immediate verbal communication is necessary.

What the Treating Physician Needs to Know

- If the specific diagnosis of chondrosarcoma of the petrous apex can be made with a high degree of confidence
- Full extent of the tumor both within bone, intracranial and extracranial
- Specific anatomic relationship to surrounding anatomic structures
- Best surgical approach based on the extent of disease
- Factors that might complicate a particular surgical approach such as a high jugular bulb and variations in the mastoid

Answer

1. A combination of surgery and radiotherapy can be offered to this patient. Several basic surgical approaches have been developed. CT and MR imaging are pivotal in planning the surgery. These approaches may be combined to balance potential morbidity against the need for adequate exposure. CT image–guided and MRI-guided surgery allows a real-time assessment of the progress of the procedure. Such guidance provides continuous monitoring of the location of the ICA, IAC, and inner ear relationship to the probe.

A transmastoid approach is only useful to obtain tissue for diagnosis.

The middle fossa approach is via a subtemporal craniotomy. The labyrinth and carotid artery obstruct complete extirpation of more caudal and medial disease.

The transcochlear approach is an extension of the translabyrinthine approach wherein the facial nerve is reflected posteriorly and the bony cochlea is drilled out and this exposure continued to the petrous portion of the carotid artery.

The transnasal approach uses advanced image guidance and an endoscopic anterior skull base approach, allowing treatment for more medial lesions.

Cranial nerve function may not return back to normal.

Radiation as primary therapy may halt the growth of a chondrosarcoma. It can be delivered by stereotactic technique in a lesion less than 3 cm in maximum dimensions. Proton beam radiation may be used where available and is the preferred method of radiation therapy.

Radiotherapy is also used as an adjunct therapy to control the growth of even gross residual tumor that may be left behind in an effort to reduce potentially unacceptable morbidity of a gross total removal.

LEARN MORE
See Chapters 125 and 39 in *Head and Neck Radiology* by Mancuso and Hanafee.

CASE 3.22

CLINICAL HISTORY *A 67-year-old male patient presented with suboccipital, ear, and upper neck pain. He had completed radiotherapy 9 months ago for tonsil carcinoma. CECT images are shown below:*

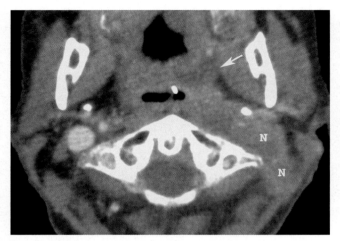

FIGURE **3.22A**

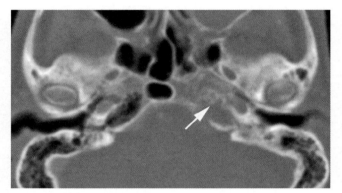

FIGURE **3.22C**

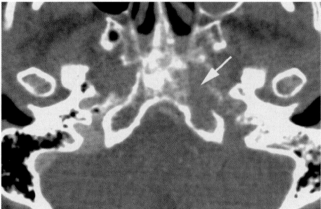

FIGURE **3.22B**

FIGURE **3.22D**

FINDINGS CT reveals likely recurrent disease at the primary site (arrow) and metastatic and cervical, retrostyloid (parapharyngeal) and retropharyngeal nodes (*N*) and invasion of the clivus and the petrous apex. Bone windows (Fig. 3.22D) show the related lytic and permeative changes of the clivus (Fig. 3.22B) and petrous apex (arrows in Fig. 3.22C,D).

DIFFERENTIAL DIAGNOSIS Chondrosarcomas, lymphoma and PTLD, leukemia and plasma cell dyscrasias, nasopharyngeal and other failed cancers, and skull base osteomyelitis

DIAGNOSIS Recurrent tonsil carcinoma metastatic to retropharyngeal and parapharyngeal lymph nodes and extranodal spread to the skull base

DISCUSSION CT and MRI are complementary in evaluating a suspected malignant lesion in the petrous apex. MR delineates the soft tissue extent better, and CT delineates the bony involvement and destruction. In this patient with a known previously treated tonsillar carcinoma, there is clear evidence of metastatic adenopathy as well as local recurrence with direct extension to the skull base and the left petrous apex. Here, cranial nerves V and VI are at risk, although at this time the patient was clinically negative for cranial nerve deficits. More posterior extension can involve cranial nerves VII and VIII and eventually the labyrinth. The other tumor that most commonly demonstrates similar findings is nasopharyngeal carcinoma. Skull base osteomyelitis can be difficult to distinguish from malignancy, especially if those infections have an indolent clinical course.

Question for Further Thought

1. What is the role of nuclear medicine imaging in malignant-appearing lesions of the petrous apex?

Reporting Responsibilities

If a possible malignant tumor or a possible infection rather than tumor is discovered, verbal communication of that unexpected finding would be wise. Other complicating features such as obstructive hydrocephalus or threatening mass effect on the brainstem should be communicated verbally.

What the Treating Physician Needs to Know

- Whether the specific diagnosis of a malignancy of the petrous apex can be made with a high degree of confidence
- Is the mass likely a process primary in the petrous apex and skull base or likely due to spread from pharyngeal cancer, perineural cancer spread, or secondary to distant metastatic disease or other systemic malignancy or process?
- Is an alternative diagnosis such as skull base osteomyelitis possible or likely?
- Full extent of the tumor both within bone, intracranial and extracranial
- Specific anatomic relationship to surrounding anatomic structures
- Best approach for tissue sampling by imaging guidance or surgery

- Suggestions for further imaging that might help establish an alternative diagnosis and/or may identify the lesion as part of a systemic process

Answer

1. Radionuclide studies may be used to search for other metastatic lesions or evidence of lymphoma, leukemia, or plasma cell dyscrasias in an effort to refine the differential and/or look for a site suitable for tissue sampling. Whether FDG-PET or bone scanning agents are more appropriate for such a search will depend on the clinical circumstances.

   A return of "inflammatory tissue" when tissue is sampled suggests peritumoral reactive changes but also raises the strong possibility of skull base osteomyelitis or even Wegener's granulomatosis. Gallium or white blood cell imaging can confirm infection.

> **LEARN MORE**
> See Chapters 126 and 42 in *Head and Neck Radiology* by Mancuso and Hanafee.

CASE 3.23

CLINICAL HISTORY *A 48-year-old male patient with a history of non-Hodgkin lymphoma presented with acute onset of facial nerve paralysis on the left. MRI was performed at presentation (Fig. 3.23A,B) and 3 weeks later (Fig. 3.23C,D). Images are shown below:*

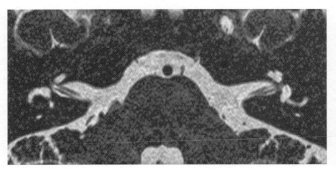

FIGURE **3.23A**

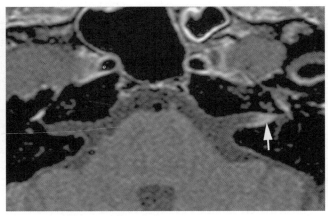

FIGURE **3.23C**

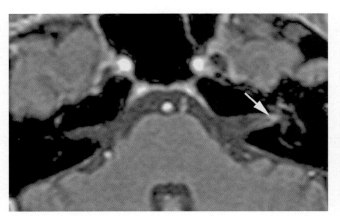

FIGURE **3.23B**

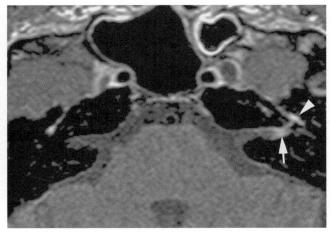

FIGURE **3.23D**

FINDINGS

Figure 3.23A,B. MRI shows no thickening of the facial nerve on a 3D steady-state image (Fig. 3.23A). Enhancement of the facial nerve in the IAC fundus, labyrinthine and first genus, and proximal tympanic segment is seen in Figure 3.23B.

Figure 3.23C,D. A follow-up MR after 3 weeks shows increased enhancement in the IAC fundus on the left as well as enhancement of the right geniculate ganglion and proximal tympanic segment with clinically unilateral facial palsy.

Further analysis revealed involvement of nerve root C7 causing arm weakness and a cutaneous recurrence of NHL.

DIFFERENTIAL DIAGNOSIS Infectious/inflammatory neuritis (e.g., viral, granulomatous, Lyme, sarcoidosis), perineural tumor spread (e.g., due to parotid neoplasm or skin cancer),

and rarely an acute (infarct, bleed) or subacute (multiple sclerosis) brainstem event will present as only facial nerve palsy.

DIAGNOSIS Neurotropic lymphoma mimicking Bell's palsy

DISCUSSION Bell's palsy is an acute-onset lower motor neuron palsy involving the facial nerve, likely to be a viral neuritis or an ischemic event incited by nerve swelling due to an inflammatory viral neuritis. The palsy could be partial or complete.

Bell's palsy *must never* be confused with a facial nerve palsy of slow, progressive, or "stuttering" onset. Also, recurrent or persistent peripheral facial nerve palsy or palsy associated with spasticity should not be considered a Bell's palsy until it is proven—by a very carefully executed imaging evaluation—not to be due to a structural lesion of the facial nerve.

When the clinical presentation is atypical, imaging is warranted. In this patient, although the presentation was typical, imaging was performed due to prior history of lymphoma. Abnormal enhancement along the entire course of the facial nerve, especially in the IAC fundus, suggested lymphoma infiltration of facial nerve. Repeat imaging showed increasing enhancement confirming the suspicion.

Question for Further Thought

1. What is the role of imaging in Bell's palsy?

Reporting Responsibilities

There should be a prompt, preferably verbal, report about whether the nerve appears abnormal in a manner consistent with a viral neuritis and that the study excludes a causative structural lesion with a very high degree of confidence. A causative parotid mass or thickening of the nerve distal to the stylomastoid foramen is often due to parotid cancer or perineural spread of skin cancer. Such cases should be directly communicated.

What the Treating Physician Needs to Know

- Are the findings consistent with the clinical suspicion of Bell's palsy?
- Does the imaging exclude a structural lesion from the seventh nerve nucleus to its peripheral site of innervation with a high degree of confidence?

Answer

1. Most treating physicians will not image a patient with acute onset of peripheral facial nerve palsy because about 75% of these palsies will be transient and will begin to recover in 4 to 6 weeks whether or not they are treated with steroids or antiviral medications and show no atypical subsequent characteristics such as recurrence of weakness.

   MRI should be done first since it most confidently excludes causative pathology at all segments. MRI is more sensitive than CT for excluding intra-axial pathology such as demyelinating disease, pia-arachnoid diseases, and small neoplasms of the nerve that might involve the cisternal segment or the segment within the IAC as well as perineural spread of cancer. CT is much less sensitive than MRI. MRI will usually be normal. It may show minimal enlargement and increased enhancement of the affected facial nerve, especially in the perigeniculate region, that may persist up to 1 year. At times this is actually a normal variation. Therefore, early imaging sometimes leads to excessive anxiety about normal variations or minor findings.

> **LEARN MORE**
> See Chapters 127 and 27 in *Head and Neck Radiology* by Mancuso and Hanafee.

CLINICAL HISTORY *A 1-year-old girl was referred to imaging since the primary care pediatrician noticed no expressions on the right side of the face. Although the parents had noticed it earlier, it recently became obvious. There was also some delay in milestones and one episode of seizure.*

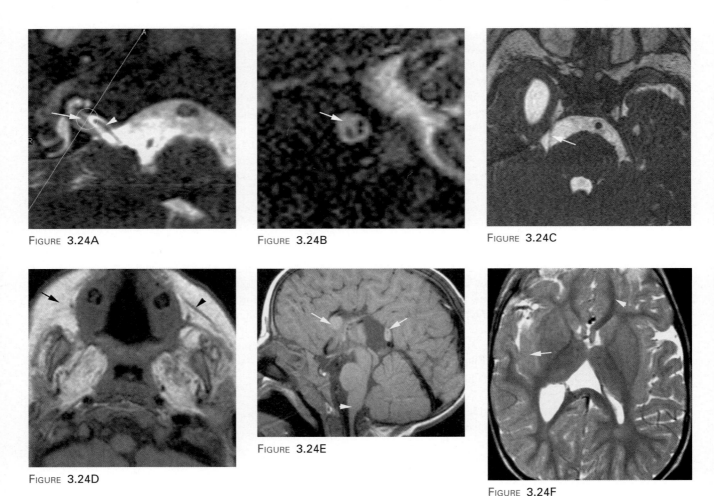

FIGURE **3.24A**

FIGURE **3.24B**

FIGURE **3.24C**

FIGURE **3.24D**

FIGURE **3.24E**

FIGURE **3.24F**

FINDINGS

Figure 3.24A. 3D steady-state image showing the typically normal cochlear nerve (arrow) and a vascular loop (arrowhead). Line "A" shows the plane of the oblique sagittal reformation in (Fig. 3.24B).

Figure 3.24B. 3D steady-state image showing the absent facial nerve (arrow) with the divisions of cranial nerve VIII (arrowheads).

Figure 3.24C. 3D steady-state image showing a small trigeminal nerve (arrow).

Figure 3.24D. T1W image showing lack of development or atrophy of the muscles of facial expression more on the right (arrow) than the left (arrowhead) and almost absence of the muscles of mastication.

Figure 3.24E. Malformations of the corpus callosum (arrows) and brainstem (arrowheads).

Figure 3.24F. T2W image showing gray matter migrational abnormalities (arrow).

RELEVANT EMBRYOLOGY The development of the facial nerve within the temporal bone is intimately linked to that of the middle and inner ear since the primordia of the facial and cochleovestibular nerves begin in very close proximity at the beginning of gestation. The development of the nerves will then be affected by that of the otic capsule and maturation of the first and second branchial arches as the latter relate to the development of temporal bone and the face, especially the mandible. More proximally, disorders of rhombencephalic development can lead to absence or hypoplasia of the facial nerve, usually in association with other cranial nerve absence or hypoplasia, craniofacial anomalies, and other genetic anomalies.

DIFFERENTIAL DIAGNOSIS Isolated facial nerve aplasia

DIAGNOSIS Unusual variant of Moebius syndrome

DISCUSSION Moebius syndrome is a rare genetic disorder. The exact mechanism altering the genome is not certain. Patients present with facial nerve weakness that is typically bilateral. Hypoplasia of the tongue is common. Cranial nerves III, IV, and VI are occasionally involved; cranial nerve V involvement is rare. The genetic errors result in aplasia and hypoplasia of cranial nerves and brainstem dysgenesis. Failure of the nerves to form properly causes lack of proper induction of associated mesodermal elements such as the development of their bony canals and, more distally, muscles of facial expression. Other associated anomalies of the brain can be seen. The craniovestibular nerve is typically normal, and there are no hearing problems.

This is an unusual case since there is only involvement of the right side. Associated brainstem and partial corpus callosum anomalies are noted. The cause of seizure is most likely due to gray matter heterotopia.

Question for Further Thought

1. What is Duane syndrome?

Reporting Responsibilities

Disorders of cranial nerves are reported routinely unless a posterior fossa tumor or some treatable infectious or inflammatory condition producing the cranial nerve deficit is identified. The urgency of reporting in the latter situation is governed by the nature and extent of the condition identified on the imaging study and the acuity dictated by clinical findings such as rate of progression of symptoms, fever, and state of consciousness.

What the Treating Physician Needs to Know

- Does the imaging exclude a structural lesion from the seventh nerve nucleus to its peripheral site of innervation with a high degree of confidence?
- If there is a lesion, what segments of the facial nerve are involved?
- Are there findings that suggest a specific causative condition?
- If so, is the condition likely to be a congenital or developmental condition?
- If so, is it likely a surgical lesion?
- Is the facial nerve present?
- Is the condition likely syndromic? Bilateral? Associated findings?
- Are there any findings that suggest the condition is one that requires urgent or emergent intervention?

Answer

1. Duane syndrome is limitation of abduction of the eye and variable degree of limited adduction as well as retraction of the eye with narrowing of the palpebral fissure. The sixth nerve nucleus and nerve are absent or hypoplastic, and the lateral rectus muscle is usually also partially innervated by a branch of the third nerve. This results in opposing muscle being innervated by the same nerve. Duane syndrome can be associated with Moebius syndrome.

> ### LEARN MORE
> See Chapter 128 in *Head and Neck Radiology* by Mancuso and Hanafee.

CLINICAL HISTORY *A 42-year-old female patient presented with bilateral peripheral facial nerve dysfunction and ocular dysmotility. MR imaging was performed. Selected images are shown below:*

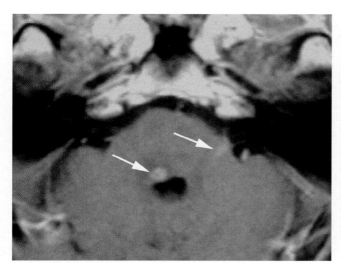

FIGURE **3.25A**

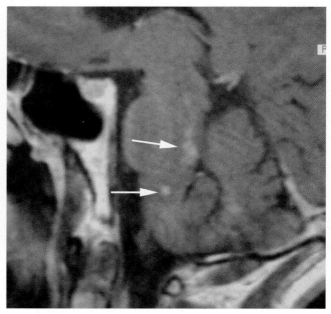

FIGURE **3.25C**

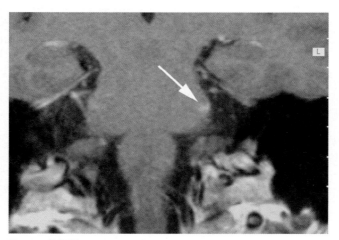

FIGURE **3.25B**

FINDINGS

The following CE T1W images show focal enhancing brainstem lesions:

Figure 3.25A. Image shows the right facial nucleus and left facial nerve root entry zone.

Figure 3.25B. Image confirms the left facial nerve root entry zone.

Figure 3.25C. Image shows the dorsal brainstem.

DIFFERENTIAL DIAGNOSIS Lyme disease and multiple sclerosis

DIAGNOSIS Viral brainstem encephalitis

DISCUSSION Bilateral facial nerve palsy and associated ocular dysmotility cannot be Bell's palsy. Bell's palsy is an acute-onset unilateral lower motor neuron palsy involving the facial nerve, likely to be a viral neuritis or an ischemic event incited by nerve swelling due to an inflammatory viral neuritis. Imaging is warranted whenever the clinical presentation is even minimally atypical. In this patient, due to an enhancing lesion in the brainstem, Lyme disease and multiple sclerosis was the primary working differential in both cases. Imaging was not typical for multiple sclerosis, as no periventricular lesions were seen and CSF analysis showed no evidence of multiple sclerosis markers; however, other parameters were consistent with a subacute inflammatory process and several years of follow-up showed no new episodes resulting in neurologic deficits or new MRI findings. Titers for Lyme disease were also negative.

Question for Further Thought

1. What is the role of nuclear medicine imaging in facial nerve palsy?

Reporting Responsibilities

The reporting should be prompt and preferably verbal. Middle ear disease and meningitis causing nerve palsy should be communicated emergently.

What the Treating Physician Needs to Know

• Does the imaging exclude a structural lesion from the seventh nerve nucleus to its peripheral site of innervation with a high degree of confidence?
• If a lesion is present, what segments of the facial nerve are involved?
• Are there findings that suggest a specific causative condition?

• Is the disease likely to be an infectious or noninfectious inflammatory condition?
• Do imaging findings suggest a likely high yield site for tissue sampling?
• Are there any findings that suggest the condition is one that requires urgent or emergent intervention?

Answer

1. If a disease process such as NOE or skull base osteomyelitis is established as the cause of facial nerve deficit, radionuclide studies may be used to monitor the response of the disease to specific antimicrobial therapy. Radionuclide studies are nonspecific in these diseases and are not generally useful for initial diagnosis.

LEARN MORE
See Chapters 129 and 13 in *Head and Neck Radiology* by Mancuso and Hanafee.

CLINICAL HISTORY *A 47-year-old female patient presented with tinnitus. On inspection, bulging of the posterior wall of the EAC was seen. The facial nerve function was normal. CT and MR images are shown below:*

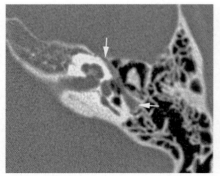

FIGURE **3.26A**

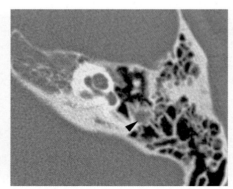

FIGURE **3.26B**

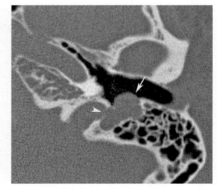

FIGURE **3.26C**

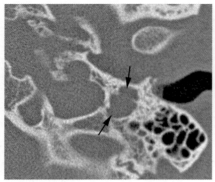

FIGURE **3.26D**

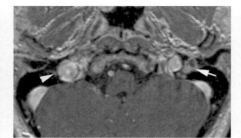

FIGURE **3.26E**

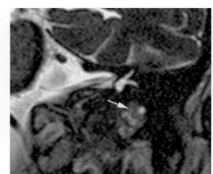

FIGURE **3.26F**

FINDINGS

Figure 3.26A. The tympanic segment of the facial nerve slightly enlarged on axial images.

Figure 3.26B–D. There is a lobulated mass along the mastoid segment causing remodeling of the surrounding bone and erosion of the posterior wall of the EAC (arrow) and the jugular plate (arrowhead).

Figure 3.26E. Axial postcontrast T1W image show inhomogeneous enhancement in the mastoid segment due to necrosis compared to the normal facial nerve (arrowhead).

Figure 3.26F. Coronal T2 also shows variable signal intensity.

DIFFERENTIAL DIAGNOSIS Facial neurofibroma and perineural tumor spread

DIAGNOSIS Facial nerve schwannoma of the tympanic and mastoid segment

DISCUSSION Nerve sheath tumors will most commonly arise along the facial nerve intratemporal segment, usually somewhere between the labyrinthine portion and the descending facial canal. These lesions might extend to the labyrinthine segment and canalicular segments but are usually diagnosed before such extension has occurred. Nerve sheath tumors beyond the stylomastoid foramen are also less common. Patients usually present with slow-onset facial nerve palsy due to slow and chronic compression. Extension to the middle ear may cause conductive hearing loss. Further growth may lead to inner ear symptoms or a mass bulging into the EAC, as seen in this patient. Tearing may be abnormal if the greater superficial petrosal nerve is involved, and involvement of the chorda tympani may alter taste and cause palatal sensory deficit.

MRI should be done first since it most confidently excludes causative pathology of all facial nerve segments (i.e., brainstem, cisternal, exit canal/foramen, extracranial) from its brainstem nucleus to the parotid gland. MRI is more sensitive than CT for excluding intra-axial pathology such as demyelinating disease, pia-arachnoid diseases, and small neoplasms of the nerve that might involve the cisternal segment or the segment within the IAC as well as perineural spread of cancer. CT is also done for similar reasons but is less sensitive to evaluate pathology in the cisterns and IAC. It demonstrates bony remodeling better than MR.

Neurofibromas are rare and may be seen in association with NF1 or NF2. They are more homogenous in appearance on MRI than schwannoma. Bony remodeling is not seen with perineural tumor spread; the bony facial canal will be either normal or frankly eroded.

Question for Further Thought

1. How is this condition treated?

Reporting Responsibilities and What the Treating Physician Needs to Know

- Does the imaging demonstrate a structural lesion from the seventh nerve nucleus to its peripheral site of innervation with a high degree of confidence?
- If a lesion is present, what segments of the facial nerve are involved?
- Are there findings that suggest a specific causative condition?
- Is that cause likely to be a benign tumor?
- Are there any findings that suggest an alternate condition that may require urgent or emergent intervention?
- If there is no structural lesion, is there a clue to an alternative diagnosis, and is there any other imaging that might prove useful in medical decision making?

Answer

1. The role of surgery has evolved with the growing power of imaging studies. Previously, surgical resection and repair was recommended for most patients with facial nerve tumors. Now that MRI demonstrates tumors of the facial nerve before they have caused profound paralysis, a more conservative approach has emerged. Currently, resection and repair is reserved for patients with severe facial paralysis. Resection alone is performed with patients who have any evidence of a compressive neuropathy since the likelihood of preserving the integrity of the nerve is higher in these patients.

   Radiotherapy will only infrequently be used to treat a facial-origin nerve sheath tumor. Such an intervention will not facilitate recovery from established palsy and may worsen already compromised facial motor function.

> **LEARN MORE**
> See Chapters 130 and 29 in *Head and Neck Radiology* by Mancuso and Hanafee.

CLINICAL HISTORY *A 59-year-old male patient presented with right-sided facial weakness for 6 weeks that was slowly progressive. Selected images from CT and MR are shown below:*

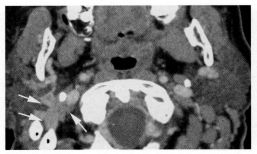

FIGURE **3.27A**

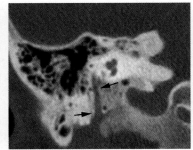

FIGURE **3.27B**

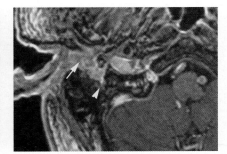

FIGURE **3.27C**

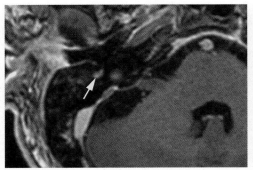

FIGURE **3.27D**

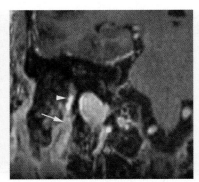

FIGURE **3.27E**

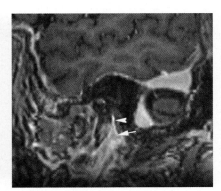

FIGURE **3.27F**

FINDINGS

Figure 3.27A,B. CT showing an infiltrative enhancing lesion extending from the digastric groove to the retrostyloid parapharyngeal space causing CN VII and XI deficits (Fig. 3.27A). The descending facial nerve canal shows neither remodeling nor erosion (Fig. 3.27B).

Figure 3.27C–F. Axial 3D T1W CE images reformatted in (Fig. 3.27E,F). In (Fig. 3.27C), the process surrounds (arrow) and infiltrates (arrowhead) the stylomastoid fat pad. In (Fig. 3.27D), perineural disease involves the descending facial canal (arrow). In (Fig. 3.27E,F), coronal and sagittal reformations, respectively, show the infiltrating process at the stylomastoid fat pad (arrows) and spread more proximally along the mastoid segment of the facial nerve to the second genu.

DIFFERENTIAL DIAGNOSIS Perineural tumor spread from skin cancer, facial nerve neurofibrosarcoma, and malignant schwannoma

DIAGNOSIS Perineural tumor spread along the facial nerve due to parotid adenoid cystic carcinoma

DISCUSSION Imaging is warranted in this patient since the clinical presentation is not acute-onset facial palsy as is

seen in Bell's palsy. Given the withheld clinical history of prior treatment for adenoid cystic cancer, a recurrence with perineural tumor spread was clinically suspected. Imaging with both CT and MR confirmed that suspicion. The definite diagnosis required biopsy, which was accomplished simply with CT guidance.

MRI should be done first for the evaluation of a peripheral facial nerve deficit since it most confidently excludes causative pathology at all segments of the nerve from its brainstem nucleus to the parotid gland. MRI is more sensitive than CT for excluding intra-axial pathology such as demyelinating disease, pia-arachnoid diseases, and small neoplasms of the nerve that might involve the cisternal segment or the segment within the IAC as well as perineural spread of cancer.

Typically, tumor spreads along the facial nerve from a peripheral primary site to obliterate the stylomastoid fat pad and grow along the facial canal to possibly as far proximally as the brainstem and meninges. The facial nerve fibers will eventually become atrophic and cease to function because they have been replaced by tumor. The muscles of facial expression comprising most of the bulk of the superficial aponeurotic system (SMAS) will go through the process of denervation atrophy. The muscles may enhance acutely and subacutely and then decrease in bulk and become fat replaced.

Question for Further Thought

1. What are the treatment options?

Reporting Responsibilities

If a parotid mass or findings suggestive of perineural spread of cancer are identified as a possible etiology, direct communication is strongly advised.

What the Treating Physician Needs to Know

- Does the imaging demonstrate a structural lesion from the seventh nerve nucleus to its peripheral site of innervation with a high degree of confidence?
- If a lesion is present, what segments of the facial nerve are involved?
- Are there findings that suggest a specific causative condition?
- Is the disease likely to be a malignant condition?
- Do imaging findings suggest a likely high yield site for tissue sampling?
- Are there any findings that suggest the condition is one that requires urgent or emergent intervention?

Answer

1. Radiotherapy may be the only form of treatment in patients with perineural tumor spread. Chemotherapy can be added to further improve the effectiveness of palliative treatment. Surgery generally does not have any role other than obtaining tissue for diagnosis, with most of that now obtained through imaging-guided fine needle aspiration and core biopsies rather than open surgery.

> LEARN MORE
>
> See Chapters 131 and 22 in *Head and Neck Radiology* by Mancuso and Hanafee.

CASE 3.28

CLINICAL HISTORY *A 21-year-old male patient presented with spasms of the left face (hemifacial spasm) for 6 months that were slowly progressive. CT and MR images are shown below:*

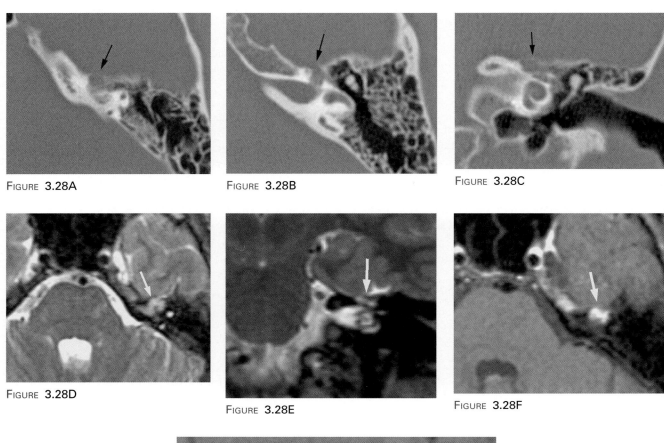

FIGURE **3.28A**

FIGURE **3.28B**

FIGURE **3.28C**

FIGURE **3.28D**

FIGURE **3.28E**

FIGURE **3.28F**

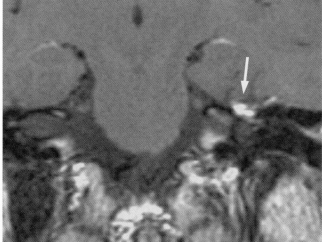

FIGURE **3.28G**

FINDINGS

Figure 3.28A–C. Axial (Fig. 3.28A,B) and coronal (Fig. 3.28C) CT. There is widening of the facial canal at the anterior genu and bone erosion with indistinct margins. There is spiculated calcification ("honeycomb appearance").

Figure 3.28D–G. MRI findings reveal a high signal intensity mass on an axial (Fig. 3.28D) image with uniform enhancement (Fig. 3.28F,G).

DIFFERENTIAL DIAGNOSIS Schwannoma of facial nerve, meningioma

DIAGNOSIS Facial nerve hemangioma

DISCUSSION Hemangiomas account for a substantial percentage of the rare occurrence of a benign mass of the facial nerve. Even a small-sized hemangioma can cause facial cranial nerve impairment. Although the symptoms may mimic a schwannoma, this discrepancy between tumor size and severity of symptoms favors the diagnosis of hemangioma. Hemangiomas will arise along the facial nerve, most commonly from the first genu and less commonly at the second genu, and along the descending facial canal. This tendency parallels the trend of the prominence of the perineural vascular plexus at these sites along the facial canal. Compression with axonal injury and/or demyelination of the nerve will interfere with its function, causing hyperexcitability that results in hemifacial spasm or diminished function causing facial weakness.

The facial nerve canal will typically appear to be focally expanded at the site of origin. Spread beyond the facial canal is most common at the first genu where the malformations spread within bone along the course of the greater petrosal nerve. They may be hyperintense on T1 and T2W images and avidly enhance on contrast administration. CT may demonstrate a pattern of punctate or subtle, spiculated calcification or ossification.

Hemangioma must always be considered especially in lesions of the anterior genu and the CT carefully evaluated for bone findings or internal pattern of calcification that will differentiate hemangioma and facial nerve schwannoma in some cases. Use of such data related to bone and calcification may not differentiate hemangioma from the meningiomas that occur in this region.

Questions for Further Thought

1. How is this condition treated?
2. What are some relevant caveats in making a medical decision to treat small facial nerve lesions?

Reporting Responsibilities

In slowly progressive disease or in patients with only hemifacial spasm, routine reporting typically suffices. If another unexpected structural lesion such as cancer or aneurysm is encountered, then verbal communication is the best course of action.

What the Treating Physician Needs to Know

- Does the imaging demonstrate a structural lesion from the seventh nerve nucleus to its peripheral site of innervation with a high degree of confidence?

- If a lesion is present, what segments of the facial nerve are involved?
- Are there findings that suggest a specific causative condition?
- Is that cause likely to be a hemangioma or other vascular lesion?
- If vascular, is it possibly life threatening, such as an aneurysm?
- Are there any findings that suggest an alternate condition that may require urgent or emergent intervention?
- If there is no structural lesion, is there a clue to an alternative diagnosis, and is there any other imaging that might prove useful in medical decision making?

Answers

1. Previously, mass lesions were often apparent only after they had resulted in significant motor dysfunction. Surgery is the only practical option in such cases. Hemangiomas may be treated by observation only, depending on whether the facial nerve weakness is progressive; however, they typically occur in younger individuals, will progressively enlarge, and will be removed. Surgery has a more favorable outcome in younger, healthier patients.

2. In the era of modern imaging, many of these lesions are discovered at a time when they may be treated by stereotactic radiosurgery without histologic confirmation. This means that at some point a hemangioma is very likely to be treated with radiotherapy, presuming it is a small nerve sheath tumor. Stereotactic radiation of a hemangioma may further worsen motor function and unlike surgery offers no proven hope for significant recovery. Radiotherapy should be delayed until the likelihood of a nerve sheath tumor is established in small (3- to 5-mm) lesions since those might actually be due to inflammatory enhancement of the nerve and the enhancement may resolve without specific therapy. Such findings might also require further testing such as Lyme titers and syphilis screening before radiotherapy is initiated. Abnormal nerve and perineural enhancement might also progress in a manner more consistent with perineural spread of carcinoma or neurotropic lymphoma and ultimately lead to a different prognosis and treatment plan.

> LEARN MORE
>
> See Chapters 132 and 9 in *Head and Neck Radiology* by Mancuso and Hanafee.

CLINICAL HISTORY *A 46-year-old woman presented 10 days after acute-onset right SNHL. She also complained of tinnitus and vertigo for 2 days. She was treated medically but was slow to respond to treatment. MRI was performed 5 weeks after onset of SNHL.*

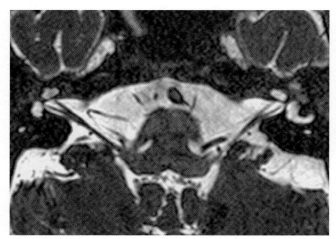

FIGURE **3.29A**

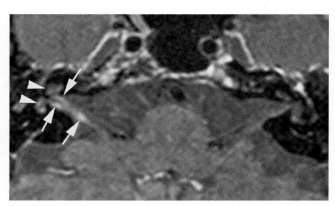

FIGURE **3.29B**

FINDINGS Steady-state 3D images show no definite abnormality of the CVN (Fig. 3.29A). The CE T1W image in (Fig. 3.29B) shows focal enhancement along the nerve (arrows) and of the labyrinth (arrowheads).

DIFFERENTIAL DIAGNOSIS The differential diagnosis for this combination of clinical presentation and imaging findings is limited and includes viral infection or early small tumor. Purulent bacterial infection of the CVN and labyrinth is usually either secondary to meningitis or from middle ear infection. NOE and skull base osteomyelitis from other unusual organisms can also involve the labyrinth as well as the CVN, if extensive. Lyme disease may result in CVN dysfunction as a presenting complaint; however, CVN symptoms will more commonly be overshadowed by the facial nerve presentation of this disease when that region of the central nervous system is involved. Syphilis, schistosomiasis, *Cryptococcus*, and tuberculosis can cause CVN dysfunction, but these diseases will commonly involve more than one cranial nerve as a manifestation of chronic meningitis.

DIAGNOSIS This is a presumptive viral infection of the CVN that resolved without intervention.

DISCUSSION MRI should be performed first since it is more sensitive and most confidently excludes causative pathology at all segments from the brainstem to the inner ear. CT can be used as an additional test, especially if bony involvement is suspected.

This case illustrates the insensitivity of steady-state images to such findings as seen above and that contrast should be used in CVN investigations. It also demonstrates why a small single nodular enhancement such as seen in this case should never be considered a nerve sheath tumor until the study is shown to remain abnormal after about 12 weeks. Even at that point, persistent enhancement should include a consideration of inflammatory etiologies of a more chronic nature than viral inflammation.

Question for Further Thought

1. What posttreatment imaging findings can be expected?

Reporting Responsibilities

Routine reporting usually suffices unless the lesion is one that suggests an aggressive disease process such as an infection or meningeal carcinomatosis.

In very small (3- to 5-mm) enhancing lesions, one must take great care to suggest that these may be focal inflammatory changes and that an absolute presumption of tumor is not appropriate. A proper range of possible inflammatory conditions should be mentioned in the report to stimulate an appropriate workup. It is also prudent to suggest that the study be repeated in 4 to 12 weeks depending on the clinical circumstances, such as CSF sampling results, to see if the enhancement resolves on its own if a specific inflammatory or infectious cause cannot be established. The possibility of Lyme disease, perhaps even in nonendemic areas, should always be included in the reported differential diagnosis.

What the Treating Physician Needs to Know

- Whether a structural lesion involving the CVN, CPA dura, or leptomeninges is producing the patient's symptoms
- If a lesion is present, what segments of the CVN are involved?
- Is the membranous labyrinth involved?

- Are there findings that suggest a specific causative condition?
- If the lesion is enhancing, might it be inflammatory or infectious?
- Are there any findings that suggest a condition, inflammatory or otherwise, that may require urgent or emergent intervention?
- If there is no structural lesion, is there a clue to an alternative diagnosis, and is there any other imaging that might prove useful in medical decision making?

Answer

1. The CVN or labyrinthine enhancement, if previously present, will resolve. Complete resolution may take a year or more. If there was an associated labyrinthitis, MRI might show replacement of the fluid signal in the labyrinth with low signal material due to fibrous or fibro-osseous changes; the latter may appear on CT as indistinctness of the modiolus and spiral lamina or filling in of the cochlea and vestibular chambers with calcification and/or ossification.

LEARN MORE

See Chapters 133 and 13 in *Head and Neck Radiology* by Mancuso and Hanafee.

CASE 3.30

CLINICAL HISTORY *A 51-year-old male patient presented with one episode of vertigo. He also had been having continuous tinnitus for a few hours before onset of the vertigo. Audiometry demonstrated high-frequency SNHL. Selected MR images are shown below:*

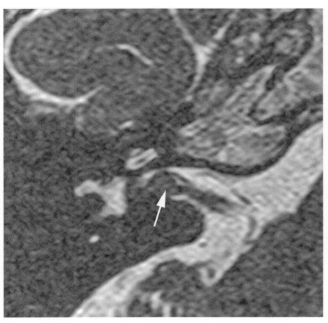

FIGURE 3.30A

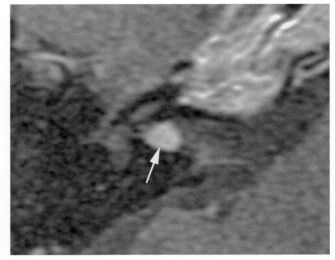

FIGURE 3.30B

FINDINGS

Figure 3.30A. 3D steady-state sequence shows a small lesion in the lateral third of the right IAC (arrows) near Scarpa's ganglion.

Figure 3.30B. Postcontrast T1W MR shows a small intracanalicular globular enhancement.

DIFFERENTIAL DIAGNOSIS Infectious (viral, Lyme) inflammation, other rare inflammatory/reactive diseases (e.g., Masson's vegetant hemangioendothelioma, metastasis (usually not focal), meningioma

DIAGNOSIS Intracanalicular vestibular schwannoma

DISCUSSION These CVN tumors are typically schwannomas that almost exclusively arise from its vestibular division. Schwannomas or neurofibromas associated with NF1 or NF2 make up a small percentage of these lesions. Meningiomas of the CPA and affecting the CVN account for less than 10% of these tumors. Meningiomas may be associated with NF2 and mosaics. The most important imaging differential is a meningioma, which in most cases has a dural tail on postcontrast T1W sequence. Meningiomas only rarely involve the fundus of the canal.

Smaller tumors can be clinically silent or may be very symptomatic. Larger tumors usually become symptomatic due to mass effect on the brainstem and cerebellum leading to ipsilateral upper and lower extremity dysfunction, ataxia and gait disturbances, causing other cranial nerve dysfunction, such as the facial and/or trigeminal nerves, and symptoms of increased intracranial pressure may occur.

To begin with, as in this case, the tumor is entirely intracanalicular. It then grows to fill the IAC and reaches the porus acoustics, at which point it protrudes into the CPA cistern, giving a typical ice-cream cone appearance. Further growth lead to mass effect with a widening ipsilateral CPA cistern. Cystic necrosis is common in larger tumors. Generally, the tumor grows at 1 to 3 mm per year. Sudden increase in mass effect is usually secondary to intratumor hemorrhage.

Imaging of these tumors requires the highest spatial resolution, especially for small intracanalicular schwannomas. MRI is the preferred modality, and CT is additional/adjunct to evaluate bony remodeling/erosion of the IAC. Any MRI protocol for this tumor is incomplete without inclusion of 3D steady-state sequence and 1-3 mm sectin thickness post contrast acquisitions.

Questions for Further Thought

1. What treatment options can be offered to this patient?
2. What is the role of surveillance?

Reporting Responsibilities

Routine reporting usually suffices unless the lesion is one that suggests an aggressive disease process such as an infection or meningeal carcinomatosis. In very small (3- to 5-mm) enhancing lesions, one must take great care to suggest that these may be focal inflammatory changes and that an absolute presumption of tumor is not appropriate. It is also prudent to suggest that the study be repeated in 4 to 12 weeks to see if the enhancement resolves on its own if a specific inflammatory or infectious cause cannot be established. In larger lesions that compress the brainstem and/or cause hydrocephalus, the need for direct communication may rise to an urgent or even emergent level.

What the Treating Physician Needs to Know

- Whether there is a structural lesion producing the patient's symptoms that is pointing to the CVN or CPA as a source
- If the lesion is an enhancing mass, what is the diagnosis—the most common being either vestibular schwannoma or meningioma?
- If the lesion has an entirely cystic-appearing mass, what is the diagnosis—the most typical being either an epidermoid or arachnoid cyst?
- If surgery is considered, whether the lesion involves the inner ear, the IAC, and/or the CPA
- Are there any findings that suggest an alternate condition or complication that may require urgent or emergent intervention?
- If there is no structural lesion, is there a clue to an alternative diagnosis, and is there any other imaging that might prove useful in medical decision making?

Answers

1. Initially, the patient may be treated medically for symptomatic relief. As the tumor is entirely intracanalicular, surgery is generally not preferred. Stereotactic radiosurgery is the preferred treatment for this patient. The goal of stereotactic radiosurgery is to eliminate or arrest tumor growth. Because of the unknown long-term effects, it may not be used in young patients. Large tumors with brainstem or cerebellar compression are a contraindication for radiosurgery because posttreatment edema may increase compression.

2. Surveillance following surgery and radiosurgery is a fairly routine practice. This is accomplished with MRI. If a "wait and scan" policy is chosen, periodic imaging is necessary since the development of symptoms does not correlate with tumor growth. No standards exist regarding the timing of follow-up examinations. This is done as often as every 6 months if growth is found on prior studies. It should be done at no greater than 2-year intervals until the growth rate is well established on serial exams.

> **LEARN MORE**
> See Chapters 134 and 29 in *Head and Neck Radiology* by Mancuso and Hanafee.

CASE 3.31

CLINICAL HISTORY *A 28-year-old male patient presented with progressively increasing pulse synchronous tinnitus for the last 6 months and headaches for 2 weeks. Audiometry demonstrated a mild SNHL.*

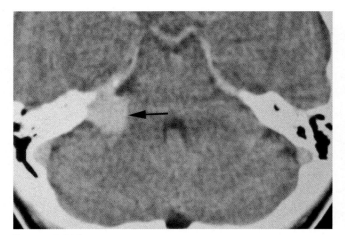

FIGURE **3.31A**

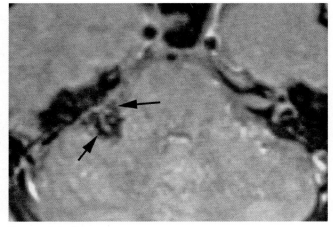

FIGURE **3.31C**

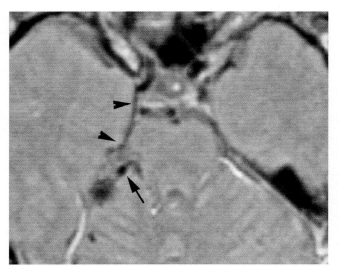

FIGURE **3.31B**

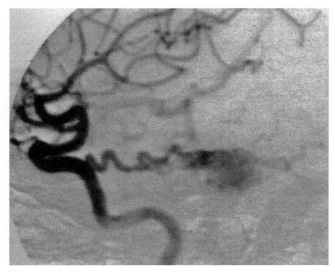

FIGURE **3.31D**

FINDINGS

Figure 3.31A. CECT shows an enhancing lesion in the CPA cistern (arrow) with a possible dural base.

Figure 3.31B,C. MRI shows that the lesion consists of enlarged tortuous vessels, presumably fed by the artery of the free margin of the tentorium (arrow and arrowheads).

Figure 3.31D. Catheter angiography confirms an arterialized mass.

DIFFERENTIAL DIAGNOSIS Meningioma, schwannoma, metastasis, hemangiopericytoma

DIAGNOSIS High-flow dural arteriovenous malformation along the right tentorium and CPA cistern

DISCUSSION Other than pulse synchronous tinnitus or listening for a bruit, there are no clinical signs and symptoms, except perhaps for the rare occurrence of palpable transcranial enlarged vessels, to suggest that a lesion in this region is of vascular etiology. Imaging, therefore, has a critical role in the diagnosis as well as either a direct role in and/ or guiding therapy. MRI may be very helpful as a diagnostic finding since flow voids may be recognized. In smaller vascular lesions, steady-state 3D sequences can help screen, perhaps better than even advanced CT angiography, for potential vascular compression and related nerve irritation. MR angiography can be helpful but is not able to assess the angioarchitecture and flow dynamics as well as the catheter angiography. Advanced CT angiography may fulfill these needs sometimes better than catheter angiography.

In this case, the postcontrast CT has an appearance that very closely mimics a meningioma. Failure to recognize the true nature of this mass would have led to an unnecessary craniotomy and a risk of disastrous bleeding.

Question for Further Thought

1. What might be the best treatment option for this patient?

Reporting Responsibilities

If a vascular malformation is discovered, it is wise to communicate this verbally to assure that there is no misunderstanding about the nature of the lesion and to determine whether surgery is indicated at that time. Such added consideration might lead to an endovascular approach to therapy. Also, a potential misadventure that might result from the lesion not being recognized as highly vascular until the time of surgery might be avoided. If an aneurysm is discovered, this should also be reported verbally.

What the Treating Physician Needs to Know

- Whether there is a structural lesion producing the patient's CVN symptoms that is pointing to the nerve or CPA as a source
- If the lesion is an enhancing mass, what is the diagnosis—the most common tumor being either schwannoma (IAC,

CPA) or meningioma (CPA)—and are there atypical features for those common lesions that suggest a vascular malformation or aneurysm?
- If the study is suspicious for a vascular lesion, what should be the next and safest study that is likely to be definitive?
- If there is no structural lesion, is there a clue to an alternative diagnosis, and is there any other imaging that might prove useful in medical decision making?
- For vascular compression syndromes, does any vessel fit a profile that may be reasonably predictive of this problem as a cause of CVN symptoms?

Answer

1. The best treatment option would be endovascular embolization of the feeding vessels. This patient was treated by embolization with coils and Onyx. Treatment was successful, and the patient's symptoms were completely relieved.

> **LEARN MORE**
> See Chapters 135 and 9 in *Head and Neck Radiology* by Mancuso and Hanafee.

CLINICAL HISTORY *Postoperative CT in a patient with a recent cochlear implant, with suboptimal hearing after the procedure.*

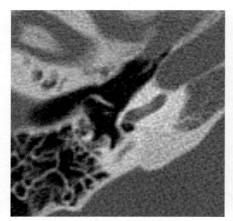

FIGURE **3.32A**

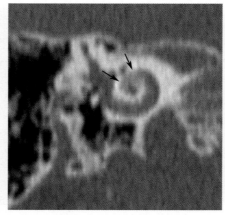

FIGURE **3.32B**

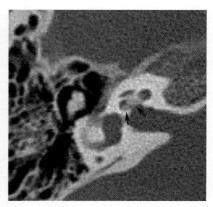

FIGURE **3.32C**

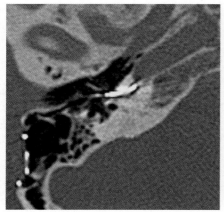

FIGURE **3.32D**

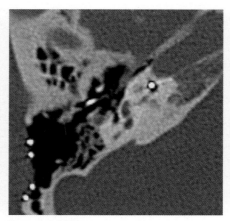

FIGURE **3.32E**

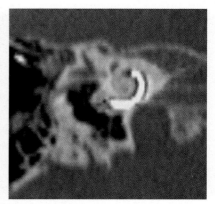

FIGURE **3.32F**

FINDINGS Incomplete insertion—preoperatively unrecognized perimodiolar ossification (within Fig. 3.32 A–C) the second turn of the cochlea (arrows in Fig. 3.32 B and C) has led to incomplete insertion of the electrode array (Fig. 3.32E,F).

DIFFERENTIAL DIAGNOSIS None

DIAGNOSIS Incomplete cochlear implant insertion due to postmeningitis perimodiolar ossification

DISCUSSION This patient developed deafness secondary to meningitis. The case illustrates the importance of preoperative MRI in detecting obliteration of the cochlea and vestibule, especially in patients who have had history of meningitis. This patient did not have a preoperative MRI. Thus, the findings of early labyrinthitis ossificans in the second turn of the cochlea were unrecognized preoperatively, possibly due to improper window and level setting used while reviewing images.

This case supports the strategy of using both CT and MRI to detect early ossification of the labyrinth, especially in the prelingual deaf, to help assure the best surgical results. Other postoperative complications that can be detected with imaging are misplacement, kinking, or poor contact of the electrodes or their becoming dislodged as well as breaks in connections within the device and CSF leak.

Question for Further Thought

1. What is the role of imaging in pretreatment evaluation?

Reporting Responsibilities and What the Treating Physician Needs to Know

Preoperative assessment:

• Anatomic variants of the mastoid and middle ear that might alter the surgical access

• Are there any signs of infection, increasing the risk of postoperative sepsis or meningitis?

• Whether the cochleovestibular system is normally developed

- If there is a developmental anomaly of the inner ear, is there a higher risk of gusher?
- Whether the cochlea is patent
- Is the cochlear nerve hypoplastic or absent?
- Are there any abnormalities along the entire auditory pathway that might contraindicate or alter the prognosis of treatment by cochlear implantation?

Postoperative assessment:

- Is the cochlear implant positioned within the inner ear?
- Are there any signs of complications that might cause malfunction, or can dysfunction be anticipated by alterations in frequency mapping?

Answer

1. Imaging with CT/MRI allows the visualization of the entire auditory pathway. MRI is more complete than CT as a single test in this regard, lacking only the bone detail of the latter. Imaging results may alter the choice of side of implantation or suggest the more appropriate electrode selection.

   It is clear that CT and MRI render complementary information in the preoperative assessment of cochlear implant candidates. The issue is what is truly necessary for medical decision making.

The surgeon needs to be informed about the patency of the cochlea and any cochlear and vestibular anomalies or bone dysplasias as well as any retrocochlear disease. Anatomic variations, especially those of the facial nerve or along the usual mastoid and middle ear approach to the preferred round window insertion site, that might alter the surgical approach should be noted.

CT provides information about the bony labyrinth, the vestibular aqueduct, and anatomic variants of the mastoid and vascular structures.

MRI will identify cochlear and retrocochlear soft tissue abnormalities, such as cochlear fibrosis in labyrinthitis, otospongiotic foci in otosclerosis, absence or extreme atrophy of the cochlear nerve, and brain pathology along the auditory pathways.

LEARN MORE

See Chapter 136 in *Head and Neck Radiology* by Mancuso and Hanafee.

CLINICAL HISTORY *A 52-year-old heavy smoker presented with right-sided otalgia. On examination, no abnormality was noted in the right ear, TMJ, or parotid gland. Additional clinical tests were also performed. The patient was then referred to radiology for imaging. CT was performed with an "otalgia" protocol. A selected CT image is shown below:*

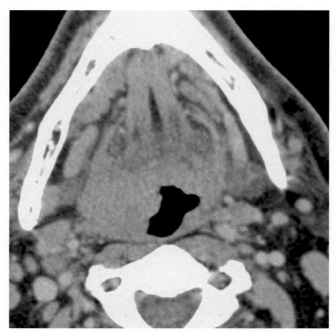

FIGURE **3.33**

FINDINGS

Figure 3.33. An infiltrating submucosal mass in the right tongue base is seen. There is no temporal bone abnormality.

DIFFERENTIAL DIAGNOSIS The differential diagnosis is most useful and helpful when it is discussed based on the nerve segments.

In the cisternal segment, intracranial or transcranial extra-axial tumors can cause glossopharyngeal neuropathy, by far the most common being paraganglioma, schwannoma, and meningioma.

In the foraminal and skull base segment, lesions include nasopharyngeal carcinoma (due to direct spread or retropharyngeal adenopathy) and paragangliomas. Less common lesions are skull base or retropharyngeal nodal metastases as a site of failure of nonnasopharyngeal SCCa, chordomas or chondrosarcoma, and medial extension of NOE. The lesions in the above segments most commonly involve multiple lower cranial nerves.

In the peripheral segment, from the skull base to the hyoid bone, lesions of the retrostyloid parapharyngeal space or carotid sheath will account for most glossopharyngeal neuropathies. The overwhelming majority will be due to a paraganglioma or a rare glossopharyngeal nerve–origin neurogenic tumor that is almost always a benign schwannoma.

More typically, a neurogenic tumor will be of vagal origin and secondarily compressing cranial nerve IX. Compressive neuropathy from Eagle syndrome (gross elongation, enlargement, and calcification of the stylohyoid ligament) can cause referred otalgia.

In the distal or end organ segment, the most common structural cause of a glossopharyngeal nerve pain pattern is SCCa or lymphoma of the palatine tonsil, glossotonsillar fossa, or tongue base seen in patients with throat pain or referred otalgia. These are sometimes entirely submucosal cancers that can only be found with CT or MRI and confirmed with endoscopic biopsy guided by the imaging.

DIAGNOSIS Submucosal tongue base cancer causing referred otalgia

DISCUSSION Referred otalgia is a very important symptom in upper aerodigestive tract disease, and it will most commonly come to imaging if progressive. Once TMJ syndromes, the salivary glands, and similar sources of pain that may have a periauricular location have been excluded clinically, it is important that these patients also have a complete clinical evaluation of the nasopharynx, oropharynx, and hypopharynx as well as otoscopy by an experienced otolaryngologist. Depending on this initial triage, they may be referred for imaging.

Otalgia may come from middle ear disease caused by eustachian tube dysfunction such as that caused by nasopharyngeal carcinoma. Referred otalgia may be via cranial nerve IX from the tongue base or tonsil or via cranial nerve X from the pyriform sinus. The cause, if found, may be a carcinoma at one of these sites. Progressive, possibly referred, otalgia must be viewed with a very high index of suspicion even in light of negative upper aerodigestive tract endoscopy, especially in the smoking/drinking population.

Within the jugular foramen, cranial nerve IX gives off its auricular or tympanic branch (Jacobson's nerve), supplying sensory fibers to the middle ear. Several branches supply sensation to the middle ear and bony eustachian tube, the posterior oropharynx and soft palate, sensation and taste to the posterior third of the tongue. Hence, imaging is focused on all of these regions when patients present with "referred otalgia."

Question for Further Thought

1. How might a patient with otalgia be imaged?

Reporting Responsibilities

In general, there is often little or no risk associated with the benign conditions that produce or mimic a lower cranial neuropathy; thus, no urgent communication is required. A likely cancer should be verbally communicated.

Special circumstances that require urgent or emergent direct communication with the referring treatment provider might include discovery of a vascular malformation, highly vascular tumor, or aneurysm when it is known an immediate surgical plan is place for biopsy of removal of the mass in question. For this reason, no submucosal mass of the pharynx should be biopsied—whether or not associated with signs or symptoms possibly due to a lower cranial neuropathy—without prior imaging.

What the Treating Physician Needs to Know

- If there is a structural cause for the neuropathy
- Is more than one nerve potentially involved?

- What is the likely diagnosis?
- If there is an alternative explanation for the symptoms or signs of the glossopharyngeal neuropathy affecting the end organ of innervation
- Does the disease process pose an immediate threat to the patient?
- Degree of confidence of a negative study excluding significant causative pathology

Answer

1. Patients with glossopharyngeal neuropathy and referred otalgia require a complete CECT study that will usually include temporal bone and posterior skull base reconstructions with the same technique used to study primary temporal bone problems and high-detail images from the posterior fossa to the bottom of the pyriform sinus. Detailed views of the entire oropharynx are also required. MR may be used for the investigation of a glossopharyngeal neuropathy if the lesion is likely intracranial; however, MRI is more likely to be degraded in the pharynx below the hard palate due to motion artifacts and does not definitively exclude smaller skull base lesions. However, the evaluation of otalgia requires images to the bottom of the pyriform sinus since it is uncertain if otalgia may be referred via Arnold's nerve (from cranial nerve X) or Jacobson's nerve from cranial nerve IX. MR images through the pyriform sinus are generally less optimal in quality compared to CT. Both studies may be necessary in some cases. It is reasonable to begin with MRI, if that is preferred, keeping in mind the potential pitfalls if the study is negative and then supplementing with CT as necessary.

LEARN MORE
See Chapters 137, 21, and 23 in *Head and Neck Radiology* by Mancuso and Hanafee.

CLINICAL HISTORY *A 48-year-old male patient presented with hoarseness of the voice of 5 weeks duration. Direct laryngoscopy demonstrated left vocal cord palsy. The chest radiograph was normal. Selected CT images are shown below:*

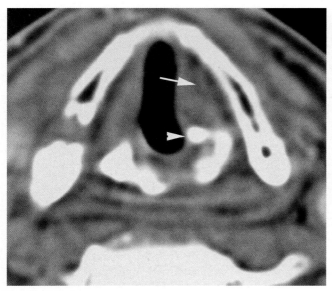

FIGURE **3.34A**

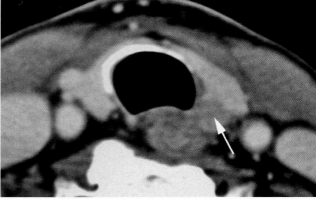

FIGURE **3.34B**

FINDINGS A paralysis of the left vocal cord (Fig. 3.34A) is manifest as a medialized, partially atrophic left vocal cord seen in association with an anterior and medial position of the vocal process of the arytenoid. A mass is seen (arrow in Fig. 3.34B) involving the recurrent laryngeal nerve in the tracheoesophageal groove.

DIFFERENTIAL DIAGNOSIS Various pathologies, from skull base to end organ innervation, can cause vocal cord paralysis. From the skull base to the carotid bifurcation, the pathologies include paraganglioma, meningioma and benign vagal-origin schwannoma, nasopharyngeal carcinoma (due to direct spread or retropharyngeal adenopathy), and untreated cervical nodal metastasis as well as recurrent metastatic nodal neck disease.

Below the bifurcation of the carotid supraclavicular lesions and masses like lymphoma can cause vagal neuropathy. In such tumors the sympathetic chain inferior cervical ganglion and the brachial plexus may also be involved. However, the more common lesion at his level of the neck is either primary thyroid cancer (as in this patient) or metastatic lymph nodes from thyroid cancer, esophageal cancer, or tracheal adenoid cystic cancer infiltrating the recurrent laryngeal nerve in the tracheoesophageal groove.

Thoracic pathologies that can cause vagal nerve palsy include those of the aortic arch such as an aneurysm and/or dissection and malignant mediastinal lymphadenopathy.

DIAGNOSIS Thyroid carcinoma involving the recurrent laryngeal nerve in the tracheoesophageal groove

DISCUSSION Once laryngeal cancer is excluded by indirect or direct laryngoscopy and a chest film is obtained to exclude obvious lung or mediastinal pathology, one must decide whether to take the imaging evaluation any further. The imaging studies then essentially become an evaluation of a vagal and/or recurrent laryngeal nerve neuropathy. If the vocal cord paresis is accompanied by a deficit in one or more of cranial nerves IX, XI, or XII, then the posterior fossa, skull base, and deep spaces down to the posterior belly of the digastric muscle must be covered. If the only other deficit is of the cervical sympathetics (Horner syndrome), then the lesion may lie between the skull base and thoracic inlet and other accompanying symptoms such as brachial plexopathy helps direct the exam.

If the only symptom is hoarseness and the only sign is an atrophic, paralyzed, or paretic true cord, a cause is most frequently not found by imaging; however, the cause may be found as a submucosal mass or other derangement within the larynx or adjacent hypopharynx. The vocal cord paresis may be the only sign of conditions as diverse as vagal cisternal segment compression due to a posterior fossa meningioma, a subtle mass in the thyroid gland or mediastinum causing compression or infiltration of the recurrent laryngeal nerve in the tracheoesophageal groove or aortopulmonary window, or even an aortic dissection in the absence of chest pain.

Question for Further Thought

1. How might one proceed as an imaging consultant when imaging is negative?

Reporting Responsibilities

Benign conditions that produce or mimic a lower cranial neuropathy require no urgent communication. A likely cancer as in this patient should be verbally communicated. Special circumstances that require urgent or emergent direct communication with the referring treatment provider might include discovery of a vascular malformation, highly vascular tumor or aneurysm when it is known an immediate surgical plan is place for biopsy of removal of a mass in question. Other vascular pathologies such as carotid or aortic dissection, life-threatening intracranial abnormality such as hydrocephalus, or brainstem compression need to be communicated immediately. The report should contain a complete assessment of the extent of the lesion causing the neuropathy, including suggestions for possible means of histologic confirmation by imaging-guided biopsy if the mass is not accessible for standard clinical biopsy approaches.

What the Treating Physician Needs to Know

- If there is a structural cause for the neuropathy
- Is more than one nerve potentially involved?
- What is the likely diagnosis?
- If there is an alternative explanation for the symptoms or signs of the neuropathy affecting the end organ of innervation

- Does the disease process pose an immediate threat to the patient?
- Degree of confidence of a negative study excluding significant causative pathology

Answer

1. Sometimes no structural lesion is identified in a patient with a specific cranial neuropathy. Imaging studies in patients with signs and symptoms of a potential cranial neuropathy such as otalgia or vocal cord paralysis will more often than not be negative. The most important thing to remember is to make sure that the study is of good quality and has been performed with the right protocol for the suspected pathology.

   When the studies are negative, the patient is reassured. If the symptoms become worse or an additional cranial neuropathy declares itself or becomes suspect, the patient should be followed with another imaging exam. Multiple cranial nerve deficits almost always will have a structural cause that can be identified with imaging.

> LEARN MORE
> See Chapters 138 and 22 in *Head and Neck Radiology* by Mancuso and Hanafee.

CLINICAL HISTORY *A 55-year-old female patient presented with a progressively worsening right shoulder droop for 2 months. She then developed intermittent hoarseness for 2 weeks before the clinical examination showing spinal accessory nerve palsy. Selected CT images are shown below:*

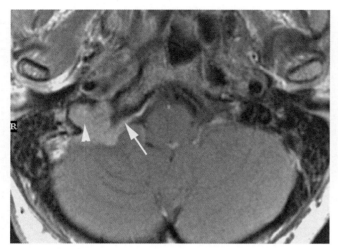

FIGURE **3.35A**

FIGURE **3.35C**

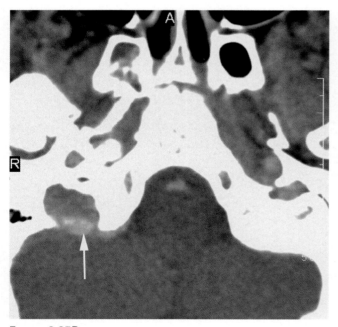

FIGURE **3.35B**

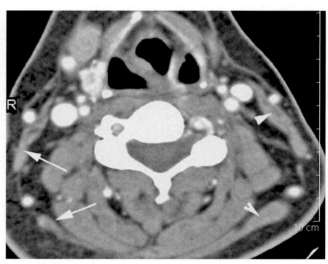

FIGURE **3.35D**

FINDINGS

Figure 3.35A. CE T1W image shows an enhancing mass spreading along the dura and involving the cranial nerve XI in the cistern (arrow) and the jugular fossa (arrowhead).

Figure 3.35B. CECT shows the involvement of the jugular fossa.

Figure 3.35C. CECT through the upper retrostyloid parapharyngeal space shows the mass also potential compress-ing cranial nerve XI (arrow) as it courses extracranially relative to the jugular vein.

Figure 3.35D. CT shows atrophy of the sternocleidomastoid and trapezius muscles (arrows) compared to the opposite side.

DIFFERENTIAL DIAGNOSIS The specific pathologies that involve the cranial nerves are variable but can be grouped by three broad mechanisms of disease, including primary neurogenic tumors, pathology that causes a particular point of compressive neuropathy, and infiltrating neuropathies. It is essential to first determine the specific localization of the offending pathology. Following that, a morphologic evaluation of the disease process will almost always lead to a specific diagnosis or a very short list of possibilities. Spinal accessory neuropathy is almost always associated with other cranial nerve deficits.

The cranial nerve nucleus segment is typically diseased due to intra-axial brain tumors, demyelinating disease, vascular disease, and rarely some unusual infectious disease.

The cisternal segment is most often involved by intracranial or transcranial extra-axial tumors, by far the most common being schwannoma and meningioma (as in this patient). Uncommon pathologies include dural and leptomeningeal diseases such sarcoidosis, lymphoma and leukemia, and meningeal carcinomatosis. Lymphoma actually might involve any segment.

Lesions in the foraminal/skull base segment most commonly produce the jugular fossa syndromes. These include schwannoma, neurofibroma, transcranial meningioma, nasopharyngeal carcinoma (due to direct spread or retropharyngeal adenopathy), and paragangliomas. Other less common lesions are skull base metastases or retropharyngeal nodal metastases as a site of failure of nonnasopharyngeal SCCa, chordoma, chondrosarcoma, and hemangiopericytoma.

The above segments are virtually never the site of origin for an isolated spinal accessory neuropathy.

In the peripheral segment (from the skull base to the hyoid bone), lesions of the retrostyloid parapharyngeal space or carotid sheath will account for most spinal accessory neuropathies. The overwhelming majority will be due to a paraganglioma or a rare spinal accessory nerve–origin neurogenic tumor that is almost always a benign schwannoma. More typically, a neurogenic tumor will be of vagal origin and secondarily compressing the cranial nerve XI. Occasionally, perineural tumoral invasion or untreated nodal metastases will cause spinal accessory neuropathy.

DIAGNOSIS Transcranial meningioma causing spinal accessory neuropathy

DISCUSSION Although one of lower cranial nerve symptoms may dominate the clinical presentation, more than one will often be involved following careful clinical testing; multiple nerve involvement is usually the case when a spinal accessory neuropathy is present. In this patient, by history, it appears that she was just beginning to have vagal nerve involvement.

Isolated spinal accessory nerve neuropathy, short of that related to surgical sacrifice, is uncommon. Pathologic processes usually involve the IX, X, XI complex. Isolated spinal accessory nerve pathology will cause dysfunction of the sternocleidomastoid and/or trapezius muscle and eventually some degree of atrophy.

Question for Further Thought

1. How might one approach, as a consultant, imaging of a spinal accessory neuropathy?

Reporting Responsibilities
Benign conditions need no special communication. A likely cancer should be verbally communicated. Special circumstances such as hydrocephalus, mass effect on brainstem and tonsillar herniation, vascular malformations, aneurysm, and dissection will need urgent verbal communication with the referring physician.

What the Treating Physician Needs to Know

- If there is a structural cause for the neuropathy
- Is more than one nerve potentially involved?
- What is the likely diagnosis?
- If there is an alternative explanation for the symptoms or signs of the neuropathy affecting the end organ of innervation
- Does the disease process pose an immediate threat to the patient?
- What is the degree of confidence of a negative study excluding significant causative pathology?

Answer

1. Patients with spinal accessory neuropathy require a complete CECT study that includes temporal bone and posterior skull base reconstructions with the same technique used to study primary temporal bone problems and high-detail images from the posterior fossa to the mandibular angle. A survey of the neck may be required.

   MR may be used for the investigation of a spinal accessory neuropathy if the lesion is likely intracranial; however, MRI may be more likely to be degraded in the pharynx below the hard palate due to motion artifacts and does not definitively exclude smaller skull base lesions.

> **LEARN MORE**
> See Chapters 139 and 31 in *Head and Neck Radiology* by Mancuso and Hanafee.

CLINICAL HISTORY *A 43-year-old male patient presented with tongue fasciculations and early tongue atrophy. On examination, there was mild deviation of the tongue toward the left side. Selected MR images done with contrast are shown below:*

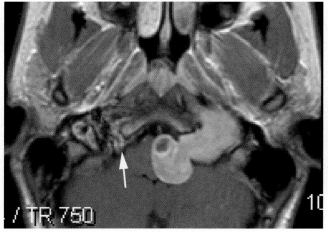

FIGURE **3.36A**

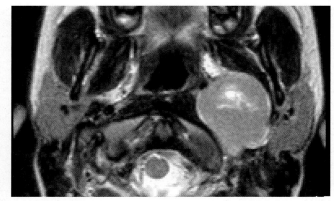

FIGURE **3.36C**

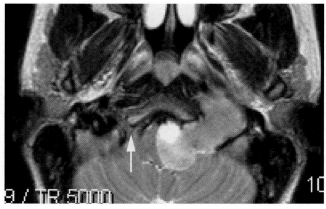

FIGURE **3.36B**

FINDINGS CE T1W (Fig. 3.36A) and T2W (Fig. 3.36B) images show a mass from the brainstem and into the hypoglossal canal with expansive growth in the retrostyloid parapharyngeal space (T2W image in Fig. 3.36C). The arrows in Figs.3.36 A and C show the noraml hypogloddal canal and nerve with its vascular plexus.

DIFFERENTIAL DIAGNOSIS The cranial nerve nucleus segment is typically diseased due to intra-axial brain tumors, demyelinating disease, vascular disease, and rarely some unusual infectious disease.

The cisternal segment is most often involved by intracranial or transcranial extra-axial tumors, by far the most common being schwannoma (as in this patient) and meningioma. Uncommon pathologies include dural and leptomeningeal diseases such as sarcoidosis, lymphoma and leukemia, and meningeal carcinomatosis.

Lesions in the foraminal/skull base segment most commonly produce the jugular fossa syndromes. These include schwannoma, neurofibroma, transcranial meningioma, nasopharyngeal carcinoma (due to direct spread or retropharyngeal adenopathy), and paragangliomas. Other less common lesions are skull base metastases or retropharyngeal nodal metastases as a site of failure of nonnasopharyngeal SCCa, chordoma, and chondrosarcoma.

In the above segments, usually multiple cranial nerves are involved.

In the peripheral segment (from the skull base to the hyoid bone), lesions of the retrostyloid parapharyngeal space or carotid sheath will account for most hypoglossal neuropathies. The overwhelming majority will be due to a paraganglioma or a rare hypoglossal nerve–origin neurogenic tumor that is almost always a benign schwannoma. More typically, a neurogenic tumor will be of vagal origin and secondarily compressing cranial nerve XII. Occasionally, untreated or failed nodal metastases will cause the hypoglossal neuropathy. Recurrent metastatic nodal neck disease may do this as well.

DIAGNOSIS Schwannoma of the hypoglossal nerve

DISCUSSION Hypoglossal neuropathy may be an isolated situation. When more than one nerve is affected and possibly associated with other symptoms or neurologic deficits, localization may be much easier and a very "directed" and concise imaging evaluation is possible. A hypoglossal neuropathy will generally require a study only from the low posterior fossa to the hyoid bone.

Seventh nerve dysfunctions cause fasciculation of the tongue and eventually atrophy. The protruded tongue will deviate toward the side of the lesion in the case of a nuclear or infranuclear lesion and away from the side of the lesion in the case of a unilateral supranuclear lesion and dysarthria. Sometimes an atrophic tongue will be seen and no structural cause can be found. In this patient, the large transcranial mass has typical imaging features of a schwannoma.

Question for Further Thought

1. How, as a consultant, might you advise the ordering provider to approach a patient with hypoglossal palsy with a negative imaging study?

Reporting Responsibilities

A mass compressing the brainstem (as in this patient) should be urgently communicated. Benign conditions need no special communication. However, cancer, recurrent cancer, vascular malformation, highly vascular tumor, or aneurysm should be verbal communicated, especially if surgery or biopsy is contemplated.

What the Treating Physician Needs to Know

- If there is a structural cause for the neuropathy
- Is more than one nerve potentially involved?
- What is the likely diagnosis?
- If there is an alternative explanation for the symptoms or signs of the neuropathy affecting the end organ of innervation
- Does the disease process pose an immediate threat to the patient?
- What is the degree of confidence of a negative study excluding significant causative pathology?

Answer

1. Sometimes no structural lesion is identified in a patient with a specific cranial neuropathy. If the patient was imaged initially with CT, then MRI should be done. If imaged initially with MR, then CT should be done.

   Multiple cranial nerve deficits almost always will have a structural cause that can be identified with imaging. Imaging studies in patients with signs and symptoms of a potential cranial neuropathy such as tongue weakness will more often than not be positive. This is much truer of hypoglossal neuropathy than those of cranial nerves IX through XI and even the cervical sympathetics.

   When both studies are negative, the patient is reassured. If the symptoms become worse or an additional cranial neuropathy declares itself or becomes suspect, the patient should be followed with another imaging exam.

LEARN MORE
See Chapters 140 and 29 in *Head and Neck Radiology* by Mancuso and Hanafee.

CASE 3.37

CLINICAL HISTORY   *A 35-year-old male patient was in a motor vehicle collision. In the emergency room, he complained of neck pain and headache. On examination, the emergency room physician noticed left-sided Horner syndrome. He therefore ordered CT angiography of the head and neck. Selected images are shown below:*

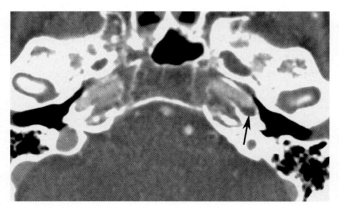

FIGURE **3.37A**

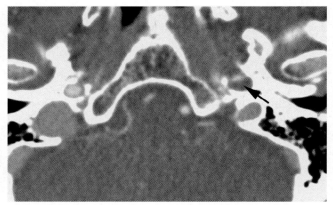

FIGURE **3.37B**

FINDINGS

Figure 3.37A,B. CECT images show a lucent zone in the vertical and proximal horizontal segment of the carotid canal (arrows).

DIFFERENTIAL DIAGNOSIS Distal cervical internal artery thrombus, vasculitis, infiltrative process in the carotid canal of skull base or soft tissue origin

DIAGNOSIS Posttraumatic dissection of the distal cervical internal carotid causing Horner syndrome

DISCUSSION The cervical sympathetics can be involved along with lower cranial nerves IX through XII or as an isolated finding (isolated involvement is more common). The tendency for the cervical sympathetics to be affected as an isolated finding is in part due to the deficit often being caused by devascularization due to a carotid dissection or brainstem thromboembolic disease secondary to vertebral artery dissection or other posterior circulation vaso-occlusive etiologies.

Horner syndrome is often associated with structural pathology; however, a structural cause may not be found since the signs and symptoms of Horner syndrome are caused by many medications. Imaging is an important part of the workup and must be focused properly by the clinical data. The cause will turn out to be neoplastic in many cases when a nonvascular etiology is established by imaging.

Common general clinical presentations that may involve the varying segments of the cervical sympathetic plexus and various conditions are outlined below:

• Central Horner will often have obvious accompanying somatosensory and/or motor symptoms. This segment is typically diseased due to intra-axial cord tumors, syringo-hydromyelia, ischemia, demyelinating diseases, and rarely

some unusual infectious disease. More central disease can also be located in the region of the cavernous sinus, suprasellar cistern, and orbital apex, although this "central location" anatomically actually represents interruption of the more distal oculosympathetic pathway.

• Clinically, in the foraminal/skull base segment, the patient presents with multiple lower cranial nerve palsy in addition to Horner syndrome. Most typically, skull base or retropharyngeal nodal disease from nasopharyngeal cancer or nonnasopharyngeal primary or skull base metastases, chordoma, and chondrosarcoma will be the source of a Horner syndrome at this location. Benign lesions do not often produce a Horner syndrome unless they are of sympathetic plexus origin. Carotid dissections in the carotid canal can produce a Horner syndrome by interrupting the distal carotid plexus blood supply.

• In the peripheral segment from the skull base to the carotid bifurcation, lesions of the retrostyloid parapharyngeal space of the carotid plexus or superior cervical ganglion will account for most sympathetic neuropathies. The majority will be due to a schwannoma of the sympathetic chain or a carotid dissection. If a patient presents with acute-onset Horner syndrome with headache, otalgia, or neck pain—this is virtually always secondary to a carotid and occasionally a vertebral artery dissection. Sympathetic neurogenic tumors are second only to vagal origin in frequency. Occasionally, other neurogenic tumors such as a cervical neuroblastoma (in children) or the more mature ganglioneuroma will present as a Horner syndrome.

• Below the bifurcation of the carotid, the lesion causing a Horner syndrome is most typically an infiltrating cancer in the supraclavicular fossa or a carotid or vertebral artery dissection. Primary esophageal and thyroid cancer, metastatic adenopathy to level 6 and supraclavicular/upper mediastinal nodes, perineural spread of breast cancer, or lymphoma can involve the sympathetics. Horner syndrome and brachial plexopathy will be due to a thoracic inlet lesion, such as superior sulcus lung cancer invading the extrapleural soft tissues. Horner syndrome and hoarseness may be due to a lesion anywhere from the carotid canal to the thoracic inlet.

Questions for Further Thought

1. Describe the clinical deficits of Horner syndrome and related anatomy of the head and neck sympathetic pathways.
2. How is Horner syndrome imaged?

Reporting Responsibilities

The most immediate risk associated with Horner syndrome is a thromboembolic complication to the brain if it is caused by a carotid or vertebral dissection. A carotid (as in this patient), vertebral, or aortic dissection and/or aneurysm or other vaso-occlusive disease and any related causative conditions or complications should be urgently and directly communicated. If an unsuspected malignancy is detected, it should also be promptly communicated, especially if a biopsy is planned.

What the Treating Physician Needs to Know

- If there is a structural cause for the neuropathy
- Is more than one nerve potentially involved?
- What is the likely diagnosis?
- If there is an alternative explanation for the symptoms or signs of the neuropathy affecting the end organs of innervation
- Does the disease process pose an immediate threat to the patient?
- Degree of confidence of a negative study excluding significant causative pathology. This is particularly important in Horner syndrome, where the study is often expected to be positive and a negative study might lead to another test or some plan for imaging as well as clinical surveillance.

Answers

1. Horner syndrome is clinically diagnosed when a constellation of signs is observed, including ptosis, miosis, pupillary lag, anhydrosis, and enophthalmos. This is due to interruption of the oculosympathetic supply to the eye. Detailed anatomy of the pre- and postganglionic pathways is critical to understand the rationale of imaging protocols and also to know the various pathologies that can lead to this condition.

   First-order neurons originating from the hypothalamus synapse in the pons or spinal cord and exit at C8-T1-T2 as second-order preganglionic neurons. The preganglionic sympathetic plexus ascends medial to the common carotid artery from the thoracic inlet while giving off essentially no branches in the infrahyoid neck (or at least below the carotid bifurcations) but getting its blood supply from the carotid artery.

   These nerves follow a course over the apex of the lung and ascend to synapse in the superior cervical ganglion. They exit as third-order postganglionic neurons to form sympathetic plexuses around the ICA and ECA. Lesions arising below T1 may spare the eye. These postganglionic fibers along the ICA enter the cavernous sinus and reach the orbit via the superior orbital fissure along with branches of V1. The other ganglia and nerves of the cervical sympathetic plexus do not carry oculosympathetic supply and hence are not relevant to the current discussion.

2. For patients with Horner syndrome, a complete study will most often include high-detail CECT images from the suprasellar region to the hyoid bone and a survey from the hyoid to the thoracic inlet and upper chest. Detailed temporal bone and posterior skull base reconstructions with the same technique used to study primary temporal bone problems and bone algorithm reconstructions of the orbital apex and juxtasellar central skull base region should be included.

   In a given patient imaging for a potential isolated Horner syndrome may be tailored by variables such as chest x-ray findings, history of smoking, or associated acute onset of the Horner and associated headache, otalgia, and/or neck pain. Usually, a more simple approach is to use an inclusive protocol that studies the posterior fossa, skull base, neck, larynx, thyroid, and upper thorax definitively in all cases with CECT unless there is a strong triggering factor that allows a less comprehensive approach.

   CECT should be done with a definitive CT angiography protocol since a carotid or vertebral artery dissection may be the root cause of Horner syndrome. Such a detailed negative study can reassure the patient and referring physician that no treatable cause has been left uncovered; however, these studies are often positive if there is a true Horner syndrome. MR may be used for the investigation of a Horner syndrome if the lesion is likely of central origin. MRI and MR angiography may be used primarily, if desired, if the same anatomic coverage and principles of examination design are applied.

LEARN MORE

See Chapters 141 and 11 in *Head and Neck Radiology* by Mancuso and Hanafee.

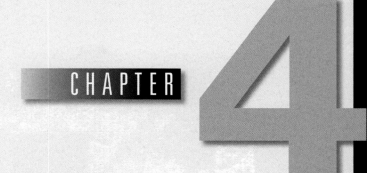

CHAPTER 4

The Suprahyoid Neck

CLINICAL HISTORY *A 45-year-old woman with gradually progressive fullness in the right side of throat that on examination was seen as a submucosal bulge at the palatine tonsil region.*

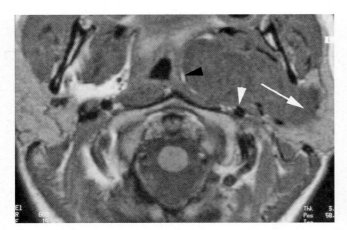

FIGURE **4.1A**

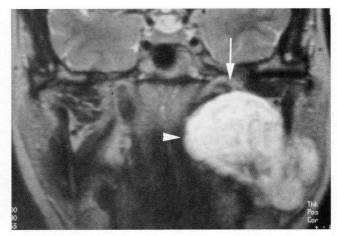

FIGURE **4.1C**

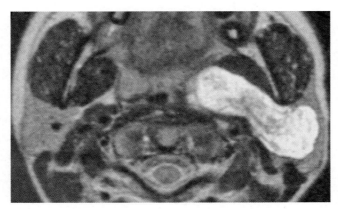

FIGURE **4.1B**

FINDINGS

Figure 4.1A. T1W contrast-enhanced (CE) image shows the mass growing through the stylomandibular tunnel (white arrow), displacing the structures of the retrostyloid parapharyngeal space (RSPS) (white arrowhead), and preserving the parapharyngeal fat (black arrowhead). The lesion is well demarcated, except maybe at its lateral border, where there might be some concern whether there is invasion of the parotid gland.

Figure 4.1B. T2W image shows relatively bright signal. The vectors of growth are as indicated in (Fig. 4.1A).

Figure 4.1C. T2W coronal image shows the proximity of the mass to the skull base. This proximity is an important aspect of surgical planning (arrow). There is also loss of the parapharyngeal fat but no definite evidence of the invasion of the superior constrictor of the pharynx (white arrowhead); this information being useful to anticipate the need for possible pharyngeal construction.

DIFFERENTIAL DIAGNOSIS About 90% of masses presenting as if they are primarily arising in the prestyloid parapharyngeal space (PSPS) will be benign glandular epithelial tumors of minor salivary gland or deep lobe parotid origin. Malignant glandular epithelial lesions (e.g., adenoid cystic carcinoma) of the same origin are unusual but are the next most common mass. All other lesions such as branchial apparatus cyst, slow-flow vascular malformations, sarcoma, leiomyoma, and rhabdomyoma are rare.

DIAGNOSIS Benign mixed tumor (pleomorphic adenoma) centered in the PSPS and inseparable from the deep lobe of the parotid gland.

DISCUSSION The suggested approach to a meaningful (differential) diagnosis would be as follows:

- Determine whether the process involves a single space or multiple spaces.
- If single, which space—in this case, it would be centered or of origin in the PSPS based on making the observations

with regard to vectors of structural displacement and "travel" of the mass.

- In case of a PSPS mass, determine if it is separable from the deep portion of the parotid gland, establish the proximity to the skull base, the inferior extent, and relationship to the superior constrictor muscle.
- Make observations regarding the likely aggressiveness of margins of the mass, transcompartmental spread, and its internal morphology.
- Identify associated findings such as lymphadenopathy or perineural spread.

The odds of a proper diagnosis can be further improved by knowledge of the relative frequency of pathology. Ninety percent of the masses presenting as primarily originating from the PSPS will be benign glandular epithelial tumors of minor salivary gland or deep lobe parotid origin, making all other lesions uncommon. Malignant glandular epithelial lesions of the same origin are the next most common mass and should be considered, for example, when the internal matrix shows a relatively low signal on T2W images.

Many of these lesions will be discovered incidentally during an imaging examination for unrelated pathology. Since most lesions in this space are benign, watchful waiting may be considered, especially in small lesions and/or in older patients or those at risk for significant complications during a major surgical procedure. A benign lesion should grow no faster than 1 to 3 mm in greatest short axis dimension in 1 year; typically, this benign growth rate is more like 1 mm per year. An interval of 3 months between the baseline and the first follow-up study, preferably magnetic resonance imaging, is acceptable. If a benign biopsy would lead to a wait and scan strategy, then imaging-guided biopsy can make a substantial contribution.

All masses presenting submucosally should be imaged before they are biopsied!

Most typically, however, the mass will be removed surgically.

Questions for Further Thought

1. Should and can this mass be biopsied?
2. List the three most common masses in this space.
3. Is watchful waiting with imaging surveillance an option in a smaller mass of this type?

Reporting Responsibilities

- When a mass is discovered incidentally, direct communication is mandatory given the small but definite risk of a possible malignant lesion. In this case, the mass and diagnosis was expected and reporting was routine.

- If in the preoperative setting or prior to a biopsy an unexpectedly high vascular lesion or, more importantly, an aneurysm is discovered, then direct and confirmed communication is necessary.

What the Treating Physician Needs to Know

- Is the mass of PSPS origin?
- Could the PSPS be only secondarily involved?
- Is the mass likely aggressive or nonaggressive? Is it transspatial?
- Full extent of the mass relative to the skull base, major vessels, facial nerve (deep portion of the parotid), other cranial nerves, and surrounding spaces and the likelihood of the mass being densely adherent to or invading the pharyngeal constrictors

These findings will help determine the surgeon's approach. Some surgeons will deliver the mass by a cephalad approach through the submandibular space if it is 1 cm or more from the skull base and away from the facial nerve.

- Associated findings such as perineural spread or adenopathy that might aid in formulating a differential diagnosis
- Most likely etiology
- If the mass is safely accessible for imaging-guided biopsy, if desired

Answers

1. All parapharyngeal space/submucosal masses should be imaged before performing a biopsy to rule out highly vascular lesions or aneurysms. About 90% of the masses primarily arising from the PSPS will be benign; however, surgeons may want a definite pathologic diagnosis before going to surgery; lesions in the PSPS space usually can be biopsied relatively easy.
2. Benign mixed tumor, malignant glandular epithelial lesions, slow-flow vascular malformations
3. A wait and scan strategy can be considered in small benign (preferably biopsy-proven) lesions with a slow growing rate (annually 3 mm or less), especially in elderly patients and those at risk for significant complications during a major surgical procedure.

> **LEARN MORE**
>
> See Chapters 143 and 22 in *Head and Neck Radiology* by Mancuso and Hanafee.

CLINICAL HISTORY *A 55-year-old woman presented after her dentist noted a pharyngeal wall bulge during a routine visit.*

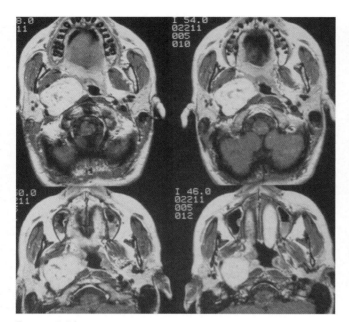

FIGURE 4.2A

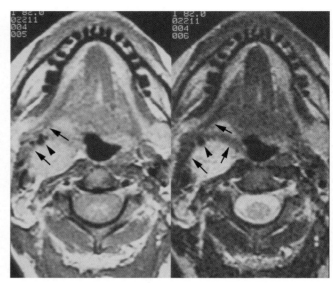

FIGURE 4.2C

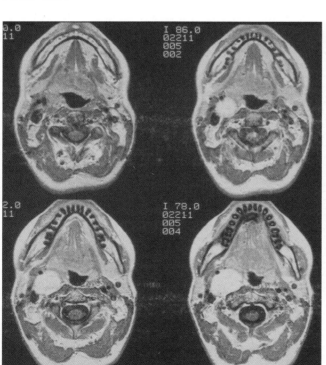

FIGURE 4.2B

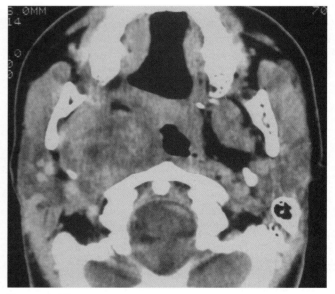

FIGURE 4.2D

FINDINGS

Figure 4.2A,B. CE contiguous T1W images show a well-demarcated mass in the RSPS.

Figure 4.2C. Proton density and T2W pair of images show the displacement of the carotid artery (arrowhead) and styloid musculature (arrows) anteriorly and splaying of the internal carotid artery and jugular.

Figure 4.2D. Contrast-enhanced computed tomography (CECT) images show the mass but the relationships to the surrounding structures to a much lesser extent than the magnetic resonance (MR) images.

DIFFERENTIAL DIAGNOSIS An RSPS mass separating the carotid artery and the jugular vein and displacing the styloid process and musculature laterally and anteriorly will most likely be a neurogenic tumor (originating from cranial nerves IX through XII) or a paraganglioma.

DIAGNOSIS Schwannoma of the RSPS

DISCUSSION A small mass within the RSPS may be discovered incidentally on studies done for other purposes. Most lesions will be discovered because someone, whether the patient or a health care provider, notices an upper neck mass or submucosal bulge along the oropharyngeal wall, usually at about the level of the palatine tonsil.

Less frequently, a lesion is discovered because of symptoms related to the mass such as pain and cranial neuropathy (e.g., hoarseness, dysphonia, Horner syndrome).

The suggested approach to a meaningful (differential) diagnosis would be as follows:

- Determine whether the process involves a single or multiple spaces
- If single, which space—in this case, it would be centered or of origin in the RSPS based on making the observations with regard to vectors of structural displacement and "travel" of the mass.
- In case of an RSPS mass, establish the proximity to the skull base at the carotid canal and jugular fossa, the relation to the major vessels and cranial nerves, and the degree of vascularity.
- Make observations regarding the likely aggressiveness of margins of the mass, transcompartmental spread, and its internal morphology.
- Identify associated findings such as lymphadenopathy or perineural spread.

The odds of a proper diagnosis can be further improved by knowledge of the relative frequency of pathology. About 90% of masses presenting as if they are primarily arising in the RSPS will be benign and either neurogenic in origin or a paraganglioma. This makes all other lesions such as transcranial neurogenic tumors, meningiomas, and hemangiopericytomas uncommon or rare. It may be difficult to tell metastatic retropharyngeal adenopathy from primary RSPS pathology unless there is an obvious primary cancer or a history of treated, usually head and neck region, cancer.

Secondary involvement from a deep neck abscess, necrotizing otitis externa or other skull base osteomyelitis, and prevertebral abscess might explain a more infiltrating process.

Since these lesions may be biopsied as part of the medial decision making, it is important to prevent potentially disastrous complications by ruling out aneurysms or highly vascular lesions.

Depending on the diagnosis, different therapeutic approaches will be considered. Most often, RSPS masses will be removed. However, sometimes a wait and scan strategy can be adopted (e.g., in elderly patients with a slow-growing benign mass).

Questions for Further Thought

1. Describe how this mass displaces the surrounding structures and deduce the space of origin based on these findings.

2. List the two most common masses in this space.
3. Should and can this mass be biopsied?

Reporting Responsibilities
When a mass is discovered incidentally, direct communication is mandatory given the small but definite risk of a possible malignant lesion. If in the preoperative setting or prior to a biopsy an unexpectedly highly vascular lesion or, more importantly, an aneurysm is discovered, then direct, confirmed communication is necessary.

In this case, the mass was expected, appeared benign, and was not of vascular origin or hypervascular; thus, it was reported routinely.

What the Treating Physician Needs to Know
- Is the mass of RSPS origin?
- Could the RSPS be only secondarily involved?
- Is the mass likely aggressive or nonaggressive? Is it transspatial?
- Full extent of the mass relative to the skull base, major vessels, cranial nerves, and surrounding spaces; the likelihood of the mass being densely adherent to or invading the pharyngeal constrictors
- Associated findings such as perineural spread or adenopathy that might aid in the differential diagnosis
- Most likely etiology
- If the mass is safely accessible for imaging-guided biopsy

Answers
1. The carotid artery and jugular vein are separated by the mass. The carotid artery is displaced anteriorly, the jugular vein posteriorly and laterally. The constrictor muscles are displaced medially. Posteriorly, the mass compresses the paravertebral muscles on the right side. The deep lobe of the parotid gland is displaced. There is no widening of the stylomandibular tunnel. This is an almost typical presentation of an RSPS mass. Classically, the carotid artery would have been displaced anteriorly and medially.
2. Paraganglioma (glomus jugulare and vagale) and neurogenic tumors (schwannoma and neurofibroma)
3. About 90% of the masses primarily arising from the RSPS will be benign; however, most surgeons will want a definite pathologic diagnosis before going to surgery. Lesions in the RSPS usually can be biopsied relatively easy, but highly vascular lesions or aneurysms need to be excluded by imaging first.

LEARN MORE
See Chapters 144 and 29 in *Head and Neck Radiology* by Mancuso and Hanafee.

CASE 4.3

CLINICAL HISTORY *A young adult male presenting with facial pain.*

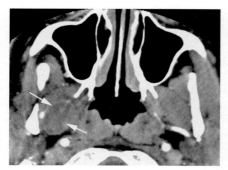

FIGURE 4.3A

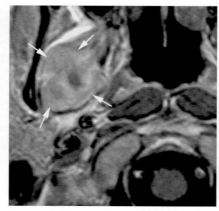

FIGURE 4.3B

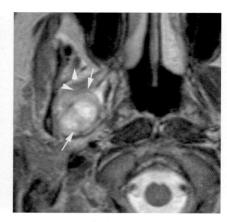

FIGURE 4.3C

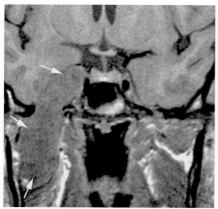

FIGURE 4.3D

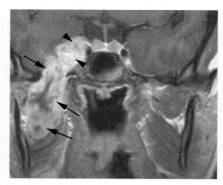

FIGURE 4.3E

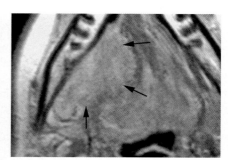

FIGURE 4.3F

FINDINGS

Figure 4.3A. CECT image shows a mass within the masticator space (MS) (arrows).

Figure 4.3B. T1W CE image shows the mass confined to the MS. Its margins are well circumscribed, and the mass enhances.

Figure 4.3C. T2W image shows the borders of the mass along the expected position of the mandibular division of the trigeminal nerve (arrows) and secondary atrophy of masticator musculature (arrowheads).

Figure 4.3D,E. Coronal T1W noncontrast (Fig. 4.3D) and CE (Fig. 4.3E) images show the tubular mass extending from the region of the cavernous sinus through the region of the foramen ovale and into the MS (arrows).

Figure 4.3F. T1W CE image shows the rhabdomyosarcoma primary arising from the floor of the mouth (arrows).

DIFFERENTIAL DIAGNOSIS Neurogenic tumor, sarcoma, (transcranial) meningioma, vascular malformation, perineural spread

of cancer cutaneous and other primary sites; uncommon to rare: fibromatoses, lymphoma, paraganglioma, pseudotumor

DIAGNOSIS Floor of the mouth rhabdomyosarcoma with intracranial perineural spread and related skull base invasion

DISCUSSION Clinically, when these masses become large enough to cause symptoms, they can produce pain and trismus. Pain might be referred to the periauricular region by the auriculotemporal nerve. Benign or malignant lesions may manifest as trismus through altered jaw mechanics. MS masses may also present as motor neuropathy of V3 with denervation atrophy of the MS muscles. Incidentally noted asymmetry in the masticator muscles might be due to benign masseteric hypertrophy.

The suggested approach to a meaningful (differential) diagnosis would be as follows:

• Determine whether the process involves a single or multiple spaces. In this case, the mass is actually transspatial, going from the floor of the mouth to the trigeminal cistern—the conduit being the lingual nerve and eventually the mandibular division of the trigeminal nerve.

- If a single space is involved, which space? This is not applicable in this case.
- Identification of associated findings such as intracranial and transcranial or perineural spread and associated lymphadenopathy. In this case, it is important to look for retropharyngeal and cervical adenopathy even though the incidence is relatively low.
- Observations regarding the likely aggressiveness of margins of the mass and its internal morphology typically are more comprehensively demonstrated on MR images.

Knowledge of the various pathologies affecting the MS and their relative frequency may help, further improving the odds of a proper diagnosis.

The MS is common secondarily involved in several common inflammatory conditions such as dental abscess and more rare inflammations such as reactive fibromyositis and pseudotumor. Mucosal-origin neoplastic conditions such as oral cavity, sinonasal and nasopharyngeal cancers, and lymphoma may also involve the MS, infratemporal fossa (ITF), and buccal space (BS). The MS is also a secondary site of involvement in transcranial tumors and lesions of the central skull base.

One should be familiar with the appearance of pseudomasses such as V3 denervation atrophy, symmetric masseter and pterygoid muscle hypertrophy, and accessory parotid glandular tissue.

All primary MS/ITF and BS masses are relatively uncommon.

Most masses presenting as if they are primarily arising in the MS/ITF will be either neurogenic in origin or due to a sarcoma or lymphoma. This makes all other tumors uncommon or rare. Transcranial meningiomas and even gliomas represent intracranial lesions that may present in this space.

Most lesions will be biopsied prior to further treatment planning. An aneurysm must definitely be excluded before any biopsy or surgical approach to the mass.

Questions for Further Thought

1. Describe in which space the lesion is centered and how the mass relates to the surrounding structures.
2. What neoplastic lesion most commonly involves this space?
3. Describe the contents of this space.

Reporting Responsibilities

In this case, the discovery of the mass in the floor of the mouth raises the issue of malignancy with perineural spread, and such a concern generally requires direct communication. The original plan for a cavernous sinus biopsy was in place, and the report and consultation offered imaging-guided biopsy as an alternative.

The main elements of the report should include the following:

- Space of origin
- Distance of the top of the mass from the skull base or extent of the skull base or transcranial spread
- Relationship the mass to the mandible
- Relationship of the mass to the deep portion of the parotid gland and main trunk of the facial nerve
- Relationship to V3
- If the findings suggest a diagnosis other than the common benign masses that arise in the MS such as a malignant tumor, transspatial mass, or one arising from another space or source
- Whether there are important associated findings such as transcranial or perineural spread
- Whether computed tomography (CT)-guided biopsy or other imaging studies would help to further clarify the findings

What the Treating Physician Needs to Know

- Likely diagnosis and degree of confidence in that diagnosis
- Full extent of the mass
- Relationship of the mass to critical surrounding anatomy
- If any more data needs to be collected with imaging assistance
- *Posttreatment imaging:* Suspicion for tumor recurrence versus expected posttreatment changes

Answers

1. MS mass. The mass displaces the lateral and medial pterygoid muscles as it grows superiorly along the lingual and mandibular nerves through the oval foramen into the trigeminal ganglion and cistern. There are denervation changes of the pterygoid muscles. The fat between the MS and the PSPS is compressed but still clearly visible. Laterally, the mass abuts the mandible; posteriorly, there is no sign of invasion of the parotid gland.

2. All primary lesions such as neurogenic tumors, sarcomas, and lymphoma as well as slow-flow vascular malformations; transcranial meningiomas or gliomas are uncommon to rare. Secondary involvement by inflammatory conditions such as dental abscesses (especially those of the lower second/third molar) and mucosal-origin neoplastic conditions are more common.

3. Mandible, muscles of mastication, branches of the mandibular division of the trigeminal nerve (V3), maxillary arteries and veins and their branches and tributaries

LEARN MORE

See Chapters 145, 21, and 35 in *Head and Neck Radiology* by Mancuso and Hanafee.

CLINICAL HISTORY *A 48-year-old man with poorly controlled diabetes presenting with trismus and facial pain.*

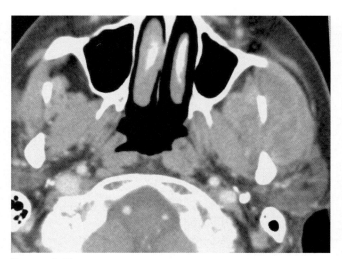

FIGURE **4.4A**

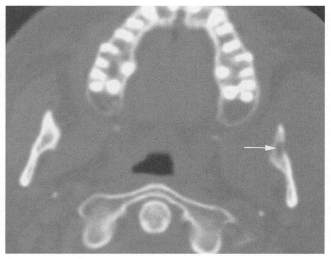

FIGURE **4.4C**

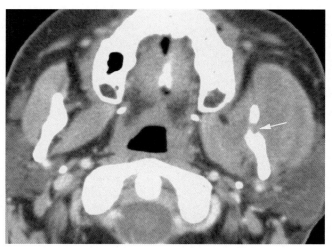

FIGURE **4.4B**

FINDINGS

Figure 4.4A,B. CECT images showing extensive and slightly heterogeneous swelling within the MS although the margins are well circumscribed.

Figure 4.4B,C. In (Fig. 4.4B), there is a suggestion of mandibular erosion (arrow) confirmed in the bone windows of the same CT scan in (Fig. 4.4C).

DIFFERENTIAL DIAGNOSIS *Inflammatory:* Abscess, cellulitis, phlegmon (bacterial, fungal, actinomycosis); neoplastic sarcoma, lymphoma, metastasis

DIAGNOSIS MS phlegmon secondary to chronic bacterial osteomyelitis of the mandible secondary to dental disease in a diabetic patient

DISCUSSION The clinical presentation will nearly always suggest an infectious/inflammatory problem based on fever and swelling. Additionally, the patient may present with pain and trismus. Otalgia is also a common complaint.

The MS is commonly secondarily involved in several inflammatory conditions such as dental abscess; spread of inflammatory salivary gland disease, especially of the parotid gland; and spread of necrotizing otitis externa and other more uncommon causes of skull base osteomyelitis. Secondary central skull base and transcranial spread from these processes via the MS is also possible.

It is important to recognize the "inflammatory" rather than "neoplastic" nature of the presenting pathology since occasionally an indolent infection may mimic one of the fibromatoses, a reactive fibrous (fibromyositic) process, lymphoma, or sarcoma. This usually is not an issue since the presenting clinical symptoms are almost always obvious.

The initial evaluation of a likely infection in the MS should determine whether it is of dental origin or nondental origin. Nondental causes, although less common, include those of the sinus or skin. Special attention is mandatory in the event of fungal infections, most typically in immunocompromised or diabetic patients, since the diagnosis of an aggressive sinus infection can be based on only early infiltration of the retroantral fat pad in light of otherwise nonaggressive antral disease.

This should be followed by a detailed analysis of the spaces involved and identification of associated findings such as osteomyelitis, vascular thrombosis, and intracranial spread.

Drainage and/or debridement will frequently be part of the therapeutic measures. If so, it is of great importance that *all* of the involved spaces should be drained by the safest and most dependable approach.

Questions for Further Thought

1. Describe the mass and its probable cause/origin.
2. What consideration(s) is/are essential when planning drainage?

Reporting Responsibilities

In general, determining the source, extent, and possible etiology of MS/ITF infection/inflammation is the goal of the study at the time of initial imaging. The referring provider will be expecting immediate direct communication. In this case, the result was discussed with the attending oral and maxillofacial surgeon.

The main elements of the report should include the following:

- Likely source/site of initial nidus if infection
- Primary space of origin
- All spaces involved
- Specific etiologic agent, if suggested by the pattern of disease
- Relationship of the infection to the mandible, maxilla, and skull base as appropriate
- Complicating factors such as vascular thrombosis and intracranial spread

- If the findings suggest a diagnosis other than infection
- Whether CT-guided tissue sampling or other imaging studies would help to further clarify the findings

What the Treating Physician Needs to Know

- Likely diagnosis and degree of confidence in that diagnosis
- Full extent of the infection or inflammatory changes
- Relationship of the infection to critical surrounding anatomy
- If any more data needs to be collected with imaging assistance
- If alternative imaging such as a bone/gallium scan might be useful in monitoring therapy
- *Posttreatment imaging:* Suspicion for recurrent or residual infection or source of ongoing infection versus successful drainage, debridement, and/or management of associated complications

Answers

1. An infiltrating mass surrounding a focus of bone erosion in the mandible. The mass extends mainly into the masticator muscle but also into the pterygoid musculature. The fat in the MS is obliterated compared to the contralateral side. There is no involvement of the surrounding spaces. The mass is centrally faintly hypodense but difficult to delineate. There is no definite rim enhancement.

2. Patients with uncontrolled diabetes are more prone to aggressive infections, as in this case of poor dental care causing osteomyelitis and spread of the infection to the MS.

3. It is of great importance that *all* of the involved spaces should be drained by the safest and most dependable approach.

> **LEARN MORE**
> See Chapters 146 and 16 in *Head and Neck Radiology* by Mancuso and Hanafee.

CASE **4.5**

CLINICAL HISTORY *Two patients with masses behind the pharynx, one in the retropharyngeal space (RPS) and the other in the prevertebral space. Which is which, and what is your diagnosis?*

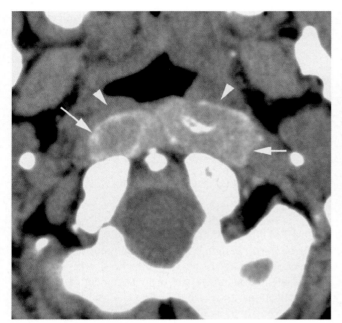

FIGURE **4.5A**

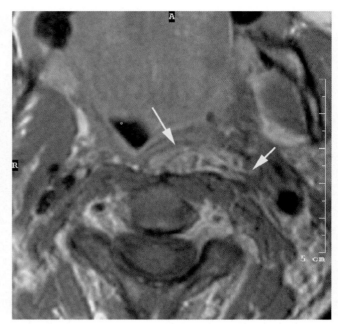

FIGURE **4.5C**

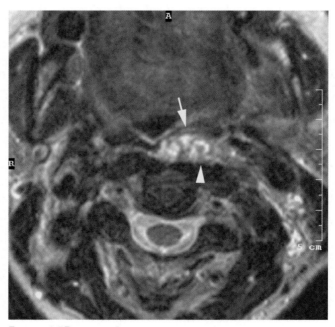

FIGURE **4.5B**

FINDINGS

Figure 4.5A. Noncontrast CT study in a patient with an incidentally discovered prevertebral space process. The process conforms to the musculature within the prevertebral space (arrows) and compresses the RPS (arrowheads).

Figure 4.5B,C. A patient with a mass principally involving the RPS. In (Fig. 4.5B), a T2W MR image shows the

same findings. Notice the displacement of the pharyngeal wall musculature anteriorly (arrow) and the malformation respecting the plane of the prevertebral fascia and muscles. In (Fig. 4.5C), CECT shows a component of the mass in the RPS spreading to involve the RSPS (arrows) and respecting the attachments of the prevertebral fascia (arrowheads).

DIAGNOSIS Advanced case of calcific tendonitis of the prevertebral muscles (Fig. 4.5A); RPS and deep neck venolymphatic malformation (Fig. 4.5B,C)

DISCUSSION The suggested approach to a meaningful differential diagnosis would be as follows:

- Determine whether the process involves single or multiple spaces.
- If single, which space—in this case, it would be centered or of origin in the RPS based on making observations with regard to vectors of structural displacement and "travel" of the mass.
- Identify associated findings such as perineural spread and associated lymphadenopathy.
- Observe regarding the likely aggressiveness of margins of the mass and its internal morphology, typically more comprehensively demonstrated on MR images.

These are unusual cases of masses presenting posterior to the pharynx. The exercise is to recognize the difference between the two spaces and the diagnostic implications of proper identification of the space of origin. In reality, most RPS masses above the hyoid are due to some secondary disease in the retropharyngeal lymph nodes. When due to inflammatory disease, the clinical situation may well dictate the correct interpretation of retropharyngeal adenopathy. It may be difficult to tell metastatic retropharyngeal adenopathy from primary RSPS pathology unless there is an obvious primary cancer or a history of treated, usually head and neck region, cancer. In the event of retropharyngeal adenopathies and an unknown primary cancer, careful inspection of the pharynx may reveal a clinically occult, submucosal primary lesion. Those aside, all other RPS masses are uncommon to rare.

Questions for Further Thought

1. What is your first concern when asked or when considering to biopsy an RPS mass?
2. Describe the contents of the RPS.

Reporting Responsibilities

When these studies are done to evaluate a patient with a pain pattern that could be related to the spine and/or pharynx, the discovery of such a mass should initiate direct communication. If the process has any potential to cause spinal cord compression, verbal contact must be escalated to urgent or emergent.

The main elements of the report should include the following:

- Space of origin
- Relationship of the mass to the skull base and upper cervical spine to help decide whether an approach to removal might be across the nasopharynx, the oropharynx, or through the neck
- Relationship of the mass to the RSPS, sympathetic trunk, cranial nerves IX through XII, and the carotid artery and jugular vein
- If the findings suggest a diagnosis other than a benign condition of the RPS or prevertebral space such as a malignant tumor, transspatial mass, or one actually arising from another space or source such as the spine
- Whether there are important associated findings such as transcranial or perineural spread or retropharyngeal or cervical adenopathy or those that suggest a possibly rapidly progressive infection
- Whether CT-guided biopsy or other imaging studies would help to further clarify the findings

What the Treating Physician Needs to Know

- Likely diagnosis and degree of confidence in that diagnosis
- If there is likelihood of imminent neurologic compromise
- Full extent of the mass
- Relationship of the mass to critical surrounding anatomy
- If any more data needs to be collected with imaging assistance
- *Posttreatment imaging:* Suspicion for tumor recurrence versus expected posttreatment changes

Answers

1. Aneurysm and tortuous carotid artery should be excluded.
2. The contents of the RPS are fat and fibrous tissue, lateral retropharyngeal nodes (of Rouviere) and medial retropharyngeal nodes, small blood vessels, and capillary lymphatics.

> **LEARN MORE**
> See Chapters 147 and 13 in *Head and Neck Radiology* by Mancuso and Hanafee.

CLINICAL HISTORY *A 5-year-old boy presenting with fever, neck pain, and odynophagia.*

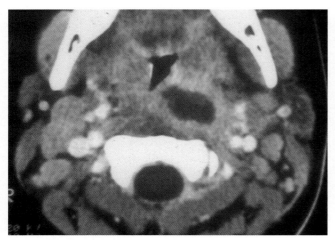

FIGURE 4.6A

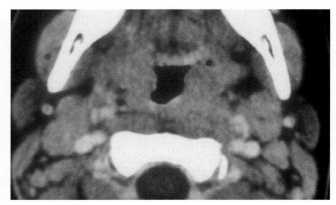

FIGURE 4.6B

FINDINGS

Figure 4.6A,B. A rim-enhancing cystic mass anterior to the prevertebral muscles, medially to the carotid artery at the expected site of the lateral retropharyngeal (*RP*) lymph node on the left. The retrostyloid and prestyloid retropharyngeal spaces appear edematous. There appears to be edema on the right in the RPS (*RPS*). The delineation of the prevertebral muscles is partially lost. Multiple, mainly level 2, enlarged lymph nodes are present bilaterally. The image posttreatment (nonsurgical) in (Fig. 4.6B) shows complete resolution.

DIFFERENTIAL DIAGNOSIS None in this clinical setting

DIAGNOSIS Pyogenic, suppurative retropharyngeal adenitis (RPA) *without* abscess

DISCUSSION The suggested approach to a meaningful differential diagnosis would be as follows:

- Determine whether the process involves single or multiple spaces. Infections are inherently capable of transspatial spread.
- If single, which space—in this case, it would be centered or of origin in the RPS based on making observations with regard to vectors of structural displacement and spread of the inflammation. In this case, the changes are almost all confined to the RPS.
- Observe regarding the morphology of the presumptive inflammatory process. CT alone is typically adequate in pharyngeal-origin infections; in this case, the morphology of the changes supports an inflammatory etiology.
- Identify associated findings such as lymphadenopathy—in this case, the main RPS finding is the presumptive suppurative lymph node.

Infections of the RPS can result in significant morbidity and mortality. Timely diagnosis and proper treatment are critical in preventing sequelae such as airway obstruction, mediastinitis, carotid artery aneurysm, and cavernous sinus thrombosis.

The RPS is a frequent secondarily involved site in common inflammatory conditions such as infectious pharyngitis due to various organisms, most commonly bacteria. One must be very judicious, especially in adults, to be sure that the process in the RPS is *not* one that is secondary to a pre- and/or paravertebral infection secondary to diskitis/vertebral osteomyelitis.

The most common infection that comes to imaging and affects this level of the RPS is RPA with or without suppuration secondary to bacterial pharyngitis. This is a disease mainly of young children but can be seen in young adults. True retropharyngeal abscess, aside from that due to penetrating trauma, iatrogenic trauma, or some other cause of pharyngeal perforation, is uncommon. Reactive RPS edema is common and frequently not directly due to inflammation.

Common clinical presentations in adults include fever, odynophagia, and dysphagia. Otalgia is possible. Children with swallowing problems may present with "feeding difficulties."

The most common RPS infection to come to imaging by far is suppurative RPA *without* abscess. Occasionally, those pus-containing nodes become so large that they constitute an abscess physiologically. Such nodes rarely rupture to produce a *true* RPS abscess. Otherwise, RPS abscess is rare and may be due to upper pharyngeal perforation. Infection or abscesses may spread from other suprahyoid spaces and may be related to skull base osteomyelitis.

The airway must be controlled and the patient treated with intravenous antibiotics. Retropharyngeal suppurative lymphadenopathy must not be mistaken for a "retropharyngeal abscess" since it is an infection that almost always responds completely to antibiotics and does not require surgical interventionist, whereas an abscess will usually be drained. Surgical drainage of suppurative retropharyngeal lymph nodes may be required for those patients with persistent or enlarging nodes that are unresponsive to aggressive antibiotic therapy and perhaps those that *exceed 3 cm in maximum axial short axis dimension* and/or appear likely to rupture. Of course, immediate surgical drainage may become necessary in patients with airway compromise.

Questions for Further Thought

1. What is of primary importance when evaluating an RPS abscess?
2. Why is the differentiation between a suppurative RPA node and a true RPS abscess so important?

Reporting Responsibilities

The diagnostic radiologist must be immediately available and in verbal contact with the treating physicians in almost all cases of suspected RPS infection, especially if it arises in a diabetic or otherwise immunocompromised patient. This is done mainly to ensure proper communication about the airway status and whether there is likely drainable pyogenic abscess or a life-threatening condition such as rapidly spreading necrotizing infection.

It is also essential to accurately communicate whether the process is suppurative RPA that can almost always be cured with antibiotics. In this case, there was direct communication with both the pediatric and otolaryngology services so that both understood this disease would likely be controlled with intravenous antibiotics and not require surgical drainage.

What the Treating Physician Needs to Know

- Likely diagnosis and degree of confidence in that diagnosis
- Whether the patient is in any imminent danger
- Full extent of the infectious process
- Relationship of the infection or inflammation to critical surrounding anatomy
- If any more data needs to be collected with imaging assistance
- *Posttreatment imaging:* Suspicion for recurrent or persistent infection versus expected posttreatment changes

Answers

1. Since there is a direct extent of the RPS to the mediastinum, an abscess should always be evaluated to above and below its obvious gross extent as seen on the images since it can become segmentally less conspicuous, especially at the thoracic inlet and at the skull base.
2. Suppurative RPA will almost always promptly (within 24 to 72 hours) respond to intravenous antibiotics, sparing young children unnecessary invasive procedures, whereas true retropharyngeal abscesses will almost always be drained.

LEARN MORE
See Chapters 148 and 13 in *Head and Neck Radiology* by Mancuso and Hanafee.

CHAPTER 5

Infrahyoid Neck and Cervicothoracic Junction (Thoracic Inlet)

CASE 5.1

CLINICAL HISTORY *A 78-year-old man presented with intermittent swallowing difficulties and dysphagia. There was prior history of aspiration pneumonia. On clinical exam, a mass was suspected laterally on the right in the neck.*

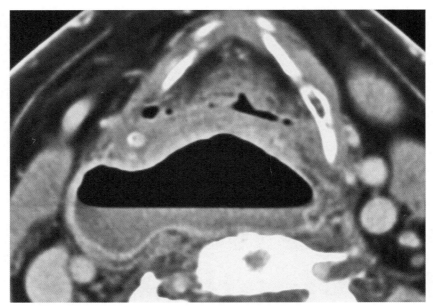

FIGURE **5.1A**

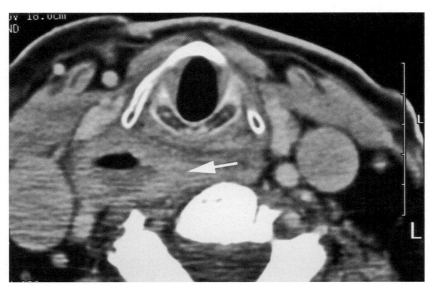

FIGURE **5.1B**

FINDINGS Contrast-enhanced (CE) axial computed tomography (CT) image through the level of the upper supraglottis (Fig. 5.1A) and postcricoid hypopharynx (Fig. 5.1B) demonstrates a rim-enhancing mass on the midline anterior to the vertebral column and extending to the right side of the neck. There is an internal air–fluid level (arrow) and a thick minimally enhancing and relatively well-demarcated wall.

DIFFERENTIAL DIAGNOSIS Zenker's diverticulum, duplication cyst, abscess, branchial apparatus cyst

DIAGNOSIS Large Zenker's diverticulum

DISCUSSION A reasonable approach to a lateral neck mass would combine the method of considering a space or compartment of origin, the incidence of every type of relevant pathology, and some etiologic considerations, such as developmental origins. One must be familiar with the full range of pathology possible because patients with neck masses of uncertain etiology sometimes present confusing clinical problems and/or physical findings that can be greatly simplified by good-quality, well-interpreted images.

In this case, the lesion seems to originate from the midline, most probably the visceral compartment, and extends to the right side in the neck. This makes branchial and thymic apparatus cysts unlikely; however, in this developmental category, it might be reasonable to consider a communicating foregut duplication cyst.

Based on the location, the pharynx/pharyngeal wall is very likely involved. The air–fluid level suggests a connection with the aerodigestive tract or gas-forming bacteria. The latter is less likely since the patient did not present with any signs of infection or inflammation and since there is the absence of surrounding edema or infiltration of the fat on the CT scan in combination with relatively sharp margins.

In case of doubt, a barium swallow study would confirm the diagnosis of Zenker's diverticulum.

Question for Further Thought

1. What are possible complications of a Zenker's diverticulum?

Reporting Responsibilities

In general, a visceral compartment and retropharyngeal condition presenting as a neck mass is typically chronic and may be reported routinely unless there is a potential airway compromise problem or if a malignancy is suspected. Many neck mass cases require direct communication with referring doctors to decide on a course of action, especially if imaging-directed biopsy is necessary.

It is especially important to communicate effectively and promptly if there is a secondary infection and in those cases to anticipate whether there may be a complicating sinus or fistula. This communication may become urgent or emergent if there is infection or findings that may herald disease in the epidural space that in turn might threaten the spinal cord.

What the Treating Physician Needs to Know

- Origin of the mass—visceral compartment versus retropharyngeal space (RPS) versus other
- Extent of the mass
- Likely diagnosis
- Any potential danger to surrounding critical anatomy
- Any airway compromise
- If further imaging would be helpful

Answer

1. Aspiration and pneumonia are possible complications of a Zenker's diverticulum.

LEARN MORE

See Chapter 150 in *Head and Neck Radiology* by Mancuso and Hanafee.

CLINICAL HISTORY *A 57-year-old man presented clinically with fever, odynophagia, and pharyngitis. Contrast-enhanced computed tomography (CECT) images are shown below:*

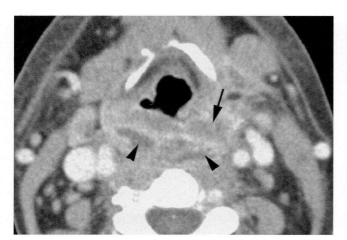

FIGURE **5.2A**

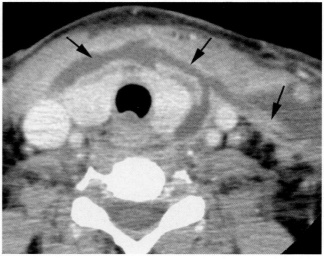

FIGURE **5.2C**

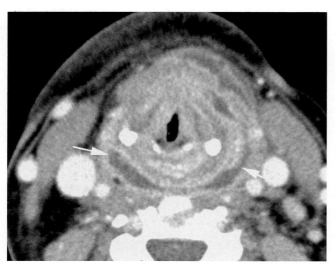

FIGURE **5.2B**

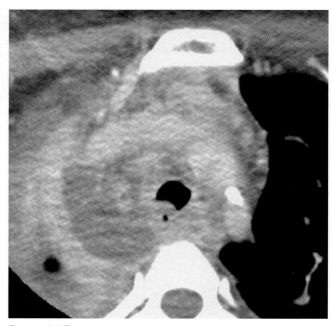

FIGURE **5.2D**

FINDINGS

Figure 5.2A. Likely purulent material spreading to the level of the hyoid within the RPS (arrowheads) while only likely edema is seen within the pharynx (arrows). This was the approximate upper level of the retropharyngeal process.

Figure 5.2B. Likely purulent material spreads extensively within the visceral compartment (arrows) and is loculated in the RPS (arrowheads).

Figure 5.2C. In the low neck, the process spreads within the visceral compartment and into the lateral compartment (arrows). There is little identifiable abnormality in the RPS.

Figure 5.2D. A large mediastinal collection is visible.

DIFFERENTIAL DIAGNOSIS Not applicable

DIAGNOSIS Pharyngitis complicated by an extensive purulent collection/abscess reaching to the mediastinum

DISCUSSION Infections of the visceral compartment and RPS can result in significant morbidity and mortality. Timely diagnosis and proper treatment are critical in preventing sequelae such as life-threatening airway obstruction, epidural abscess and cervical cord injury, mediastinitis, carotid artery aneurysm, and cavernous sinus thrombosis.

The RPS at the level of the infrahyoid neck is commonly affected, without any clinical significance, by inflammatory conditions such as infectious pharyngitis manifest only as variable amounts of RPS edema. In the infrahyoid RPS, retropharyngeal abscesses may be due to a complication of bacterial pharyngitis, penetrating trauma, iatrogenic trauma, or some other cause of pharyngeal perforation. RPS abscess is sometimes due to extension of a prevertebral space (PVS) or other deep neck abscess. Reactive RPS edema is often due to causes other than infection.

Infectious disease originating from the cervical spine must be differentiated early in the diagnostic process from that originating due to pharyngeal disease to avoid a potentially catastrophic neurologic event involving the cervical spinal cord.

The initial evaluation of a disease process in the RPS must determine whether the RPS is only secondarily involved. Infectious disease rarely begins in the RPS except for retropharyngeal suppurative adenitis or in a penetrating or perforating type of injury. The RPS may be secondarily involved by inflammation beginning in the visceral compartment or the PVS. RPS edema due to radiotherapy, venous occlusive disease, deep neck infections, and even just generalized body edema disease is a common finding and significant in most cases only in that it should not be mistaken for a more serious problem if the etiology is obvious clinically or from associated imaging findings.

The method of differential diagnosis is driven by an orderly process of relatively simple observations that may be made on the basis of magnetic resonance imaging (MRI) and/or CT studies. The process may be supplemented by imaging-directed aspiration and/or tissue sampling, which is very safe.

The suggested process is as follows:

- Determine whether the process involves single or multiple spaces.
- If single, which space is involved, based on making observations with regard to vectors of structural displacement and spread of the inflammatory process?
- Make observations regarding the morphology of the presumptive inflammatory process that may require both MRI and CT for a comprehensive evaluation.
- Identify associated findings such as a foreign body or gas or findings suggesting a PVS origin.

The most common RPS infection by far is suppurative retropharyngeal adenitis without abscess. Occasionally, those pus-containing nodes become so large that they constitute an abscess physiologically. Such nodes rarely rupture to produce a true RPS abscess. Otherwise, RPS abscesses are relatively uncommon and usually are due to hypopharyngeal or esophageal perforation or extension of a deep neck lateral compartment abscess.

Retropharyngeal abscesses that are very conspicuous in the infrahyoid neck may become relatively inconspicuous at the thoracic inlet, giving the impression that they are ending in the low neck only to again "blossom" in the mediastinum, as seen in this case.

Questions for Further Thought

1. What are the most common causes of RPS inflammatory changes?
2. What are the indications for the use of CT and MRI in RPS infections?

Reporting Responsibilities

The diagnostic radiologist must be immediately available and in verbal contact with the treating physicians in almost all cases of suspected RPS and PVS infection. In the RPS, this is done mainly to assure proper communication about the airway status, presence of a drainable pyogenic abscess, foreign body or a likely life-threatening condition such as rapidly spreading necrotizing infection. Infections that arise in a diabetic or otherwise immunocompromised patient usually require some direct communication.

What the Treating Physician Needs to Know

- Likely diagnosis and degree of confidence in that diagnosis
- Full extent of the infectious process
- Relationship of the infection or inflammation to critical surrounding anatomy
- If any more data needs to be collected with imaging assistance
- *Posttreatment imaging:* Suspicion for recurrent or persistent infection versus expected posttreatment changes

Answers

1. Most RPS inflammatory changes below the hyoid are secondary peripharyngeal changes from pharyngeal mucosal infections, mainly cellulitis/phlegmon, or other etiologies for reactive edema such as radiotherapy or vascular thrombosis.
2. In general, CT is more definitive than MRI for inflammatory conditions unless the disease is primarily related to a spinal infection. MRI should be done urgently or emergently if there is any hint that the cervical spinal cord might be threatened.

> LEARN MORE
> See Chapters 151 and 13 in *Head and Neck Radiology* by Mancuso and Hanafee.

CLINICAL HISTORY *A painless neck mass in a 15-year-old boy.*

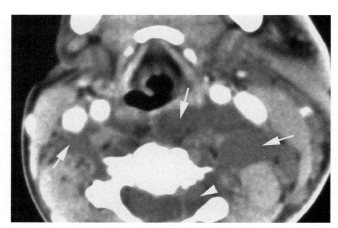

FIGURE **5.3**

FINDINGS

Figure 5.3. A hypodense multiloculated-appearing mass spreading transspatially with extension into a neural foramen, the prevertebral/paravertebral space, RPS, and lateral compartment. The origin is likely from various spinal nerve roots and possibly the sympathetic plexus (arrows). The extension into the neural foramen (arrowhead) on the left clearly identifies at least one segmental cervical nerve root of origin.

DIFFERENTIAL DIAGNOSIS Venolymphatic or vascular malformation, edema, fluid collection, neurogenic or nerve sheath tumor such as plexiform neurofibroma

DIAGNOSIS Plexiform neurofibroma

DISCUSSION The initial evaluation of a mass involving the RPS and PVS must determine whether they might be only secondary involved due to a mucosal disease or due to a transspatial process. Transspatial processes are, regardless of space of origin, masses that arise primarily in the deep spaces of the neck. The mechanisms and potential routes of transspatial spread vary. For aggressive pathologies such as cancers or diskitis and vertebral osteomyelitis, transspatial spread is a simple morphologic spread pattern to understand. It is also is a fairly intuitive pattern to understand in developmental abnormalities that affect these spaces since venolymphatic malformations simply follow vessels as they develop. In the case of the RPS and PVS, such developmental knowledge also helps to predict how nerve sheath tumors extend cross-spatial boundaries.

In general, the suggested differential diagnostic process is as follows:

- Determine whether the process involves single or multiple spaces.

- If single, in the RPS or PVS based on making the following observations with regard to vectors of structural displacement and "travel" of the mass:
  - *Laterally:* The fat between the RPS and carotid sheath will be compressed, and lateral spread in posterior compartment masses will be confined by the tough pre- and paravertebral fascial layer.
  - *Medially:* The process will occupy the midline or a paramedian position in the essentially midline RPS and may be contained primarily in the midline, somewhat contained by the prevertebral muscles in PVS-origin processes.
  - *Anteriorly:* The process will displace and/or invade the posterior muscular wall of the pharynx if it is primarily of RPS origin, and it will displace the anterior longitudinal ligament and prevertebral fascia and possibly the prevertebral muscles if of PVS, spinal origin.
  - *Posteriorly:* It will respect the plane of the prevertebral fascia if of RPS origin. If of PVS origin, it may involve the paravertebral space and its musculature, disks, vertebral bodies, and epidural space.
- Observations regarding the likely aggressiveness of margins of the mass and its internal morphology are typically more comprehensively demonstrated on magnetic resonance (MR) images.
- Identify associated findings such as lymphadenopathy, epidural disease, diskitis, or tendon and ligament calcification.

In this case, there is clearly a transspatial mass involving the lateral compartments, RPS, and PVS and extending into a neural foramen that appears to be enlarged. This favors the diagnosis of neurogenic or nerve sheath tumor such as plexiform neurofibroma. Nerve sheath tumors are clearly the type of lesion that can demonstrate transcompartmental spread since they follow nerves through anatomic gaps and across boundaries between these compartments.

Question for Further Thought

1. What is the relative frequency of RPS and PVS masses as opposed to inflammation or infection in these spaces?

Reporting Responsibilities

In general, masses of the retropharyngeal and prevertebral spaces are typically chronic and may be reported routinely unless there is a potential airway compromise problem or if a malignancy is suspected. Many of these cases require direct communication with referring doctors to decide on a course of action, especially if imaging-directed biopsy is necessary. It is particularly important to communicate effectively and promptly if there is a secondary infection and in those cases to anticipate whether there may be a complicating sinus or fistula. This communication may become urgent or emergent if the infection involves or may herald disease in the epidural space that might threaten the spinal cord.

What the Treating Physician Needs to Know

- Likely diagnosis and degree of confidence in that diagnosis
- Full extent of the mass
- Relationship of the mass to critical surrounding anatomy
- If any more data needs to be collected with imaging assistance
- *Posttreatment imaging:* Suspicion for tumor recurrence versus expected posttreatment changes

Answer

1. All of these masses are rare and sporadic.

LEARN MORE

See Chapters 152 and 29 in *Head and Neck Radiology* by Mancuso and Hanafee.

CLINICAL HISTORY *A 40-year-old adult with a prior history of alcohol and nicotine abuse presenting with a slightly tender right upper neck mass.*

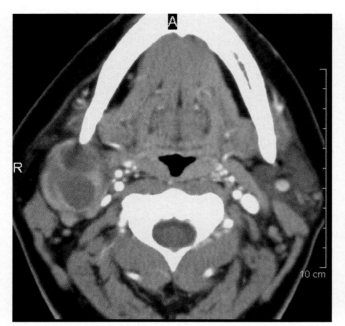

FIGURE 5.4A

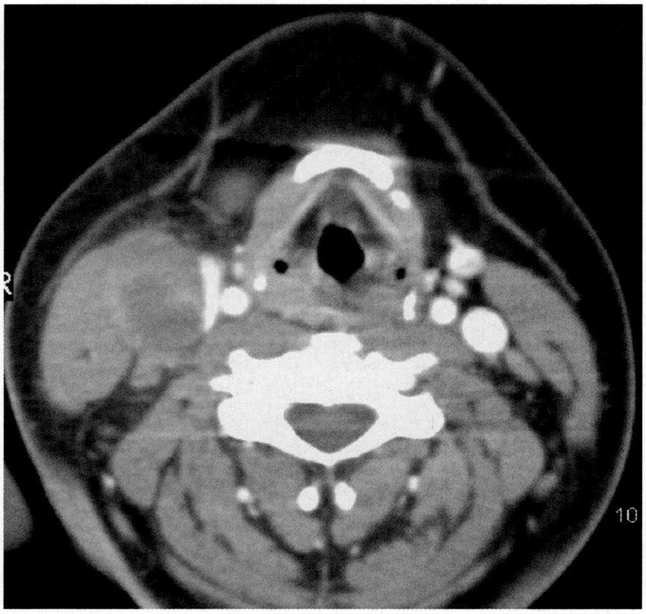

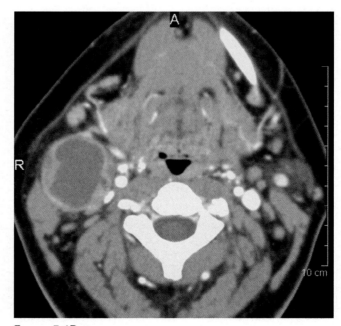

FIGURE 5.4C

FIGURE 5.4B

FINDINGS

Figure 5.4A–C. CECT showing a somewhat loculated and thick-walled–appearing cystic mass from the angle of the mandible to the mid-neck along the lateral aspect of the carotid sheath and the anterior and medial border of the sternocleidomastoid muscle, deep to the platysma and displacing the carotid artery and jugular vein medially. No definite internal fistula could be identified on the imaging study.

DIFFERENTIAL DIAGNOSIS Metastatic lymph node, infected second branchial cleft cyst, pyogenic adenopathy

DIAGNOSIS Infected second branchial cleft cyst

DISCUSSION Congenital anomalies of branchial origin affecting the neck come to imaging commonly in both the pediatric and adult population. Their embryologic origin explains the diverse appearance of these anomalies on imaging studies as well as their various clinical presentations. Anomalous branchial apparatus development results in glandular ectopia as well as various cysts, sinuses, and fistulas. These anomalies may be of branchial, thymic, and parathyroid origin.

The general mechanism of these developmental errors is incomplete obliteration of the branchial apparatus leaving buried cell rests trapped where they do not belong during the embryologic stage where they later produce branchial apparatus–related problems.

The basic classification of a branchial anomaly is by whether it is a sinus, fistula, or cyst and also according to its pouch or cleft of origin. Classification is done mainly to anticipate anatomic relationships that may be important treatment considerations, such as the course and point of pharyngeal communication of a fistula or sinus tract that has become complicated by infection so that it can be treated completely.

Branchial anomalies arise mainly from the second branchial apparatus. Cysts, as in this case, will present as a neck mass, often because they become secondarily infected. Infection implies a connection with the pharynx when there is no visible sinus tract to the skin. The mass is typically in the lateral compartment of the neck and bears some close relationship to the carotid sheath. The cysts will be deep to the superficial fascia (platysma). Cysts most typically relate to the anterior triangle but may be lateral to the carotid sheath so that those projecting more toward the posterior triangle are more likely related to the third cleft.

A history of intermittent changes in size or inflammation will suggest a branchial cleft cyst as a possible etiology, especially in children and young adults. Third apparatus cysts may present as recurrent infection in the region of the thyroid gland (the exact branchial apparatus origin of these remains somewhat controversial).

The younger the patient, the more a developmental problem will be plausible, but great care must be taken in adults. A predominantly cystic mass may be a nodal metastasis, and this possibility must be definitively excluded, especially in this case where the patient has a prior history of alcohol and nicotine abuse. Aspiration of fluid from the mass is not definitive in this regard. Moreover, a carcinoma confirmed in a cystic neck mass must never be presumed to be a cancer arising in a branchial cleft cyst. For the safety of patients, the entity "cancer arising in a branchial cleft cyst" must be considered an impossibility and the cystic mass presumed to be a nodal metastasis from cancer of the pharynx or larynx, skin (if parotid region), or thyroid if in the low neck.

Question for Further Thought

1. How would calcifications within the mass alter your differential diagnosis?

Reporting Responsibilities

Branchial apparatus developmental anomalies are generally chronic entities that may be reported routinely. An infected cyst or one that might threaten the airway requires direct, prompt communication. In an adult, a cystic mass more often will turn out to be due to a metastatic node, and a diligent search of the images for a possible primary tumor and direct communication to the referring provider are essential. Communication might include identification of the primary source or a suggestion for needle aspiration/biopsy of the mass.

What the Treating Physician Needs to Know

- Are the findings due to a branchial apparatus anomaly or possibly another condition?
- What is the arch of likely origin to anticipate a internal fistula or sinus tract location?
- If a cyst, its full extent relative to surrounding anatomy
- Is there an associated sinus or fistula? If so, what is the extent of that finding?
- Are their associated findings?
- Is the finding associated with glandular ectopias or pathology arising in ectopic glandular tissue?

Answer

1. Nodal metastasis of a papillary thyroid cancer would need to be added.

> **LEARN MORE**
> See Chapters 153 and 13 in *Head and Neck Radiology* by Mancuso and Hanafee.

CLINICAL HISTORY *A 2-year-old boy presenting with a neck mass.*

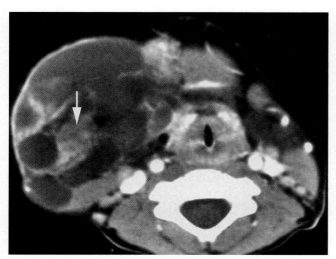

FIGURE **5.5A**

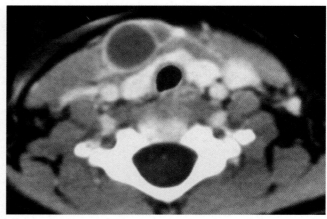

FIGURE **5.5C**

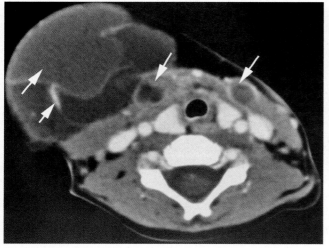

FIGURE **5.5B**

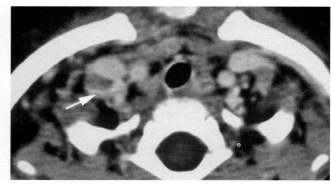

FIGURE **5.5D**

FINDINGS

Figure 5.5A–D. CECT shows an extensive, multiloculated, cystic mass extending from the upper neck to the supraclavicular fossa. Some enhancing areas and septations are present. The mass is centered primarily in the anterior cervical triangle and is bilateral. Note the transspatial spread pattern.

DIFFERENTIAL DIAGNOSIS None

DIAGNOSIS Mixed venolymphatic malformation

DISCUSSION The embryology of the lymphatic system explains the pathogenesis and imaging appearance of cervicothoracic (and other) venolymphatic malformations of the region. The tendency for all growth of these venolymphatic malformations is to involve the spaces predominantly deep to the superficial fascia and insinuate along the vessels from which they arise. In following those parent vessels the malformations also follow the cervical nerves their vessels of origin supply. This includes the possibility of following those neurovascular structures across fascial boundaries as well as around and into the various viscera of the neck that those neurovascular bundles would supply. By such developmental tendencies, isolated and relatively simple malformations as well as highly complex transcompartmental malformations become possible and their growth patterns relatively easy to understand.

A venolymphatic malformation such as seen in this case may be explained by a failure of the right paratracheal and internal thoracic lymph plexuses to join with the juguloaxillary sac during embryologic development. The mixed vascularity is due to an abnormal vessel bud retaining its original venous communication and not allowing the related mesenchyme of the venous bud to fully differentiate into a purely lymphatic structure. The malformation in that way grows while retaining some blood vessel vascular characteristics.

Removal of these lesions is usually related to functional and cosmetic issues. Because of their often insinuating growth around critical structures (e.g., carotid artery, vagus nerve), gross total excision is frequently not possible.

Question for Further Thought

1. State two reasons why such a mass would show a sudden growth.

Reporting Responsibilities

Vascular-related conditions affecting the lateral compartment may run a spectrum from those of little consequence, such as in this case, to those that might result in rapid neurologic deterioration or death—the timing of which is not necessarily predictable from the findings. Acute or hyperacute circumstances most typically are due to carotid disease and penetrating neck injuries and not operative in this case; direct communication with the referring treatment provider is essential in such high-acuity cases. In venolymphatic malformations, acute enlargement can rarely cause rapid airway compression.

What the Treating Physician Needs to Know

- Type of vascular condition and degree of confidence in that diagnosis
- Are there associated or causative factors identified, and can such findings be excluded?
- Full extent of the condition
- Is there a risk of preventable and/or functional or life-threatening complications?
- If any more data needs to be collected with imaging assistance

Answer

1. These lesions frequently enlarge rapidly because of hemorrhage or reactive lymphoid hyperplasia caused by upper respiratory infections (the lesions arise from the lymphatic system and contain immunocompetent cells). If their presence was unknown before this incident, this presentation might mimic a more aggressive process. This is especially common in the supraclavicular fossa.

LEARN MORE

See Chapters 154 and 9 in *Head and Neck Radiology* by Mancuso and Hanafee.

CLINICAL HISTORY *A young adult with tonsillitis, fever, odynophagia, neck swelling, and tenderness.*

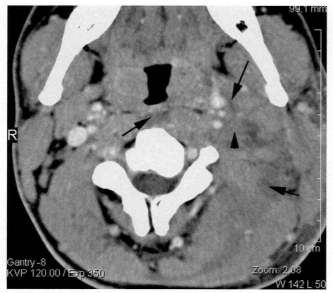

FIGURE 5.6A

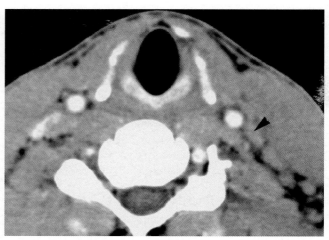

FIGURE 5.6C

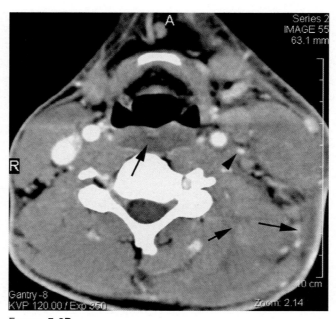

FIGURE 5.6B

FINDINGS

Figure 5.6A–C. CECT of a young adult with tonsillitis shows extensive inflammatory changes in multiple compartments in the neck (arrows), including the tonsil region, parapharyngeal space, RPS, paravertebral space, and entire lateral compartment associated with occlusion of the jugular vein (arrowheads).

DIFFERENTIAL DIAGNOSIS None

DIAGNOSIS Tonsillitis with spreading edema and secondary internal jugular vein thrombosis (Lemierre syndrome)

DISCUSSION

The initial evaluation of a disease process in the lateral compartment must determine whether the lateral compartment is only secondarily involved. Frequently, the infection in the lateral compartment is spreading from more cephalad sources such as pharyngeal and dental infections. Most of the time the source declares itself by its clinical circumstances, but sometimes the infection is so rapidly progressive or widespread at the time of presentation that only imaging identifies the source of infection.

Infectious disease occasionally begins in the lateral compartment from ruptured suppurative adenitis, an infected branchial apparatus cyst, postoperatively, or in a penetrating or perforating type of injury. The lateral compartment may be secondarily involved by inflammation beginning in the visceral compartment or the RPS and rarely the posterior compartment.

Lateral compartment edema and/or cellulitis may be generated by thrombophlebitis of the jugular venous system or carotid arteritis or may produce those conditions as a secondary effect of lateral compartment infection.

The morphology of a rapidly spreading infection may vary considerably depending on the specific organism and immune status or comorbidities of the patients.

In this case, a thrombosis of the internal jugular vein occurred as a complication of the severe tonsillitis. Jugular or even smaller tributary vein thrombosis is an extraordinarily important finding since it heralds multisystem (pulmonary, hepatic, and renal) and potentially fatal conditions due to organ failure called *Lemierre syndrome*. The venous thrombosis in this case may account for some of the neck edema, but the widespread infectious and reactive changes are more a testimony to the virulence of this infection that was eventually controlled with intravenous antibiotics.

Question for Further Thought

1. What is the pathophysiology of Lemierre syndrome?

Reporting Responsibilities

The diagnostic radiologist must be immediately available and in verbal contact with the treating physicians in almost all cases of suspected RPS and PVS infection. In the RPS, this is mainly done to assure proper communication about the airway status and presence of drainable pyogenic abscess, foreign body or a life-threatening condition such as rapidly spreading necrotizing infection. Infections that arise in a diabetic or otherwise immunocompromised patient usually require some direct communication. Potential Lemierre disease is a medical emergency and must be directly communicated to the treatment team.

What the Treating Physician Needs to Know

- Likely diagnosis and degree of confidence in that diagnosis
- Full extent of the infectious process
- Relationship of the infection or inflammation to critical surrounding anatomy
- If any more data needs to be collected with imaging assistance
- *Posttreatment imaging:* Suspicion for recurrent or persistent infection versus expected posttreatment changes

Answer

1. Pyogenic tonsillitis causes jugular vein thrombosis/thrombophlebitis; this septic thrombophlebitis can then give rise to septic microemboli that disseminate to other parts of the body where they can form abscesses and septic infarctions. The disease can lead to death caused by multisystem failure.

> LEARN MORE
> See Chapters 155 and 15 in *Head and Neck Radiology* by Mancuso and Hanafee.

CLINICAL HISTORY *An adult man presenting with a "lump" in the neck.*

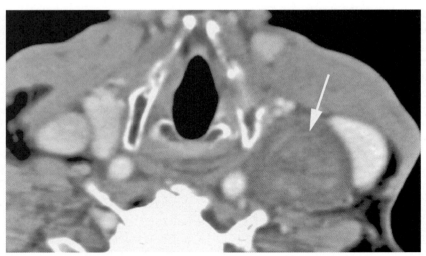

FIGURE **5.7A**

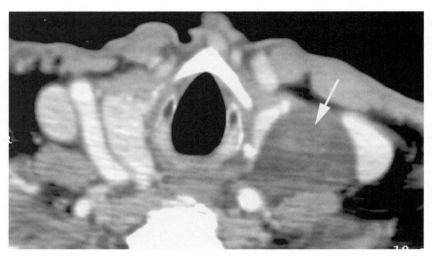

FIGURE **5.7B**

FINDINGS

Figure 5.7A,B. A lateral neck mass on the left (arrow) splays the common carotid artery and jugular vein. The mass is solid but hypodense to muscle with a sparse internal pattern of reticulated increased density and no obvious enhancement.

DIFFERENTIAL DIAGNOSIS
Neurogenic tumor (schwannoma or neurofibroma), sarcoma

DIAGNOSIS
Vagal schwannoma

DISCUSSION
The method of differential diagnosis is driven by an orderly process of relatively simple observations that may be made on the basis of MRI and/or CT studies. The process may be supplemented by imaging-directed biopsy, which is very safe and effective in this region, especially when compared to what it takes to secure a surgical sample. The suggested process is as follows:

- Determine the compartment of origin.
- If of lateral compartment origin, is there a likely specific anatomic source, morphologic pattern, or clue suggesting developmental origin that can be identified:
  - Does it relate more to the anterior or posterior triangle?
  - Is it solitary or multiple, unilateral or bilateral?
  - Is it of carotid or jugular or vagal origin?
  - Does it arise from the sternocleidomastoid muscle?
  - Is it developmental of either branchial apparatus or venolymphatic origin?

- Observations regarding the likely aggressiveness of margins of the mass and its internal morphology can also help in the differential diagnosis and suggest the relative acuity of the problem and need for enhanced communication or facilitation of the workup.

The initial evaluation of a potential nonnodal mass in the lateral compartment is highly driven by the patient age, specific clinical situation, and related likely disease category. All of these nonnodal masses are relatively uncommon and sporadic once those of branchial, venolymphatic, and visceral compartment origin are eliminated.

In this case, there should be little doubt that the mass is of neurogenic origin and shows no overt signs of malignancy.

Question for Further Thought

1. What disease of neurogenic origin would present as bilateral neck masses?

Reporting Responsibilities

In this case, routine reporting suffices. The mass is of no danger to the patient, and there is no significant acuity in this situation. Nonnodal masses of the lateral compartment may run a spectrum from those of little consequence to those that might result in rapid neurologic deterioration or death—the timing of which is not predictable from the findings. Acute or hyperacute circumstances arising in the lateral compartment most typically are due to carotid disease. Direct communication with the referring treatment provider is essential in such cases.

What the Treating Physician Needs to Know

- Type of cause of the nonnodal mass and degree of confidence in that diagnosis
- Are there associated or causative factors identified, and can such findings be excluded?
- Full extent of the mass and its relationship of the mass to critical surrounding anatomy
- Is there a risk of preventable and/or functional or life-threatening complications?
- If any more data needs to be collected with imaging assistance

Answer

1. Neurofibromatosis

> **LEARN MORE**
> See Chapters 156 and 29 in *Head and Neck Radiology* by Mancuso and Hanafee.

CASE 5.8

CLINICAL HISTORY   *A 48-year-old male patient with a right-sided, level 2 region, anterior triangle neck mass and no apparent primary tumor.*

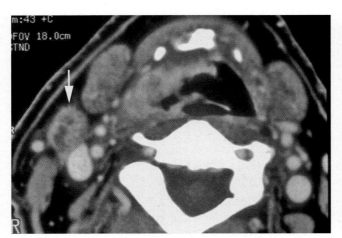

FIGURE **5.8A**

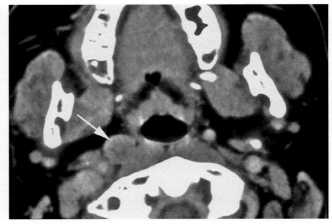

FIGURE **5.8B**

FINDINGS

Figure 5.8A. Level 2A lymph node showing early extranodal spread (arrow) as irregularity at the nodal margin extending minimally into the perinodal fat.

Figure 5.8B. Positive retropharyngeal lymph node metastasis (arrow).

DIFFERENTIAL DIAGNOSIS Inflammatory lymphadenopathy, cervical lymphoma, cervical metastatic disease

DIAGNOSIS Cervical metastatic disease due to a tongue base–vallecula submucosal and otherwise clinically unapparent primary squamous cell carcinoma (SCCa)

DISCUSSION Cervical node metastatic disease most frequently presents as a neck mass, of which the most common cause is SCCa from head and neck cancers of mucosal or skin origin, although other "solid tumors" and lymphoma can also present as cervical lymph node disease. If the origin of the neck mass is uncertain by physical examination, imaging followed by panendoscopy and fine-needle aspiration biopsy of the mass is the most effective strategy to confirm the etiology.

Management of the primary in SCCa is intimately related to the management of cervical lymph node metastasis and, unless the neck disease is very advanced, is usually controlled with the optimal use of surgery, radiation, and chemotherapy. In about 2% to 5% of SCCa cervical metastasis, the primary cannot be found by complete endoscopy, creating the dilemma of an "unknown primary." Slightly more than half of these clinically occult tumors are found with anatomic imaging—a detection rate that may be marginally improved with the addition of PET-CT.

All histologic malignancies can show lymphatic spread. The factors that increase the risk of lymph node metastasis include the following:

- Decreased degree of differentiation, which is associated with an increased invasiveness of the margins
- Increased capillary lymphatic density of the tissue involved: Once a tumor develops in a capillary lymphatic–rich area, the risk of metastasis depends on the depth of invasion; this trend is best established in the evidence base in cutaneous melanoma in skin and for SCCa of the oral tongue.
- Vascular space invasion
- Recurrent lesions
- Increasing T stage

In general, the diagnosis of metastatic SCCa in lymph nodes depends on the following:

- *Size:* The largest short axis dimension (LSAD) is typically used. This is the least useful criterion and is very limited with regard to predicting the risk of lymph node micrometastasis in otherwise normal nodes. Levels 1 and 2 should be less than 15 mm; levels 3, 4, 5, and 6 (except prelaryngeal) as well as parotid and lateral retropharyngeal groups should be less than 10 mm. Median retropharyngeal, delphian (prelaryngeal), facial, occipital, mastoid, and lingual groups or nodes that are normally not visible or distinguishable from small vessels should be less than 5 mm. In patients with ipsilateral disease, the opposite neck could be used as a control to improve size criteria accuracy. In general, nodal size criteria are not reliable for high-level clinical decision making.
- *Focal parenchymal defects:* Manifested as focal areas of decreased density/signal intensity, focal enhancement, or foci of impacted keratin debris and/or dystrophic

calcification. Central necrosis is often a late finding in nodal disease and is not specific for carcinoma and can be seen in suppurative nodes, granulomatous disease (i.e., tuberculosis), fungal infection, and lymphoma (treated or aggressive lymphoma or HIV-positive patients).

- *Node capsule penetration by the tumor:* Manifested as rim enhancement (nonspecific for early extranodal spread of cancer since it can also be seen in reactive, infected, or lymphomatous nodes), irregular nodal margins, or infiltration of the perinodal tissue. Extracapsular spread of malignancy has been associated with an approximately 50% decrease in survival. Extranodal spread can focally invade and become fixed to (manifested as a loss of a separating plane) and/or encase (≥270-degree surrounding arc of tumor) the surrounding structures. Carotid encasement and fixation to the prevertebral fascia and floor of the neck are typically incurable.

Lower neck regional disease (i.e., level 4), extranodal spread, and numerous involved lymph nodes are likely associated with an increased incidence of distant metastasis and should be further evaluated with a PET scan.

Questions for Further Thought

1. What lymph nodes should always be accounted for when evaluating head and neck malignancies and why?
2. What is a modified neck dissection?

Reporting Responsibilities

Immediate direct communication with the referring treatment provider is required in the event of a discovery of an unsuspected primary tumor or distant metastatic disease and in circumstances where it may be anticipated from imaging that a major change in medical decision making might be made. No special communication is required when cervical metastatic disease is known or suspected; nonetheless, the report must contain a complete assessment of the disease extent and all information that is relevant to treatment planning.

What the Treating Physician Needs to Know

- If the neck is N+ or N0
- Number of positive nodes and location by the current level 1 through 6 classification system
- Status of retropharyngeal and highest level 2 nodes; when applicable, status of other nodal groups including facial, parotid, and posterior neck groups
- In the treated neck, signs of satellite nodules and lymphatic obstructive changes
- Presence and extent of extranodal spread and risk for focal invasion, adherence or fixation and encasement of the surrounding structures, prevertebral fascia or floor of the neck
- Likely site of a clinically not apparent primary tumor
- Whether the pattern of adenopathy is typical for the disease at hand or suggests an anticipated situation

Answers

1. Retropharyngeal level 2 nodes above the posterior belly of the digastric muscle and deeper level 6 nodes. These nodes are not accessible by physical examination or some modified neck dissections. They have the potential to alter treatment plans and can become the site of unsalvageable failure when they are not accounted for in the initial treatment plan.

2. The classical radical neck dissection removes the superficial and deep cervical fascia as well as the enveloped ipsilateral lymph nodes, the sternocleidomastoid muscle, the omohyoid muscles, the internal and external jugular vein, the spinal accessory nerve, and the submandibular gland. A modified neck dissection is a customized more selective neck dissection where some components of the radical are not removed, causing less potential morbidity.

> ## LEARN MORE
> See Chapters 157 and 21 in *Head and Neck Radiology* by Mancuso and Hanafee.

CLINICAL HISTORY *Two febrile pediatric patients presenting with a tender upper lateral compartment neck mass.*

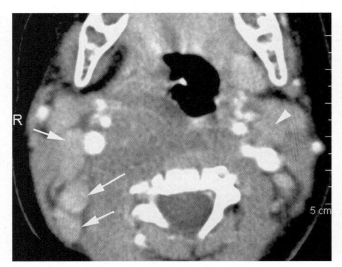

FIGURE **5.9A**

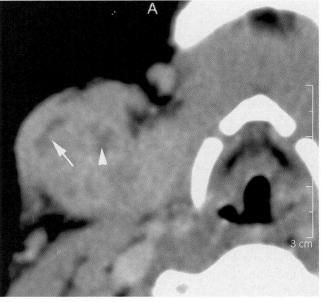

FIGURE **5.9B**

FINDINGS

Patient 1. Extensive predominantly right-sided retropharyngeal edema crossing the midline. Bilateral homogeneously enlarged lymph nodes (arrows in Fig. 5.9A), slightly more enhancing on the right side. The adenopathies are situated in level 2 and 5 on the right and level 2 on the left. The jugular vein is patent.

Patient 2. Enlarged lymph node with peripheral crescentric (arrow) and more central (arrowhead) necrotic areas and slightly unsharp borders in Fig. 5.9B.

DIFFERENTIAL DIAGNOSIS

- *Nodal:* Adenopathies due to the following:
  - Systemic disease such as lymphoma, leukemia, sarcoidosis, Castleman disease
  - Metastatic disease (head and neck or infraclavicular primary), which is very unlikely in this age group
- *Inflammatory:* Infectious and reactive
- *Nonnodal disease:* In this age group, infected branchial cleft cyst or sarcoma

DIAGNOSIS *Patient 1 Fig. 5.9A:* Pharyngitis with reactive/infectious but not obviously suppurative adenitis
   Patient 2 Fig. 5.9B: Cat scratch disease

DISCUSSION The main task is to differentiate lateral compartment neck masses as nodal and nonnodal. That done, an attempt should be made to discriminate between benign adenopathies and reactive nodes and those of primary and secondary lymph node malignancies. This may eventually require

needle biopsy or node excision. In some instances, other clues to systemic and/or inflammatory diseases may be present by way of other imaging findings, clinical evaluation, and supportive laboratory data as suggested by the age, febrile nature of the illness, and tenderness in these two patients.

Patient 1:

Reactive nodes range from incidental findings to a feature that is useful in the differential diagnosis to a situation that must be distinguished from significant treatable pathology. At times, such adenopathy must initially be distinguished from malignant adenopathy and that due to benign systemic diseases as well as other lateral compartment masses such as infected branchial apparatus cysts.

   Reactive nodes in general will enlarge and retain an otherwise normal architecture. The vascular pedicle will typically enlarge, and flow will be increased via the hilar vascular pedicle. The capsule of the lymph node may also manifest the physiologic hypervascularity of the node.

   Infectious nodes may undergo focal and diffuse architectural changes. In pyogenic infections, this will reflect a cellulitic-type or "presuppurative" phase followed by various degrees of liquefaction that tends to be central but may be more peripheral within the node. Depending on the virulence of the infection, host factors, and treatment status, there will be capsular reactive changes and perinodal inflammatory changes. At some point, the suppurative node becomes equivalent to an abscess, or purulent material can rupture from the node and produce a true deep neck abscess. Later-stage or healing changes may include dystrophic calcification.

   Viral infections will result in typically reactive-appearing nodes with little, if any, capsular or perinodal findings suggestive of infection. Lower-grade or partially treated infectious adenopathy may show a hybrid reactive-suppurative appearance.

Reactive adenopathy is very common in pharyngeal infections, both viral and bacterial, and skin infections of the face and neck. If the adenopathy is bilateral and in a young adult, both Epstein-Barr virus and HIV should be suggested as possible etiologies. In patients with HIV, the nodes may be due to lymphoma rather than the primary infection or immune reconstitution following initiation of maintenance therapeutic regimes. In immunocompromised patients, reactive-appearing adenopathy can be seen as a manifestation of posttransplant lymphoproliferative disorder.

The distribution of nodes in the neck provides significant clues about the likely source of the infectious or immune challenge within the nodes. The distribution combined with nodal morphology adds power to this analysis. Bilateral nodes are more typically seen in reactions to viral infection or in systemic disease. Unilateral or marked asymmetric adenopathy typically suggests a lateralized source.

In this case, the lymph nodes are homogeneously enlarged and show an enhancement that is greater on the side of pharyngeal infection.

Patient 2:
Frankly necrotic adenopathy is found in pyogenic bacterial infections, cat scratch disease and suppurative infections, tuberculosis, and neoplastic nodal involvement. Occasionally, the etiology of nodes that are not necrotic and go on to dystrophic calcification is never established, even following removal and definitive pathologic evaluation.

In this case, the peripheral and especially crescentric low-density areas within the nodes are fairly characteristic of cat scratch disease. The laterality suggests a lateralized source of infection, and level 1 disease suggests the skin or the face as a source in the absence of an oral cavity source.

Questions for Further Thought

1. Can reactive adenopathy be distinguished from lymphoproliferative adenopathy?
2. Does the finding of uncomplicated reactive adenopathies in young children warrant immediate action?
3. If so, name specific circumstances that might warrant immediate action.

Reporting Responsibilities

Reactive nodes typically are reported routinely unless there is a potential for a relation to a treatable medical condition or malignancy is suspected.

If the adenopathy is likely due to a suppurative infection, it should be communicated directly with the treating provider at the time of the interpretation. Direct communication is also wise if there is a potential complication of the infection such as Lemierre syndrome, which is a potential medical emergency. In Patient 1, the pharyngitis is likely pyogenic, based on the extent of reactive cellulitis, and the potential for airway problems and

Lemierre exists (but was excluded); thus, verbal communication is essential.

In Patient 2, the nodal morphology is highly suggestive of a specific infectious disease, so verbal communication is indicated to move the medical decision making in the most productive direction as rapidly as possible.

Some of these adenopathies, whether or not infectious, can mimic those due to malignancies, and direct communication at the time of interpretation may be wise if the etiology remains in doubt after consideration of the imaging findings in light of available clinical information.

Specific report content might include the following:
- Distribution of the adenopathy—groups involved, unilateral or bilateral, low neck
- Internal node morphology
- Extranodal changes
- If extranodal changes involve critical anatomic structures
- Nonnodal factors that might suggest the etiology of adenopathy

What the Treating Physician Needs to Know
- Likelihood that the nodal pathology is reactive and degree of confidence in that diagnosis
- If the degree of confidence is low, what are potential alternatives and follow-up imaging strategy?
- If infectious adenopathy, is there a clue to etiology of the infection given the distribution and morphology of the adenopathy?
- If infectious, is there any related extranodal complication?
- Is there any causative pathology visible on the study?

Answers
1. Reactive adenopathy may be distinguished from lymphoproliferative, metastatic, and infectious adenopathy with imaging in many cases based on the distribution and morphology of the pathologic nodes. However, sometimes reactive adenopathy and that due to lymphoproliferative disease may not be distinguishable on any imaging study and follow-up; thus, at least by clinical exam, it is essential to exclude a malignant etiology.
2. Reactive adenopathy is a common finding on imaging studies and in young children can be considered "physiologic."
3. In any case of pharyngitis that comes to imaging, it is essential to determine whether the jugular vein or its major tributaries are thrombosed so that the potentially life-threatening Lemierre syndrome can be detected as early as possible. Potential airway compromise must also be communicated verbally.

LEARN MORE
See Chapters 158 and 13 in *Head and Neck Radiology* by Mancuso and Hanafee.

CLINICAL HISTORY *Two young adults with cervical adenopathy.*

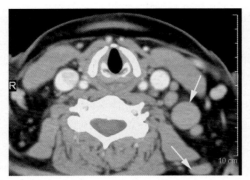

FIGURE **5.10A**

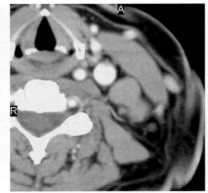

FIGURE **5.10B**

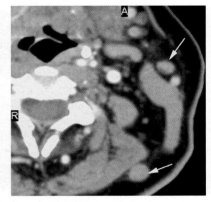

FIGURE **5.10C**

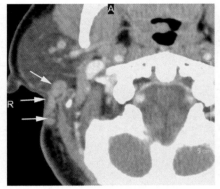

FIGURE **5.10D**

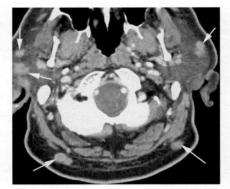

FIGURE **5.10E**

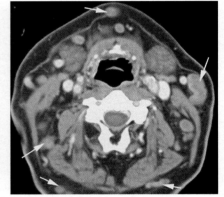

FIGURE **5.10F**

FINDINGS CECT showing nodal enlargement in almost all head and neck groups including the parotid, retromastoid, and posterior neck and level 5 nodes with a homogeneous internal morphology in Patient 1 (Fig. 5.10A–D) and minor internal morphologic low density in Patient 2 (Fig. 5.10D,E) without clear evidence of capsular or perinodal changes in either patient.

DIFFERENTIAL DIAGNOSIS *Nodal:* Adenopathies due to the following:

- Systemic disease (e.g., lymphoma, leukemia, sarcoidosis, Castleman disease)
- Metastatic disease (head and neck or infraclavicular primary)
- Reactive to infection, likely viral

DIAGNOSIS Lymphoma in both cases

DISCUSSION The main task is to differentiate benign adenopathies from reactive nodes and those of primary and secondary lymph node malignancies. This usually requires needle biopsy or node excision. In some instances, other clues

to systemic diseases may be present by way of other imaging findings, clinical evaluation, and supportive laboratory data.

In this case, the facts that the nodes are bilateral (suggesting systemic disease), that the parotid, retromastoid, posterior neck, and level 5 nodes are involved, and that nodes show a homogenous density make lymphoma a very probable diagnosis in Patient 1. In patient 2, the distribution suggests lymphoma as well even though there is some altered density within the node parenchyma.

The adenopathy of lymphoma and leukemia overlap with other diseases that may involve the head and neck nodes. The most common cause of adenopathy is infectious disease even if the exact cause of the infection is not apparent clinically and more often than not viral. Cervical adenopathy may be part of systemic diseases of uncertain etiology such as sarcoidosis and Langerhans cell histiocytosis.

Abnormal cervical nodes may also be a secondary expression of immune-mediated disease that may involve other systems such as the autoimmune rheumatoid-related diseases.

Lymphoma often involves the level 1 through 5 nodes and frequently the parotid, mastoid, and posterior neck nodes bilaterally. This disease is often asymmetric, but both necks are most often involved. This pattern of adenopathy together with the nodal internal morphology will strongly suggest lymphoma. In non-Hodgkin lymphoma, there may be extranodal disease in Waldeyer's ring and elsewhere. Leukemia, especially chronic lymphocytic leukemia, can appear the same as lymphoma. Hodgkin disease tends to involve lower neck nodes, and extranodal disease is unusual. Unilateral neck involvement is more common in Hodgkin than in non-Hodgkin lymphoma. If due to lymphoma, internal low density suggests that the disease is non-Hodgkin, has been treated, is unusually aggressive, and/or is associated with HIV infection. Rarely, solid metastases may *secondarily* involve lymphomatous nodes.

A suggested approach to potential nodal disease in the head and neck region could be as follows:

A. Is the mass of lymph node origin?

B. Is the node solitary, one of multiple abnormal nodes, or is there generalized adenopathy (bilateral disease points in the direction of systemic disease, although metastatic disease secondary to SCCa also presents with bilateral adenopathies)?

C. What specific neck groups are involved? Are other groups (retropharyngeal, facial, parotid) involved?

D. Nodal morphology:

1. Solid, minimal capsular, and hilar enhancement point to lymphoma (nonspecific), reactive adenopathy, sarcoid, and so on.

2. Focal peripheral defects in normal or enlarged nodes point to metastases from "solid" neoplasms (usually SCCa).

3. Large fluid areas in nodes indicate gross necrotic metastases or infectious disease (pyogenic, tuberculosis).

4. Any capsular involvement or extracapsular spread (important to note extent of spread)?

5. Does the extranodal spread involve the carotid, jugular, prevertebral fascia, sternocleidomastoid muscle, and so on?

E. Does the nodal morphology suggest an inflammatory rather than neoplastic cause of the adenopathy?

F. Is there another abnormality that might be associated with the adenopathy (e.g., primary site, Waldeyer's ring lymphoma, lymphoepithelial parotid lesions, or HIV)?

Questions for Further Thought

1. What should you do if needle biopsy shows SCCa?

2. How should one measure a lymph node, and is it relevant when trying to exclude metastatic disease?

Reporting Responsibilities

In these two patients, the etiology of the neck mass was uncertain and is likely due to lymphoma; thus, direct communication of the findings is the wisest course of action. An offer to sample a node via imaging guidance if node excision is not planned should also be part of the report. Based on pathologic confirmation, systemic imaging with FDG-PET, perhaps supplemented by detailed anatomic imaging, should also be suggested.

In any type of lymphadenopathy, the report must contain a complete assessment of the disease extent and all information that is relevant to treatment planning.

What the Treating Physician Needs to Know

• Whether the neck mass is nodal or nonnodal

• Location of positive nodes by current classification system reported by level and including status of other (nonnumbered) nodal groups including facial, parotid, and posterior neck retropharyngeal nodes

• Presence and extent of extranodal spread

• When applicable (not in this case of lymphoma), likely site of a clinically not apparent primary tumor

• Whether the pattern of adenopathy is typical for disease at hand or suggests an unanticipated clinical situation

Answers

1. If needle biopsy shows SCCa, a scan must include the entire pharynx and neck and a careful search made for a clinically occult primary tumor. The groups involved will suggest the most likely primary sites.

2. A node's shape on axial sections depends on its orientation to the transverse plane of the body. Shape should be taken into account since LSADs are typically used as a criterion for metastatic disease or even suggesting a node is significantly abnormal, especially in the younger pediatric age range.

LEARN MORE
See Chapters 159 and 27 in *Head and Neck Radiology* by Mancuso and Hanafee.

CASE 5.11

CLINICAL HISTORY *A 56-year-old man presenting with dysphagia and neck pain.*

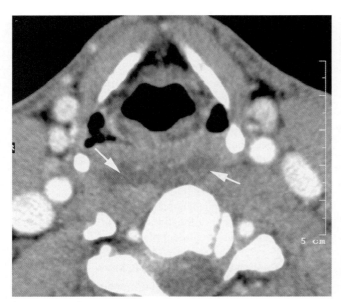

FIGURE 5.11A

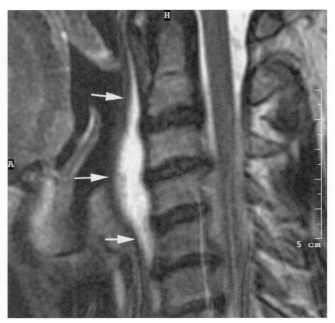

FIGURE 5.11C

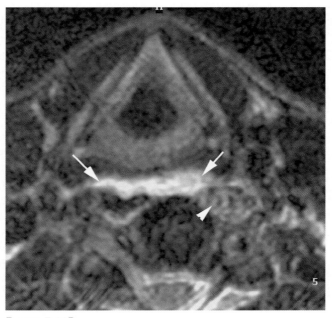

FIGURE 5.11B

FINDINGS

Figure 5.11A–C. Low density on CT (Fig. 5.11A) and hyper-intensity on a T2W MR image within the retropharyngeal and prevertebral spaces (Fig. 5.11B and C), correlating with edema within the retropharyngeal and prevertebral spaces (arrows) judging from the way it is contained near the midline and by the edema within the prevertebral muscles on the left (arrowheads Fig. 5.11C). The edema clearly displaces the pharyngeal musculature anteriorly.

DIFFERENTIAL DIAGNOSIS Reactive edema, prevertebral and paravertebral abscess, calcific and noncalcific musculotendinous and ligament inflammation. Diskitis/vertebral osteomyelitis/epidural abscess, pyogenic myositis must be excluded.

DIAGNOSIS Noncalcific musculotendonitis of the longus colli muscle group

DISCUSSION Infections of the PVS and those of the RPS can result in significant morbidity and mortality. Timely diagnosis and proper treatment are critical in preventing sequelae such as airway obstruction, epidural abscess and cervical cord injury, mediastinitis, carotid artery aneurysm, and cavernous sinus thrombosis.

The PVS is mainly involved by inflammatory pathology of the spine, usually diskitis and/or vertebral osteomyelitis or facet infection. Other posterior compartment inflammatory diseases are rare in the absence of penetrating trauma or an open surgical procedure. Differentiating PVS infections from musculoskeletal chronic inflammatory conditions is an important part of this process. Infectious disease originating from the cervical spine must be differentiated early in the diagnostic process from that originating due to pharyngeal disease to avoid a potentially catastrophic neurologic event involving the cervical spinal cord.

The suggested differential diagnostic process is as follows:

- Determine whether the process involves single or multiple spaces.
- If single, which space based on making observations with regard to vectors of structural displacement and spread of the inflammatory process?
- Make observations regarding the morphology of the presumptive inflammatory process that may require both MRI and CT for a comprehensive evaluation, especially when the PVS is the focus of the disease process, whereas CT alone is usually adequate in pharyngeal/RPS-origin infections.
- Identify associated findings such as epidural disease and diskitis or chronic-appearing vertebral body and ligament findings.

In this case, there is edema within the retropharyngeal and prevertebral spaces in the absence of signal alterations within the adjacent intervertebral disks or vertebral bodies. The patient had no fever, and no enhancing rim was noted around, nor gas within, the fluid component/edema. This basically excludes any potentially life-threatening pyogenic source of the edema. No primary cause for the edema was identified in the surrounding spaces.

This patient was diagnosed as having noncalcific musculotendonitis of the longus colli muscle group, and the findings resolved on anti-inflammatory medications. Acute or chronic determined clinically, and sometimes calcific tendinitis of the longus colli muscle is a common pathology, typically in 30- to 60-year-old adults, that produces predominantly PVS findings. This is associated with abnormal deposition of hydroxyapatite crystals. Complications of spondyloarthropathies may also present in the PVS. These inflammations of the muscle, tendon, and ligament attachments to the cervical spine are not uncommon and can mimic PVS and RPS infection/inflammation.

Question for Further Thought

1. In general, what are the relative values of using CT and MRI in PVS inflammatory conditions?

Reporting Responsibilities

Inflammatory processes affecting the PVS may result in neurologic deterioration—the timing of which is not predictable from the findings. Neurologic deterioration due to an epidural abscess can be rapid. Direct communication with the referring treatment provider and documentation of that communication is essential in such cases. Sometimes a warning against myelography should accompany such a communication due to the potential for myelography to worsen a developing or impending neurologic complication.

The main elements of the report should include the following:

- Space of origin and all spaces of involvement including the thoracic inlet and mediastinum below and the skull base above
- Is the inflammatory process likely infectious or noninfectious?
- Is there an abscess?
- Relationship of the findings to the mid to lower cervical spine to help decide whether the source of infection/inflammation is from diskitis and/or osteomyelitis
- Whether there is epidural disease or any sign of spinal canal and cord compromise
- Whether CT aspiration, tissue sampling, or other imaging studies would help to further clarify the findings

What the Treating Physician Needs to Know

- Likely diagnosis and degree of confidence in that diagnosis
- Full extent of the infectious/inflammatory process
- Relationship of the infection or inflammation to critical surrounding anatomy, including the spinal cord, carotid artery, and airway
- If any more data needs to be collected with imaging assistance
- *Posttreatment imaging:* Suspicion for recurrent or persistent infection versus expected posttreatment changes

Answer

1. In general, CT is more definitive than MRI for inflammatory conditions unless the disease is primarily related to a spinal infection. MRI should be done urgently or emergently if there is any hint that the cervical spinal cord might be threatened.

> LEARN MORE
> See Chapters 160 and 13 in *Head and Neck Radiology* by Mancuso and Hanafee.

CLINICAL HISTORY *A 20-year-old man presents with a left lower neck mass.*

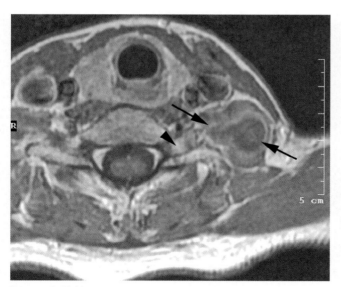

FIGURE 5.12A

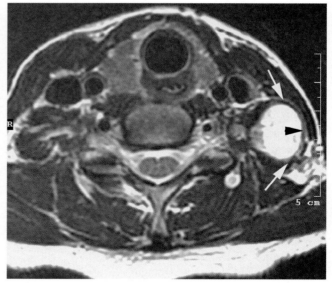

FIGURE 5.12C

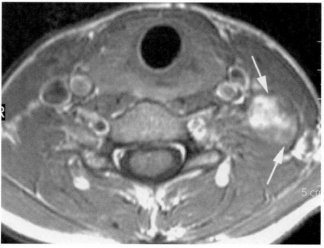

FIGURE 5.12B

FINDINGS

Figure 5.12. MRI of a well-demarcated paravertebral mass in the lower neck on the left (arrows in (Figs. 5.12A–C)). The lesion lies within the scalene muscle group and only slightly displaces the carotid sheath anteriorly and levator scapula muscle posteriorly. The mass enhances heterogeneously. The lesion extends to a neural foramen on the left (arrowhead in Fig. 5.12A).

DIFFERENTIAL DIAGNOSIS None

DIAGNOSIS Schwannoma of the brachial plexus

DISCUSSION The initial evaluation of a potential mass in the posterior compartment is highly driven by the patient age, specific clinical situation, and related likely disease category. Interpretation of imaging should first determine whether the posterior compartment is the site of origin and then whether the mass has secondarily involved the lateral or visceral compartment and related RPS as a transspatial process. Transspatial benign masses that begin in the posterior compartment are most often due to nerve sheath tumors. The mechanisms and potential routes of transspatial spread vary depending on the type of pathology. Nerve sheath tumors, for example, simply follow the cervical roots of origin.

Next, the specific structure of origin should be identified if possible, excluding vascular causes, followed by evaluating the morphology of the lesion.

The differential diagnostic process may be supplemented by imaging-directed aspiration and/or tissue sampling, which is very safe and effective in this region, especially when compared to what it takes to secure a surgical sample.

In this case, the lesion seems to grow out of a neural foramen that may appear minimally widened, as can be seen in slow-growing benign lesions. The lesion is well demarcated, is fusiform on coronal imaging (not shown) following the brachial plexus, and shows no signs of invasion into the surrounding structures. This, in addition to the signal intensities on MRI, is typical for a nerve sheath tumor/schwannoma.

Questions for Further Thought

1. List four neurologic deficits that might be associated with a lower neck mass.
2. Must imaging precede needle biopsy in the evaluation of a lower neck mass?

Reporting Responsibilities

Masses of the posterior compartment may run a spectrum from those of little or no acute consequence to those that might result in rapid neurologic deterioration due to spinal cord involvement that may not be predictable from the findings. Direct communication with the referring treatment provider is essential in the latter cases or if a mass might be malignant or vascular.

The main elements of the report should include the following:

- Site of origin and all spaces/compartments involved from the thoracic inlet and supraclavicular fossa below to the skull base above

- Whether the spinal cord is potentially involved
- Is there a risk of the mass being malignant?

What the Treating Physician Needs to Know

- Are there associated or causative factors identified, and can such findings be excluded, like multiplicity or adenopathy, that suggest a systemic disease or metastatic malignancy?
- Full extent of the mass and its relationship of the mass to critical surrounding anatomy
- Cause of the mass and degree of confidence in that diagnosis
- Is there a risk of preventable and/or functional or life-threatening complications?
- If any more data needs to be collected with imaging assistance

Answers

1. Vocal cord paralysis, Horner's syndrome, sensory and motor deficits (brachial plexus), paralyzed diaphragm
2. An aneurysm or other vascular etiology must be definitely excluded before any biopsy or surgical approach to the mass.

LEARN MORE

See Chapters 161 and 29 in *Head and Neck Radiology* by Mancuso and Hanafee.

CLINICAL HISTORY   *A 7 year old female child presenting with posterior neck mass and pain in the neck.*

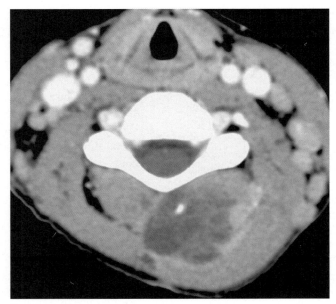

FIGURE 5.13

FINDINGS

Figure 5.13. CECT image of a left-sided mass lesion in the posterior neck compartment crossing the midline and invading the posterior spinal musculature. The lesion is mainly hypodense and focally heterogeneous but clearly has a solid enhancing peripheral nodular component on its left border. There also appear to be thinner enhancing septations within the mass.

DIFFERENTIAL DIAGNOSIS Metastasis, lymphoma, fibromatoses, malignant fibrous histiocytoma, mesenchymal sarcomas, and neurogenic malignancies.

DIAGNOSIS Angiomatoid malignant fibrous histiocytoma

DISCUSSION The initial evaluation of a potential mass in the posterior compartment is highly driven by the patient age, specific clinical situation and related likely disease category. At first one must determine whether the posterior compartment is the site of origin and then whether the mass has secondarily involved the lateral or visceral compartment and related RPS as a transspatial process. Transspatial malignant masses that begin in the posterior compartment are rare. The mechanisms and potential routes of trans spatial spread of these aggressive pathologies such as lymphoma, metastases and sarcomas are by direct invasion and/or perineural along the cervical nerve roots potentially to the epidural space and cervical spinal cord.

Next, the specific structure of origin should be identified if possible, excluding vascular causes, followed by evaluating the morphology of the lesion. The differential diagnostic process may be supplemented by imaging directed aspiration and/or tissue sampling. An aneurysm or other vascular etiology must be definitely excluded before any biopsy or surgical approach to the mass; imaging may guide biopsy away from potential risk factors such as prominent vascular structures within the mass.

In this case, the aggressive growth of the lesion (invasion of the muscles) suggests a malignant etiology. Malignant tumors are more likely to be painful than benign tumors. Metastases are relatively rare in this age group, so they should be lower on the differential list. The lesion has no unique features and it was biopsy that revealed the diagnosis of malignant fibrous histiocytoma.

Question for Further Thought

1. Describe the vectors of structural displacement and spread of a mass centered in the paravertebral space.

Reporting Responsibilities

Malignant tumors of the posterior compartment may run a spectrum from those that pose no immediate consequence to those that might result in rapid neurological deterioration due to spinal cord involvement that may not be predictable from the findings. Direct, urgent communication with the referring treatment provider is essential in the latter cases and always at the time of initial suspicion of a malignant mass.

The main elements of the report should include:

- The site of origin and all spaces/compartments involved from the thoracic inlet and mediastinum below to the skull base above
- Whether the spinal cord is potentially involved
- Risk of the mass being malignant

What the Treating Physician Needs to Know

- Are there associated or causative factors identified, and can such findings be excluded, like multiplicity or adenopathy, that suggest a systemic or metastatic malignancy
- Full extent of the mass and its relationship of the mass to critical surrounding anatomy
- Cause of the mass and degree of confidence in that diagnosis
- Is there a risk of preventable and/or functional or life-threatening complications?
- If any more data needs to be collected with imaging assistance

Answer

1. Superiorly, the process may approach the posterior skull base in the vicinity of the upper cervical spine or foramen magnum. Inferiorly, the mass may track to the supraclavicular fossa and into the upper back. Laterally, the paravertebral space is most often involved. The lateral compartment of the neck may then be secondarily involved. Medially, the process will occupy the midline or a paramedian position; it may involve the spine and neural elements. Anteriorly, the process will displace the prevertebral muscles and fascia and possibly the anterior longitudinal ligament if of PVS/spinal origin. Posteriorly, the process will involve the spinal elements and epidural space; it will expand the containing fascia toward the subcutaneous fat and skin.

LEARN MORE
See Chapters 162 and 37 in *Head and Neck Radiology* by Mancuso and Hanafee.

CLINICAL HISTORY *A 6-year-old child presenting with a low neck mass.*

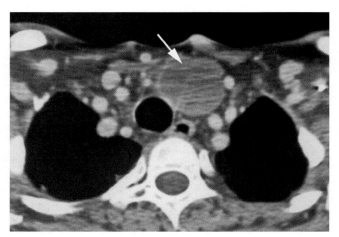

FIGURE **5.14**

FINDINGS

Figure 5.14. CECT study showing a cystic-appearing mass with a thin and not obviously enhancing rim at the thoracic inlet displacing the trachea slightly posterolaterally to the right. There is no connection with the esophagus.

DIFFERENTIAL DIAGNOSIS Tracheal diverticulum, thyroid-origin cyst, pharyngeal diverticulum, developmental malformations (branchial apparatus, venolymphatic malformation, developmental cysts), dermoid/epidermoid cyst, nodal pathology, vascular problems, cystic (degenerated) tumor

DIAGNOSIS Thymic cyst

DISCUSSION In general, the site of origin (one compartment/transcompartmental), vector on surrounding structures, and morphology of the mass itself, as well as any surrounding reactive or associated abnormalities, are the keys to an accurate diagnosis. The rate of incidence and patient factors such as age should be taken into account.

An etiologic approach based on developmental origin should be the primary diagnostic approach to pediatric patients and young adults once the thyroid is excluded as an etiology.

Thymic migration follows the path of the third branchial apparatus from the level of the carotid bifurcation in the lateral compartment to the midline in the low neck, terminating in the mediastinum so that various iterations of thymic remnants may present in the low neck and thoracic inlet. Developmental cysts are mainly related to the thymus and as such tend to be in the midline, then veering to the left.

Venolymphatic malformations are relatively common and the most ubiquitous of the transcompartmental benign masses encountered in the low neck and thoracic inlet.

Disorders of branchial apparatus development may be the source of a mass. Cervicothoracic junction masses may also be related to other branchial cleft or pouch dysgenesis, a prime example being the infected pyriform sinus tract or third branchial cleft cyst and related tracts that most frequently present as an infection in the low neck around the thyroid gland.

Duplication cysts of the foregut and neuroenteric cysts may be a rare cause of a thoracic inlet mass. More commonly, cysts and "celes" related to the pharynx, such as various diverticuli, will occur at sites of natural weaknesses at developmental boundaries between muscles or along penetrating neurovascular bundles.

Rests of germ cell layer tissue may produce epidermoid, dermoid, and teratomatous masses in the low neck and thoracic inlet. Rests of salivary gland tissue are also left within the deep spaces of the head and neck during development. These may give rise to both benign and malignant salivary epithelial tumors at virtually any neck level, but these tumors are rare at this level.

Neurologic developmental abnormalities such as those arising from neural crest remnants and dysraphisms can present as a neck mass.

In this case, a cystic mass in a median to left-sided paramedian position at the thoracic inlet in a child was highly suggestive, although not pathognomonic, of a thymic cyst.

Question for Further Thought

1. What are general considerations when planning the surgical approach?

Reporting Responsibilities

Developmental conditions are typically not of high acuity with regard to management decisions and may be reported routinely unless there is a potential airway or spinal cord compromise or if a malignancy is suspected.

The report should contain precise detail about the full extent of the mass and relationship to critical surrounding anatomic structures that might be the origin of the lesion and/or affected by surgical or other treatment. In general, the most critical of these relationships are how the mass relates to the trachea, brachiocephalic vessels, brachial plexus, and mediastinum.

It is especially important to communicate effectively and promptly if there is a secondary infection and in those cases to anticipate whether there may be a complicating sinus or fistula.

What the Treating Physician Needs to Know

- Origin of the mass
- Extent of the mass
- Likely diagnosis
- Any potential danger to surrounding critical anatomy
- Any airway compromise
- If further imaging would be helpful

Answer

1. A specific surgical approach will depend heavily on the extent and origin of the mass as determined from imaging. Decisions about how a lesion is approached depend on the site of origin and its relationship to the supraclavicular fossa, brachial plexus, and mediastinum; the latter in particular determines whether the surgical approach will require sternum splitting for adequate exposure. The relationship of the mass to the brachiocephalic vessels, particularly the carotid and vertebral arteries, may be pivotal in decision making. In general, masses that remain above the brachiocephalic vein do not require splitting of the sternum for adequate surgical exposure.

> ## LEARN MORE
> See Chapters 164 and 8 in *Head and Neck Radiology* by Mancuso and Hanafee.

CASE 5.15

CLINICAL HISTORY *A 42-year-old female patient presented with supraclavicular fullness and tenderness as well as symptoms suggesting vascular insufficiency in the right arm. She was originally diagnosed as having vasculitis.*

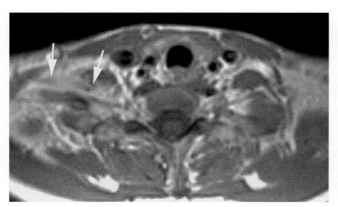

FIGURE 5.15A

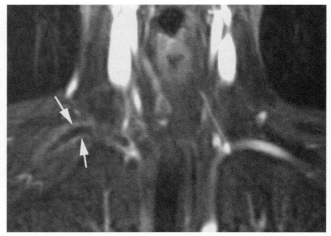

FIGURE 5.15C

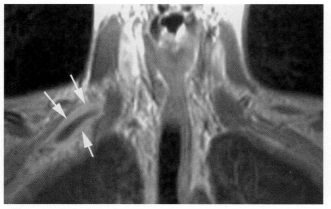

FIGURE 5.15B

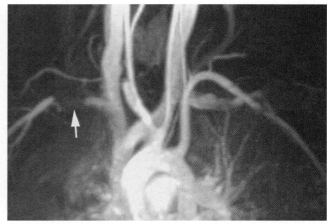

FIGURE 5.15D

FINDINGS

Figure 5.15A. T1W CE image shows enhancement within and around the scalene muscle group (arrows) but is otherwise not definitive.

Figure 5.15B. Coronal T1W CE image shows the subclavian artery wall to enhance (arrows) and that the lumen is potentially patent.

Figure 5.15C,D. Flow-sensitive gradient echo image shows that the right subclavian is actually clotted; that finding is further confirmed on the maximum projection intensity image in (Fig. 5.15D).

DIFFERENTIAL DIAGNOSIS Acute vascular thrombosis in combination with inflammation due to vasculitis, mechanical factors, post radiotherapy, infection, tumor, trauma

DIAGNOSIS Compressive vascular thoracic outlet syndrome (TOS) with surrounding inflammation resulting in vascular occlusion

DISCUSSION Vascular conditions that involve the cervicothoracic junction and brachial plexus are relatively uncommon. They are a possible source of symptoms or even a mass lesion, and a vascular etiology must be considered when a mass is accompanied by signs and symptoms of ischemia or venous occlusion. Such conditions are often lumped under the term *thoracic outlet syndrome;* however, most instances of TOS are manifested only neurologically in the form of a brachial plexopathy.

Other vascular conditions that manifest at the cervicothoracic junction include vascular malformations, vasculitis, dissection, true aneurysms, and contained leaks as well as venous thrombosis and thrombophlebitis and normal variants mimicking pathology.

In this particular case, mechanical irritation and compression resulted in inflammation that also affected the subclavian artery wall. Supposedly the mechanical compression, the inflammation, and possibly the damage to the arterial wall then resulted in an arterial occlusion.

Question for Further Thought

1. What are the surgical implications for a patient with vascular TOS?

Reporting Responsibilities

Compressive thoracic outlet conditions may be a significant acute threat to the patient when acute or subacute arterial occlusion is possible. Such cases require direct, immediate communication with referring providers to decide on any course of additional diagnostic imaging action or endovascular therapeutic interventions. Discovery of a dissection, leak, or aneurysm or high-grade stenosis most often requires prompt and direct communication.

The report should contain precise detail about the full extent of the vascular condition or mass and relationship to critical surrounding anatomic structures that might be causative. In the case of chronic TOS and in general, the most critical of these relationships are those within the zones of potential compression discussed as follows: The first and most critical of these regions is the most proximal interscalene triangle whose borders are the anterior scalene muscle anteriorly, the middle scalene muscle posteriorly, and the medial surface of the first rib inferiorly; the second region of possible constriction is the costoclavicular triangle, which is bordered by the middle third of the clavicle anteriorly, by the first rib posteriorly and medially, and by the upper border of the scapula posteriorly and laterally; the third and most distal region of possible constriction is the subcoracoid space beneath the coracoid process lying deep to the pectoralis minor tendon.

Reporting may be more routine if a benign etiology or chronic vascular condition is identified.

What the Treating Physician Needs to Know

- Likely diagnosis
- Any risk of thromboembolic complications
- Any associated vascular abnormalities such as high-grade stenosis or occlusion, dissection, aneurysm, or contained leaks
- If further imaging or endovascular intervention would be helpful

Answer

1. For vascular TOS, a specific surgical approach will depend heavily on the extent and origin of the compressive zone, if it can be determined from imaging. The zone involved and/or offending structure(s) can be resected. Recent trends have moved away from first rib resection and more toward decompression and reconstruction of the affected zone(s). The procedure is typically just a decompression, but vascular reconstruction, open and/or endovascular, may be necessary if the subclavian artery has been injured.

> ### LEARN MORE
> See Chapters 165 and 15 in *Head and Neck Radiology* by Mancuso and Hanafee.

CLINICAL HISTORY *A 61-year-old woman with prior history of breast cancer presenting with a left-sided brachial plexopathy.*

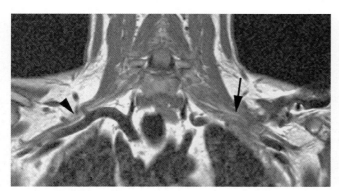

FIGURE **5.16A**

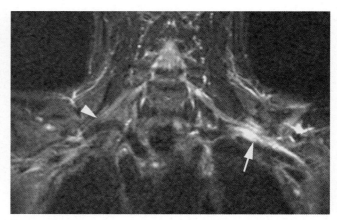

FIGURE **5.16B**

FINDINGS Coronal T1W (Fig. 5.16A) and T2W fat-suppressed (Fig. 5.16B) images showing thickening of the brachial plexus branches and infiltration of the surrounding fat on the left side (arrows) compared to the normal side (arrowheads), without mass lesion. The increased signal, as seen in (Fig. 5.16B), is compatible with related edema.

DIFFERENTIAL DIAGNOSIS Postradiation plexopathy, mechanical irritation TOS with localized tissue reactive response, infectious or other noninfectious inflammation

DIAGNOSIS Postradiation brachial plexopathy

DISCUSSION Inflammatory conditions that involve the cervicothoracic junction and brachial plexus are unusual. Inflammatory conditions generally cause the segments of the plexus involved to enlarge slightly and enhance. The surrounding tissue planes may be preserved but tend to be obscured by reactive changes during the most active phase of the disease. The surrounding planes typically return to normal. The nerves themselves may show persistent swelling and enhancement or evidence of atrophy, depending on the cause and evolution of the process.

The compression in TOS can be aggravated by a localized tissue reactive response due to mechanical irritation and/or associated vasculitis. The inflammation can also be due to other pathologic conditions or the healing process related to these conditions and anatomic variations, with the latter most commonly related to the first rib or fibrous bands.

In the post radiation situation, the trunks and perhaps roots of the brachial plexus tend to enlarge slightly and enhance. The surrounding tissue planes may be preserved but tend to be obscured by reactive changes at the time of the more active phase of the condition usually close to the time of the initial study. The nerve bundles may eventually atrophy, showing brighter than usual signal on T2W images, and the surrounding tissue planes return to normal. Even when the tissue planes return to normal, the roots may remain swollen and edematous and persistently enhance in a chronic active phase of this condition.

Infection may cause brachial plexus inflammation. Other noninfectious pathology such as fibromatoses can mimic an inflammatory condition.

In this case, the diagnosis is fairly straightforward, given the prior history of radiation therapy for breast cancer and in the absence of any mass lesion. The edema in and around the affected part of the brachial plexus correlates with ongoing inflammation. The inflammation can begin and go on for years after the initial radiation, causing a chronic, severe, and painful plexopathy that eventually can result in complete functional loss of the affected upper extremity.

Question for Further Thought

1. What is a possible next diagnostic step if no abnormality can be found within the brachial plexus in a patient with suspected brachial plexopathy?

Reporting Responsibilities

In general, brachial plexus conditions are only occasionally a significant acute threat to the patient—for example, when there is an associated acute or subacute arterial occlusion. Such cases require direct, immediate communication with referring providers to decide on any course of additional diagnostic imaging action or therapeutic interventions.

The report should contain precise detail about the full extent of the inflammatory process and any associated complications, especially if those might affect the epidural space, spinal cord, or nearby brachiocephalic vessels or produce airway compromise.

In this case, the results can be reported routinely. While the disease of the plexus as seen might conceivably be due to recurrent cancer, the morphology of disease as seen on this study would much more strongly suggest plexopathy. As a result, the wording in the report should be constructed carefully so that the patient is not unduly worried about recurrence. A suggestion for ongoing surveillance can then be guided by the clinical evolution of the disease. A follow-up study in 6 months, assuming the clinical situation remains relatively stable, can be done to reassure that the plexopathy is not related to recurrent cancer.

What the Treating Physician Needs to Know

- Likely diagnosis of inflammatory vs. neoplastic condition
- Any associated vascular abnormalities such as high-grade stenosis or occlusion, dissection, aneurysm, or contained leaks
- Any risk of thromboembolic complications
- If further imaging or endovascular intervention would be helpful

Answer

1. It is wise to remember that central neurologic pathology such as multiple sclerosis or acute disseminated encephalomyelitis may cause plexopathy-like symptoms and should be investigated accordingly.

> LEARN MORE
>
> See Chapters 166 and 13 in *Head and Neck Radiology* by Mancuso and Hanafee.

CLINICAL HISTORY *A 56-year-old man developing left-sided brachial plexopathy.*

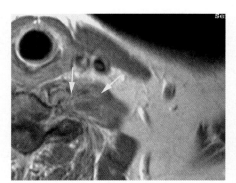

FIGURE **5.17A**

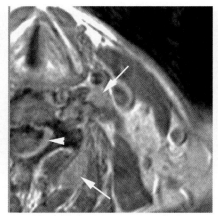

FIGURE **5.17B**

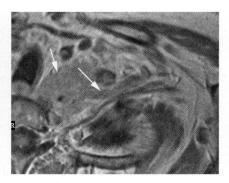

FIGURE **5.17C**

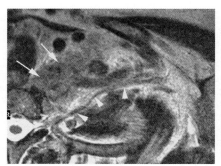

FIGURE **5.17D**

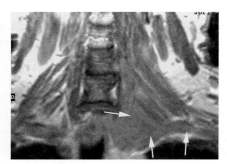

FIGURE **5.17E**

FINDINGS

Figure 5.17A–C. T1W axial images. These show a mass infiltrating the scalene muscles and the posterior compartment (arrows) as well as extending along the nerve root sheath to involve the epidural space (arrowheads).

Figure 5.17D. T2W image shows the infiltrating mass to be of signal intensity consistent with tumor (arrow) and sparing of a lower brachial plexus nerve root and trunk (arrowheads).

Figure 5.17E. Coronal T1W image shows the overall extent of the spread within and around the brachial plexus (arrows).

DIFFERENTIAL DIAGNOSIS Primary tumor (e.g., lung apex), tumor recurrence after therapy in the form of metastases and perineural spread, supraclavicular node metastases with extranodal tumor growth, postradiation plexopathy, inflammatory pathology

DIAGNOSIS Lymphoma, likely breaking out of the nodes and invading in a perineural pattern

DISCUSSION The primary imaging observation will most often be that of a mass and whether the origin of the mass is the brachial plexus. This is followed by an analysis of whether the plexus is secondarily involved or the mass secondarily involves adjacent critical structures or is associated with more remote regional (e.g., nodal) disease. A specific structure of origin aside from the plexus might be suggested based on anatomic localization. The morphology, in addition to localization and the patient's clinical history, is sometimes distinctive enough to allow a specific diagnosis.

In this case, the withheld medical history of lymphoma in combination with nodal disease and extranodal spread invading the adjacent structures including the brachial plexus leaves no room for a broad differential diagnosis. Please be aware that lymphoma may also present, as opposed to recur, in this pattern.

The general differential diagnosis when considering plexopathy due to a malignant mass lesion is quite broad. If the patient has been treated for a malignancy, the plexopathy may result from perineural recurrence of disease or metastases to adjacent nodes that then grows out of the node capsule to spread along the plexus. Both these mechanisms of failure, for instance, occur in breast and lung cancer. Primary cancers at the apex of the lung can invade the chest wall and plexus directly or metastasize to the supraclavicular nodes and secondarily invade the plexus. The same is true of metastases to the supraclavicular nodes from other malignancies originating below the clavicles. Leukemia and lymphoma can have a perineural spread pattern that affects the plexus and/or be secondary to extranodal spread of supraclavicular and low neck nodal disease. If there are bilateral masses, a systemic disease such as lymphoma should be suspected.

More slowly progressive plexopathy may due to benign or slowly progressive tumors such as those of nerve sheath origin or those in the spectrum of the fibromatoses.

Question for Further Thought

1. Give possible types of neurologic involvement in the case of a growing cervicothoracic junction mass.

Reporting Responsibilities

Brachial plexus masses are unpredictable with regard to threat to the patient but are more often "bad news" than good. They may be reported routinely unless there is a potential airway or spinal cord compromise or if a malignancy is suspected. Many of these cases require direct communication with referring providers when a mass is first discovered to decide on a next best course of action, especially if imaging-directed biopsy may help.

The report should contain precise detail about the full extent of the mass and relationship to critical surrounding anatomic structures that might be the origin of the lesion and/or affected by surgical or other treatment. The most proximal extent of spread along plexus trunks and roots must be noted in detail. If epidural space and intrathecal spread can be excluded with confidence, such exclusionary observations would be useful to report.

Other critical relationships of plexus tumors include how the mass has extended relative to the mediastinum, supraclavicular fossa and chest wall, trachea, and carotid and vertebral arteries.

Communication may need to become urgent or emergent if a tumor causes brachiocephalic vascular insufficiency or threatens the airway or spinal cord.

What the Treating Physician Needs to Know

- Origin of the mass
- Extent of the mass
- Likely diagnosis
- Any potential danger to surrounding critical anatomy
- Any airway compromise
- If further imaging would be helpful

Answer

1. Neurologic deficits such as brachial plexopathy, Horner syndrome (sympathetic chain), vocal cord weakness (vagus and/or recurrent laryngeal nerve), or a paralyzed diaphragm (phrenic nerve) are not unusual and when present suggest that the mass causing it is likely to be malignant.

LEARN MORE

See Chapters 167 and 27 in *Head and Neck Radiology* by Mancuso and Hanafee.

CLINICAL HISTORY *A 27-year-old man with severe functional loss of the right arm after a motorbike accident.*

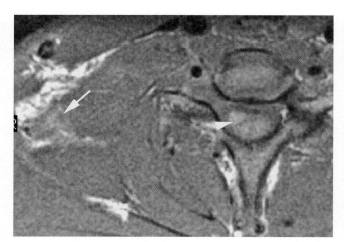

FIGURE 5.18A

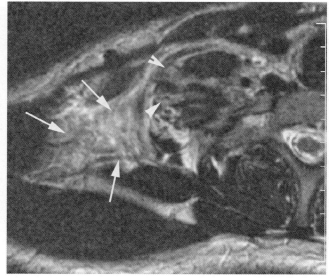

FIGURE 5.18C

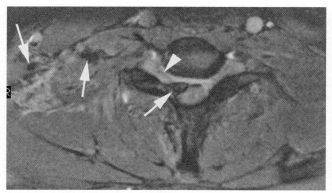

FIGURE 5.18B

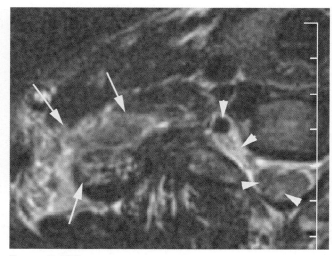

FIGURE 5.18D

FINDINGS

Figure 5.18A. T1W image shows subacute blood products along the lateral margin of the scalene muscle (arrow) and generalized swelling within that muscle group. There is a small hematoma adjacent to the root entry zone of the cervical roots at the spinal cord (arrowhead) that is more conspicuous on some of the following images.

Figure 5.18B. Fat-suppressed CE T1W image showing blood products along the roots and trunks of the brachial plexus distally to the root entry zone at the spinal cord, where there is a discreet hematoma (arrows) proximally.

An abnormal-appearing nerve root is visible within the nerve root sheath (arrowhead).

Figure 5.18C. The T2W image shows the extensive soft tissue swelling surrounding the trunks of the brachial plexus (arrows) and the swollen distal roots (arrowheads) as they emerge between the scalene muscles (arrowheads). The findings taken together suggest gross disruption of the root–trunk junction.

Figure 5.18D. The T2W image shows the extensive soft tissue swelling surrounding the trunks of the brachial plexus (arrows) as well as blood products and disrupted nerve roots within the nerve root sheath to the root entry zone, where there may be minimal cord edema (arrowheads).

DIFFERENTIAL DIAGNOSIS None

DIAGNOSIS Severe, mainly preganglionic, posttraumatic brachial plexus injury

DISCUSSION Variable brachial plexus injury can result from blunt trauma (especially in the multitrauma setting) or penetrating trauma. Traction injuries wherein the head and neck are moved violently away from the ipsilateral shoulder are most common. Shoulder dystocia during birth is a relatively common cause of such traction injury.

In traction-type injuries, it is important to establish whether the injury is proximal (preganglionic) or distal (postganglionic) to the dorsal root ganglion. Preganglionic ruptures may be central at the root entry zone junction with the spinal cord or more distal than the root entry zone but still intradural. Preganglionic root avulsion does not cause wallerian degeneration or traumatic neuroma formation but causes the cell bodies of the sensory nerves to be pulled from the cord, greatly reducing the possibility of recovery or chance of successful surgical reconstruction. The development of an injury-related pseudomeningocele strongly suggests a preganglionic injury. Postganglionic lesions are physiologically similar to peripheral nerve injuries; the healing/regenerative response of the nerve may produce a neuroma when the path of the regenerating axons is blocked by scarring. Critical factors for restoring upper arm function after brachial plexus injury are patient selection, timing of surgery, and prioritization of restoration.

In a multitrauma setting, the clinical diagnosis of brachial plexus injury might be delayed, particularly when combined with head and spinal trauma, warranting for a high index of suspicion. Imaging is essential in cases where there might be an acute vascular complication.

Later on in the nonimmediate posttraumatic setting, swelling of the plexus might occur as well as denervation edema within the denervated muscle groups followed by atrophy.

Question for Further Thought

1. What is the diagnostic role of CT and MRI in brachial plexus injuries?

Reporting Responsibilities

The diagnosis of brachial plexus injury is made clinically, so reporting is most often routine.

If there is an acute compressive hematoma and/or acute vascular complication or any threat to the spinal cord, this should be communicated verbally and emergently.

The report should contain precise detail about the cause and extent of the brachial plexus injury as outlined in the following section.

What the Treating Physician Needs to Know

- Extent of injury to the brachial plexus and cervical cord
- Whether the injury is preganglionic (proximal) and/or postganglionic (distal) relative to the nerve root ganglion
- Is there compressive pathology, either musculoskeletal or due to hematoma, that might produce neuropraxis as opposed to a nerve disruption?
- Is there an associated vascular injury?
- Is there an associated spinal injury that might be unstable?
- Is there an associated musculoskeletal injury?
- If chronic, is there evidence of a posttraumatic neuroma?

Answer

1. MRI is the primary diagnostic tool in most instances of traction, blunt, and penetrating injuries. If detailed views of the dorsal and ventral root entry zones within the thecal sac are required, then volumetric CT myelography may prove more consistently definitive than MRI in cases of subtle, preganglionic nerve root injury. MRI and volumetric CT myelography are sometimes complementary, and both may be necessary.

LEARN MORE
See Chapter 168 in *Head and Neck Radiology* by Mancuso and Hanafee.

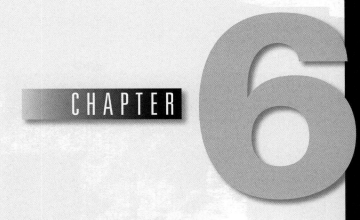

CHAPTER 6

Thyroid and Parathyroid Glands

CLINICAL HISTORY *A 46-year-old female patient with a history of an enlarging neck mass.*

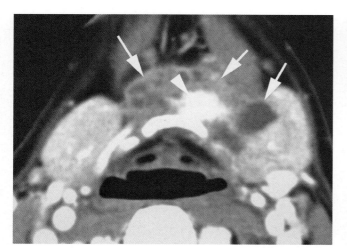

FIGURE **6.1A**

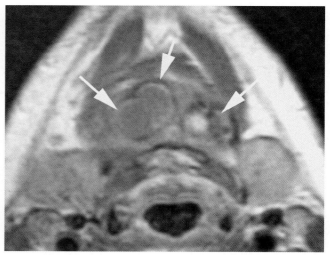

FIGURE **6.1C**

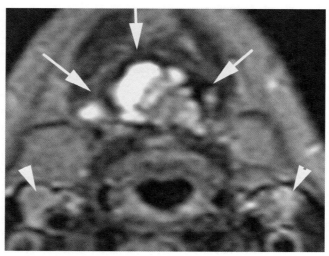

FIGURE **6.1B**

FINDINGS

Figure 6.1A. Contrast-enhanced computed tomography (CECT) study shows a complex multicystic mass invading the floor of the mouth and submandibular space (arrows). There is enhancing thyroid tissue that is markedly irregular at its margins within the multicystic mass (arrowhead).

Figure 6.1B. T2W images showing the multicystic component of the mass correlating well with the computed tomography (CT) study in (Fig. 6.1A). There appears to be a dense dark pseudocapsule at the margins of the mass, suggesting adherence to the floor of the mouth. There is bilateral level 2 metastatic adenopathy (arrowheads).

Figure 6.1C. Contrast-enhanced (CE) T1W magnetic resonance (MR) image shows the complex mass invading the floor of the mouth anterior to the hyoid bone (arrows).

DIFFERENTIAL DIAGNOSIS Not applicable

DIAGNOSIS Thyroglossal duct remnant with a thyroid carcinoma arising in ectopic thyroid tissue

DISCUSSION Thyroid developmental anomalies generally arise when the thyroglossal duct incompletely develops, obliterates, and/or descends, causing agenesis or hypoplasia of the thyroid gland, thyroid gland ectopia, or thyroglossal duct remnants. All thyroid congenital anomalies occur along the thyroglossal tract in a median/paramedian location from the foramen cecum of the tongue to the thyroid isthmus anterior to the upper trachea. They commonly present as a neck mass or are found incidentally on studies done for other indications.

Thyroglossal duct cyst (TGDC) anomalies are the most common visceral compartment abnormality to present as a neck mass. Although most frequently infrahyoid, they can also be suprahyoid or at the level of the hyoid. When infrahyoid, they lie along the laryngeal skeleton, usually superficial to the infrahyoid strap muscles, though they can project into the pre-epiglottic space. They are usually well circumscribed and generally round. The margin is nonenhancing unless there is inflammation or functioning thyroid tissue. The main contents are fluid density, but the signal intensity on MR will vary depending on the cyst content modified by substances such as colloid protein and products of bleeding. The cysts are often multiloculated and may enlarge or change abruptly anywhere along their paths with areas appearing as a tiny tract and at others as large multi- or unilocular cysts. TGDCs may be associated with incomplete descent of thyroid tissue that at risk for the same diseases that might be encountered in a normal thyroid gland including cysts, adenomas, and rarely a malignancy.

Thyroid carcinoma is rare in TGDCs. When this occurs, there is also a multifocal papillary carcinoma in the thyroid gland in at least 25% of the patients. Thyroglossal duct remnants are typically unilocular or multilocular cystic structures with a relatively small amount of solid components. If the thyroglossal tract mass is predominantly solid, then cancer should be suspected even if there are no signs of aggressive features such as local tissue invasion or metastatic lymph nodes.

Questions for Further Thought

1. What is the significance of a dark pseudocapsule surrounding a TGDC on MR?
2. How are TGDCs treated surgically?
3. Is ultrasound useful for the evaluation of thyroid developmental anomalies?

Reporting Responsibilities

Although thyroid anomalies are generally chronic entities, suspicion of an associated malignancy should be verbally communicated to the referring provider.

What the Treating Physician Needs to Know

- Are the findings due to a thyroid anomaly or possibly another condition?
- Is the finding associated with glandular ectopias or pathology arising in ectopic glandular tissue, and is there multifocal ectopia?
- Full extent of the TGDC relative to surrounding anatomy and the usual course of thyroid anlage descent
- Is there ectopic tissue in association with the TGDC?
- Are there associated findings of importance that suggest an alternative diagnosis or critical associated condition such as thyroid cancer?

Answers

1. A dark pseudocapsule surrounding a TGDC on MR is strongly suggestive of dense adherence to the surrounding structures. The finding of adherence to an adjacent structure or to the skin or lobulations will alter the surgical management and should always be sought for and reported.

2. Although ultrasound can confirm the cystic nature of the mass and perhaps if thyroid tissue is present, it will not show the full extent of an anomaly. Therefore, it is considered cost additive and not definitive for the medical decision making required.

3. The classic surgery is a complete Sistrunk procedure, which includes resection of the mid portion of the hyoid and removal of a 5- to 10-mm core of tissue between the hyoid and foramen cecum at the tongue base and a dissection continuously down to the thyroid, removing all abnormal tissue along the tract of descent. Current imaging techniques permit modification of this procedure depending on the extent of disease identified.

> ## LEARN MORE
> See Chapters 170 and 22 in *Head and Neck Radiology* by Mancuso and Hanafee.

CLINICAL HISTORY *A 62-year-old euthyroid female patient presenting with dyspnea of exertion.*

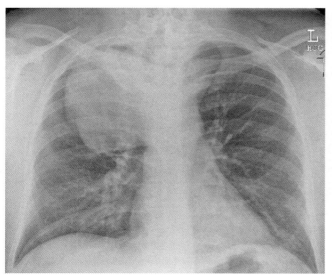

FIGURE **6.2A**

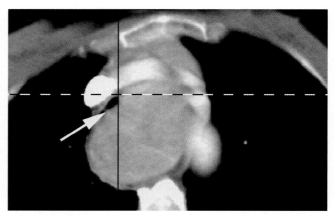

FIGURE **6.2C**

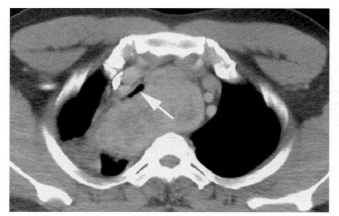

FIGURE **6.2B**

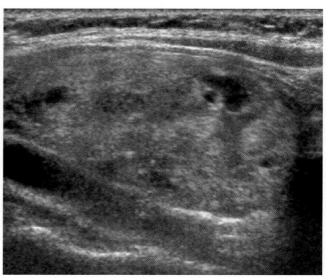

FIGURE **6.2D**

FINDINGS

Figure 6.2A. Routine chest x-ray shows likely thyroid gland enlargement.

Figure 6.2B. CECT shows a mass extending into the mediastinum, posterior and laterally to the right of the trachea, causing significant compression of the airway (arrow).

Figure 6.2C. The mass extends posterior to the left brachiocephalic trunk inferiorly into the mediastinum.

Figure 6.2D. Ultrasound shows a multinodular mass.

DIFFERENTIAL DIAGNOSIS Nontoxic thyroid gland enlargement, thyroid lymphoma, anaplastic thyroid carcinoma

DIAGNOSIS Nontoxic multinodular thyroid gland enlargement (goiter)

DISCUSSION Goiter is described as an enlargement of the thyroid gland without any associated functional derangement or malignancy. It can be uniformly diffuse or restricted to a particular area. Thyroid nodules are discrete focal growth of thyroid cells and may contribute or just coexist within an enlarged gland. They are endemic in regions deficient in iodine but are otherwise sporadic in areas with iodine-enriched diets. Goiters are more common in females and the elderly population.

Goiterogenesis is multifactorial, with genetic and environmental causes being the major players. Most patients have normal thyroid-stimulating hormone (TSH) levels since various TSH-independent growth factors are responsible for increase in the thyroid gland volume.

The goiter tissue is often heterogeneous both histologically, since it contains areas of hemorrhage, follicles filled with colloid, zones of hyperplasia, and even neoplasia, and physiologically, since some follicles have a high capacity to uptake iodine and produce thyroid hormones, whereas others lack this ability.

Goiters present as a very slow growing mass or with obstructive symptoms such as globus sensation or positional/exertional dyspnea. Acute bleeding can exacerbate these symptoms.

Imaging is done to determine the extent and consistency of the gland. Patients with nodular disease may be further investigated with fine-needle aspiration but, unfortunately, multiple nodules carry the same risk of malignancy as a single nodule. Radioiodine therapy may be useful to shrink diffusely enlarged glands. Surgery is reserved for patients who fail or are poor candidates for radioiodine therapy or for immediate relief of symptoms.

Questions for Further Thought

1. What is the importance of describing if a neck mass extends into the superior mediastinum, posterior to the brachiocephalic vessels?
2. What is the significance of vocal cord dysfunction in a patient with a presumed goiter?

3. What are the most common malignancies that mimic a goiter?

Reporting Responsibilities

Although goiters are generally chronic entities, suspicion of an associated malignancy should be verbally communicated to the referring provider.

What the Treating Physician Needs to Know

- Are the findings due to a nontoxic goiter or possibly another condition?
- Are there associated findings of importance that suggest an alternative diagnosis or a critical associated condition such as thyroid cancer?
- Full extent of a nontoxic goiter, including its relationship to the trachea, esophagus, and brachiocephalic vessels, and extent of mediastinal extension

Answers

1. If surgery is contemplated, extent up to the level and inferior to the left brachiocephalic vein usually indicates that there will need to be a sternum-splitting procedure to fully excise the mass.
2. This is a red flag that suggests the enlargement is *not* benign and the "goiter" is actually a cancer or there is a cancer within a multinodular goiter.
3. The malignancies most commonly mimicking a goiter are anaplastic thyroid cancer and lymphoma.

> **LEARN MORE**
> See Chapters 171 and 22 in *Head and Neck Radiology* by Mancuso and Hanafee.

CLINICAL HISTORY *A 58-year-old female patient with a history of a "goiter." She now presents with progressive hoarseness.*

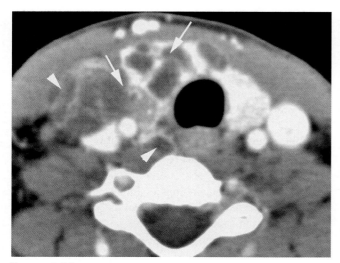

FIGURE **6.3A**

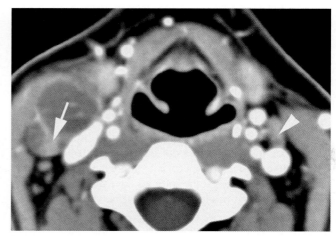

FIGURE **6.3C**

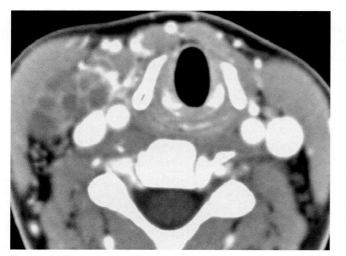

FIGURE **6.3B**

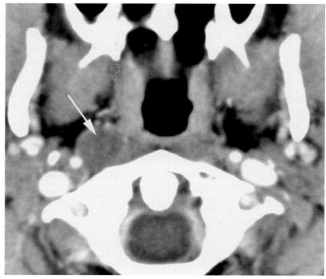

FIGURE **6.3D**

FINDINGS

Figure 6.3A. CECT shows a mass (arrows) contiguous with level 4 and 6 metastatic lymph nodes (arrowheads).

Figure 6.3B. More superiorly, there is a multicystic pattern of level 3 adenopathy.

Figure 6.3C. Upper level 4 cystic adenopathy with an enhancing mural nodule (arrow). There also is a contralateral enhancing positive node with a focal low density defect (arrowhead).

Figure 6.3D. Cystic retropharyngeal node metastasis.

DIFFERENTIAL DIAGNOSIS None

DIAGNOSIS Papillary thyroid carcinoma with cervical and retropharyngeal node metastases

DISCUSSION Thyroid nodules are commonly identified as incidental findings on examinations of the neck done for other purposes than evaluating the thyroid gland. How to manage many of these incidentally discovered nodules continues to be a complicated issue and can pose a problem from the patient's point of view and/or the referring clinician concerning the risk of cancer in one of these nodules.

Thyroid carcinoma is a relatively uncommon disease of highly variable clinical behavior; many of these cancers will never threaten the life expectancy of the patient, even if left untreated. They are more common in females worldwide and in whites in the United States.

Thyroid cancer can arise from the thyroid follicle (papillary, follicular, and anaplastic), parafollicular cells (medullary), and lymphocytes (thyroid lymphoma). Papillary and follicular lesions comprise 80% of the total group.

Papillary carcinomas most commonly present as an incidental thyroidal mass without lymph node metastasis or as lower cervical lymphadenopathy. They can cause vocal cord weakness, dysphagia, or airway symptoms.

These cancers are typically slow-growing unencapsulated tumors that are frequently multifocal and do not have a tendency toward vascular invasion. About half of the patients have gross evidence of regional lymph node metastasis at surgery, characteristically to levels 3, 4, and 6. When there is a substantial amount of neck disease, thyroid carcinoma has a particular tendency to metastasize to retropharyngeal nodes. Level 6 nodes are a common site of recurrence. Lymph node metastasis will characteristically have a cystic component and/or a densely enhancing nodule, sometimes with calcification. If a node with such morphology and distribution is present on a study, the primary is always in the thyroid even if it cannot be seen by imaging.

Extension of the primary tumor through the capsule with invasion of the surrounding viscera and distant metastasis are possible. Regressive changes such as cyst formation and psammomatous calcifications are common at imaging.

Questions for Further Thought

1. When should thyroid cancers be examined by CT or MR imaging?
2. What are recognized risk factors for the development of thyroid cancers?
3. What ultrasound features increase the probability of a nodule being malignant?

Reporting Responsibilities

Verbal communication with the referring physician is mandatory if the tumor places the airway at risk, when an anticipated tracheostomy might cross tumoral tissue, if a tumor that was not clinically suspected is discovered, or any time anaplastic carcinoma or thyroid lymphoma is suspected because of the risk of rapid dissemination and/or rapid growth with airway compromise.

What the Treating Physician Needs to Know

• Risk of malignancy of a thyroid nodule and follow-up options based on currently applicable guidelines

• If not thyroid cancer, what is the likely alternative diagnosis for a low neck mass, adenopathy, or cause of vocal cord weakness or paralysis based on imaging?
• Exact extent of the primary tumor lesion within the thyroid gland
• Evidence for invasion beyond the gland capsule to involve the laryngeal framework, trachea and esophagus, and structures of the carotid sheath
• *Neck lymph nodes:* Are they involved? Where are the pathologic lymph nodes located? Any evidence for extranodal tumor spread?
• *Posttreatment imaging:* Is there any suspicion for tumor recurrence?

Answers

1. CT and MR are most useful for the following:
   • Establishing the extraglandular extent of a tumor, especially in the following cases:
     • A cancer discovered by ultrasound is greater than 3 cm in size, because of the likelihood of capsular penetration.
     • A tumor is potentially associated with vocal cord weakness, dysphagia, or airway symptoms. MR is the primary study for establishing the local extent of a known cancer since it is superior to CT at evaluating soft tissue invasion (i.e., tracheal/esophageal wall). Invasion to the laryngeal skeleton is best evaluated with CT. Neurovascular involvement can be determined with any of the two modalities.
     • Evaluation of the extent nodal metastasis since superior mediastinal and retropharyngeal lymph nodes cannot be reliably evaluated by ultrasound. CT has a modest advantage over MR in detecting nodal disease.

2. Risk factors for the development of thyroid cancer include a thyroid mass in a child or young adult, history of neck irradiation, family history of thyroid cancer, rapid growth, lymphadenopathy, and tracer accumulation on an FDG-PET study.

3. Ultrasound features of increased risk of malignancy include the following:
   Morphology: Nodules with greater than a 25% solid component, microcalcifications, hypoechoic nodule, irregular margins, or the absence of a halo.
   Flow: Predominantly peripheral flow is suggestive of a benign nodule, while those with hypervascularity toward the center of the nodule are at a higher risk of malignancy.

> LEARN MORE
> See Chapters 172 and 22 in *Head and Neck Radiology* by Mancuso and Hanafee.

CASE 6.4

CLINICAL HISTORY *A 57-year-old female patient with a history of known chronic thyroiditis now presenting with a discrete mass in the left lobe of the gland.*

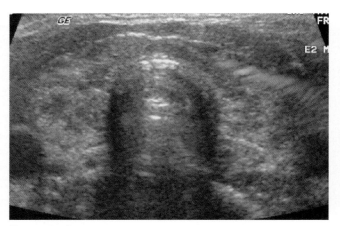

FIGURE 6.4A

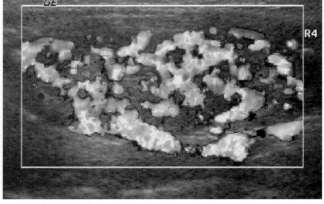

FIGURE 6.4C

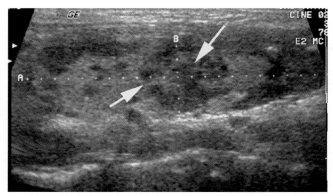

FIGURE 6.4B

FINDINGS

Figure 6.4A. Axial ultrasound image shows a slightly enlarged thyroid gland with a diffuse texture abnormality and no focal mass.

Figure 6.4B. Sagittal image shows a diffuse texture abnormality and a discrete focal nodule (arrows).

Figure 6.4C. Color flow Doppler image shows diffuse hypervascularity both within the questionable nodule and the gland—a nonspecific finding.

DIFFERENTIAL DIAGNOSIS Chronic inflammatory thyroiditis with an associated granuloma, chronic thyroiditis complicated with thyroid lymphoma, superimposed infectious thyroiditis and abscess

DIAGNOSIS Chronic thyroiditis complicated with thyroid lymphoma

DISCUSSION Chronic thyroiditis is an autoimmune disease against the thyroid gland, ultimately leading to a decrease in its function. The functional effects of chronic thyroiditis

may be seen as an incidental abnormal tracer accumulation on studies done for other reasons, especially on radionuclide studies such as those done using gallium or FDG-PET. Imaging may be done to identify a possible cause of airway and/or esophageal compressive symptoms. The late effects may be seen as a small gland on MR or CT.

Thyroid lymphoma is a sporadic disease, but the risk is much higher in patients with chronic thyroiditis. It grows in a usually highly infiltrating pattern beyond the capsule of the gland to invade any of the surrounding structures. Lymph nodes may not be involved.

Ultrasound has been used for surveillance in patients with chronic thyroiditis who may develop thyroid lymphoma as a late complication. This appears as a new texture change in a gland of already abnormal texture due to the effects of chronic thyroiditis.

Thyroid lymphoma is generally high grade and likely to be hypermetabolic on FDG studies. The suspicion of thyroid lymphoma constitutes an emergent finding due to the risk of rapid dissemination and/or rapid growth with airway compression.

Questions for Further Thought

1. What role does imaging play in the evaluation of thyroid inflammatory disease?
2. What situations may predispose the patient for the development of a life-threatening thyroid dysfunction?

Reporting Responsibilities

Immediate direct verbal communication with the referring treatment provider is required in the event of a discovery of a threatened airway or a lesion suspicious of malignancy rather than an inflammatory condition. The findings of acute thyroiditis and trauma should also be directly communicated since these conditions can potentially lead to a thyroid storm becoming a medical emergency.

What the Treating Physician Needs to Know

- If the findings are due to an inflammatory condition
- If there are associated findings that suggest an alternative diagnosis or critical associated condition such as thyroid cancer
- If there is a threat to the airway
- Are there circumstances that could lead to thyroid storm?

Answers

1. Imaging has a limited role in thyroid disease and trauma and is contributory to the disease management plan only after a complete clinical evaluation, including laboratory; otherwise, the findings can be very nonspecific.
2. Thyroiditis (usually acute) and thyroid trauma can predispose the patient to development of a life-threatening thyroid storm.

> **LEARN MORE**
> See Chapters 173 and 27 in *Head and Neck Radiology* by Mancuso and Hanafee.

CLINICAL HISTORY *A 61-year-old male patient who was found to have hypercalcemia and high parathyroid hormone levels.*

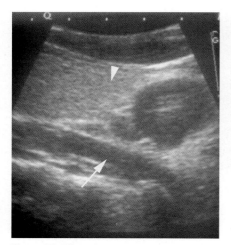

FIGURE 6.5A

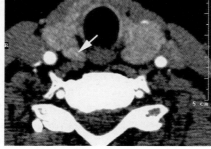

FIGURE 6.5B1

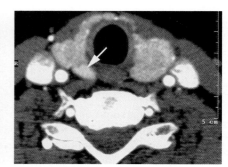

FIGURE 6.5B2

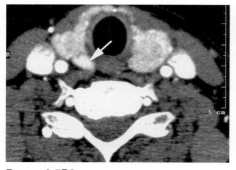

FIGURE 6.5B3

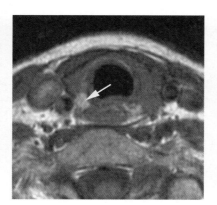

FIGURE 6.5C

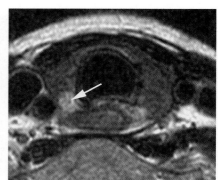

FIGURE 6.5D

FINDINGS

Figure 6.5A. Sagittal ultrasound image showing a hypoechoic nodule between the longus colli muscle and thyroid gland in a different patient, which would be about what was expected in this patient, and demonstrating the ease of using ultrasound in this condition in most patients.

Figure 6.5B. Three-phase CT study in the patient under consideration whose MR image is seen in (Fig. 6.5C,D), demonstrating progressive accumulation of contrast (from top to bottom) in the lesion (arrow).

Figure 6.5C. T1W noncontrast MR image shows a lesion with increased signal intensity relative to muscle.

Figure 6.5D. T2W MR image shows the lesion to be hyperintense relative to muscle and the thyroid gland.

DIFFERENTIAL DIAGNOSIS Parathyroid adenoma, thyroid adenoma, level 6 lymph node

DIAGNOSIS Parathyroid adenoma

DISCUSSION Hyperparathyroidism (HPT) is the excessive production of parathyroid hormone. The most common cause of HPT is a single parathyroid gland adenoma (>80%). Other causes include four gland hyperplasia (10%), double adenomas (4–5%), and carcinoma (1%).

Although most parathyroid tissues and adenomas are in the neck, they can develop anywhere from the carotid bifurcation to the lowermost positions of thymic migration in the anterior mediastinum.

The most important function of head and neck imaging in the preoperative evaluation of HPT is localizing the cause. The current approach to localization with excellent results is a logical progression from ultrasound to radionuclide studies and then CT for problem solving. MR has many limitations in the evaluation of adenomas, but it can be used in patients who cannot have iodinated contrast. Recurrent disease is best evaluated with a combination of anatomic CT and functional sestamibi exams.

Ultrasound evaluates adenomas that are in the normal parathyroid gland positions and ectopic glands inferior to the thyroid gland but above the mediastinum. Upper pole adenomas are less reliably localized when ectopic. Normal parathyroid glands are not confidently visible with ultrasound. A parathyroid adenoma appears as a well-marginated homogenously hypoechoic nodule in the region between the thyroid gland and longus colli. The fibrofatty pad that normally surrounds the gland will be compressed and may appear as a thin hyperechoic line separating the adenoma from the thyroid gland. Power Doppler imaging may identify polar vessels feeding the adenoma.

Technetium sestamibi will show a nodule that should display delayed washout compared to the thyroid gland.

CECT and MR will show a homogeneously enhancing nodule with smooth margins. Adenomas will be bright on T2W imaging and isointense to muscle on noncontrast T1W imaging. They may show necrosis.

Questions for Further Thought

1. How is HPT classified?
2. What features are suggestive of parathyroid carcinoma?

Reporting Responsibilities

In general, the disease is known or highly suspected at the time of imaging, so no special communication is required. Suspicion of a rare carcinoma might be directly communicated, but this usually is of no more risk to the patient than an adenoma.

What the Treating Physician Needs to Know

- That the study was done with a protocol that includes all potential ectopic sites

- If it is a solitary adenoma
- Exact location of the adenoma or adenomas
- Degree of confidence in localization
- If there is a chance of hyperplasia or an adenoma coexistent with hyperplasia
- If there is any indication of a rare parathyroid carcinoma

Answers

1. HPT may be classified as primary, secondary, or tertiary. Primary HPT is due to autonomously functioning adenoma(s) or carcinoma. Secondary HPT is due to glandular hyperplasia driven by the physiologic state of calcium and phosphorus metabolism that accompanies chronic renal failure. Tertiary HPT is caused by prolonged secondary HPT, which leads to autonomous production of parathyroid hormone as the glands become insensitive to calcium and phosphate levels, even after normalization of electrolyte balance after a kidney transplant.

2. Calcification and level 6 adenopathy are suggestive of malignancy at imaging. The diagnosis is based on invasion into blood vessels, the lymphatic network, and the capsule. Most of the time, those features are not evident until the permanent sections are evaluated.

LEARN MORE
See Chapters 174 and 22 in *Head and Neck Radiology* by Mancuso and Hanafee.

Major Salivary Glands: Parotid, Submandibular, Sublingual

CLINICAL HISTORY *A 13-year-old male patient with a left parotid region and upper neck mass.*

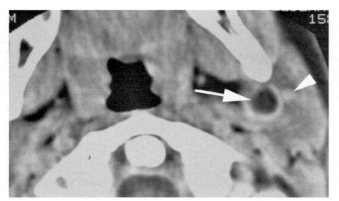

FIGURE **7.1A**

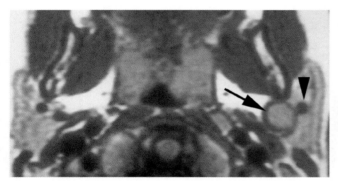

FIGURE **7.1B**

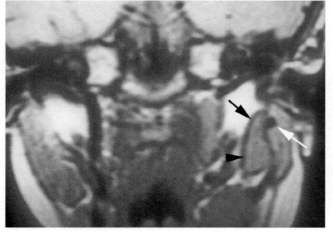

FIGURE **7.1C**

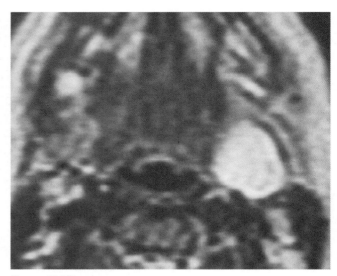

FIGURE **7.1D**

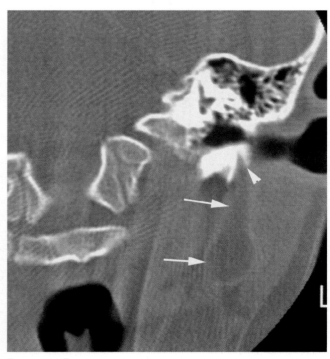

FIGURE **7.1E**

FINDINGS

Figure 7.1A,B. Contrast-enhanced computed tomography (CECT) and T1W magnetic resonance (MR) images study show a cystic tract (arrow) deep to the expected position of the facial nerve that should be lateral to the retromandibular vein (arrowhead) on higher sections through the gland.

Figure 7.1C. T1W coronal image shows the fairly typical appearance of this type of brachial apparatus cyst, with the more dilated part of the cyst seen inferiorly (arrowhead) while it tapers toward a potential tract toward the external auditory canal (black arrow) but clearly remains deep to the expected position of the main trunk of the facial nerve, which at this level in the parotid gland should lie just lateral to the retromandibular vein (white arrow).

Figure 7.1D. Bone window shows a cyst to the parotid gland (white arrow) with a portion involving the external auditory canal (white arrowhead).

Figure 7.1E. T2W image confirms the cystic nature of the mass and demonstrates its more expansile portion.

DIFFERENTIAL DIAGNOSIS Not applicable

DIAGNOSIS First branchial cleft cyst and sinus tract

DISCUSSION Developmental abnormalities that involve the parotid region are mainly those due to venolymphatic malformations and first branchial apparatus abnormalities. First branchial apparatus developmental abnormalities can present below the angle of the mandible or within or around the parotid gland. They most commonly result in fistulas and cysts.

First branchial cleft cysts have been classified into types: Bailey type 1 cysts are generally superficial in location relative to the parotid gland; Bailey type 2 cysts run through the gland usually deep to the expected position of the facial nerve main trunk.

First branchial cleft fistulas and sinus tracts will typically be near the junction of the bone and cartilage portions of the external auditory canal. These usually cannot be identified. The tympanic and styloid portions of the temporal bone, as well as the external auditory canal, may be deformed. There may be an associated epidermoid cyst.

Patients with first branchial cleft cysts present with a periparotid or upper neck mass; if there is a sinus tract to the skin, they may present with inflammation in the region of the sinus or with an infected cyst. Facial nerve dysfunction is rare.

Questions for Further Thought

1. What is the most common cause of a cystic neck mass in adults?

2. What findings are suggestive of branchial cleft cysts in children and young adults?

Reporting Responsibilities

Although branchial apparatus anomalies are generally chronic entities, immediate direct communication with the referring treatment provider is required in the event of a discovery of an unsuspected malignancy and in circumstances where it may be anticipated from imaging that a major change in medical decision making might be made.

What the Treating Physician Needs to Know

- Are the findings due to a branchial apparatus anomaly or possibly another condition such as a venolymphatic malformation or neoplasm?
- If a branchial apparatus cyst, its full extent relative to surrounding anatomy, especially the facial nerve
- Is there an associated sinus or fistula? If so, what is the extent of that finding?
- Are there associated findings principally of the temporal bone?
- Do the findings suggest a developmental condition that may be syndromic?

Answers

1. A cystic mass is far more likely to be of nodal neoplastic or inflammatory origin unless there are some characteristic associated findings to suggest a developmental cyst. This tendency clearly increases with age.

2. A history of intermittent changes in size or inflammation of a mass is mostly suggestive of a branchial cleft cyst, although venolymphatic malformations may also present in a similar fashion.

LEARN MORE
See Chapters 176 and 13 in *Head and Neck Radiology* by Mancuso and Hanafee.

CASE 7.2

CLINICAL HISTORY *A 21-year-old male patient with a 4-day history of worsening pain and tenderness in the left parotid region.*

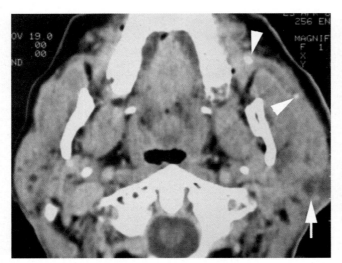

FIGURE 7.2A

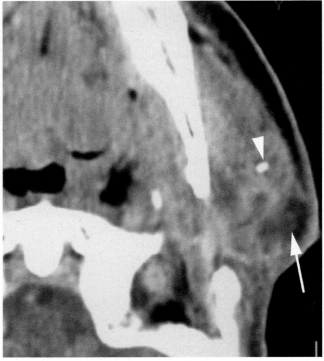

FIGURE 7.2B

FINDINGS

Figure 7.2A. CECT demonstrates stones within the dilated main parotid duct (arrowheads). The duct wall enhances. Farther back in the gland, there is a parotid abscess (arrow). Also note that the other gland enhances abnormally and shows lucent zones consistent with distal duct dilatation and/or parenchymal cysts.

Figure 7.2B. A section more inferiorly shows stones likely within the ductal system (arrowhead) and a discreet parotid abscess secondary to infection at the tail of the gland (arrow).

DIFFERENTIAL DIAGNOSIS Acute pyogenic parotitis, autoimmune parotitis, viral parotitis, chronic parotitis

DIAGNOSIS Acute, obstructive (due to sialolithiasis) pyogenic parotitis and parotid abscess superimposed on chronic parotitis

DISCUSSION Parotid inflammatory conditions can be noninfectious or infectious. Viruses (mumps, Epstein-Barr virus, HIV), bacteria, and less likely tuberculosis or fungus are causes of infectious parotid gland inflammation. They commonly present with pain, tenderness, swelling over the parotid gland, which may be exacerbated by meals, and are typically associated with lymphadenopathy and inflammatory changes in the adjacent tissues. Indolent infections frequently present as a parotid region mass/discomfort or even otalgia associated with meals. They are usually sporadic and occur most commonly in children and young adults.

Parotid infections are usually not imaged. Imaging is used to aid medical decision making because the clinical examination may be very limited. Imaging of viral infections are usually not performed unless they are unilateral, mimicking a bacterial infection. Imaging of acute or subacute pyogenic bacterial infections of the parotid gland are often performed for three main reasons: to look for a complicating abscess, to evaluate for an underlying cause, or to look for the origin of the infection if it is not certain that it is arising from the parotid gland. Studies of chronic persistent or recurrent bacterial infections are usually done to identify a cause or complicating factor such as duct obstruction or stones.

Imaging modalities of parotid gland infections include computed tomography (CT), which is the preferred study for acute/subacute processes; MR, used for the evaluation of chronic inflammatory conditions; ultrasound, which is a good initial triage instrument in experienced hands looking for ductal dilation, stones, or abscesses; or conventional sialography, mainly done for nonacute ductal pathology.

Parotid inflammatory conditions can affect the parotid parenchyma and/or the ductal system. The ductal system may predispose the gland to infections when an underlying stone, stricture, or rarely an intraductal mass causes obstruction. This manifests as ductal dilatation, periductal inflammatory changes, or even destruction of the terminal acini—the latter causing intraparenchymal cysts that communicate with the main ductal system that manifest on sialography as punctate intraparenchymal leakage of contrast material and on CT as nodular parenchymal changes. Parenchymal manifestations of parotid inflammation include diffuse/focal enhancement and fluid collections. Intraparenchymal fluid collections may be due to sialoceles or branchial apparatus cysts, which may or may not be infected, and abscesses. Infected fluid collections present in one of two ways: as a zone of fluid density within a diffusely enhancing gland or as a classic rim-enhancing fluid collection. A fluid collection with bulging contours is a sign that it is drainable.

Questions for Further Thought

1. What predisposing factors are associated with the development of parotid infections?
2. What information is suggestive of a process other than a bacterial etiology?

Reporting Responsibilities

Although these are not typically urgent studies, direct contact with the treating physician should be made in the event of a likely drainable pyogenic abscess, infections arising in a diabetic or immunocompromised patient, or infections that may pose a risk to the airway.

What the Treating Physician Needs to Know

• If the infection is intrinsic or extrinsic to the parotid gland

• If not an intrinsic parotid infection, what is the likely alternative diagnosis based on imaging?
• If extrinsic, what is the likely source?
• Is there a parotid abscess?
• Nature and extent of ductal pathology—is the system dilated or focally obstructed?
• Are there stones?
• Are there findings that suggest a diagnosis other than an infection?

Answers

1. Diabetes mellitus, dehydration, or conditions that cause decreased salivary flow, such as partial/complete obstructions and prolonged periods of no oral ingestion (as with critically ill patients in the intensive care unit), are factors that predispose to the development of parotid infections.
2. Bilateral acute parotid inflammatory findings suggest a viral infection, while bilateral chronic parotid symptoms suggest an autoimmune disease, especially if other major salivary lacrimal glands are affected.

LEARN MORE
See Chapters 177 and 13 in *Head and Neck Radiology* by Mancuso and Hanafee.

CASE 7.3

CLINICAL HISTORY *A 52-year-old female patient with a history of a xerophthalmia and xerostomia.*

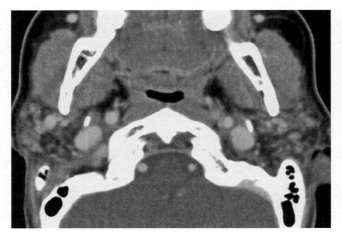

FIGURE 7.3A

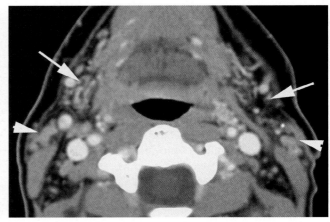

FIGURE 7.3C

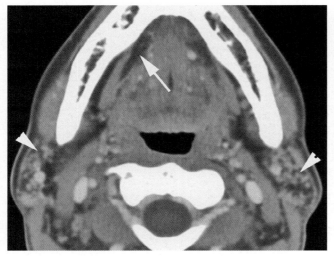

FIGURE 7.3B

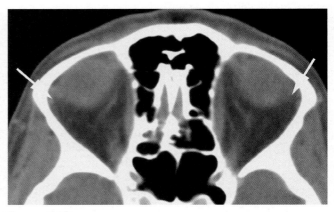

FIGURE 7.3D

FINDINGS

Figure 7.3A. CECT shows nodularity within otherwise fatty parotid glands.

Figure 7.3B. Atrophy and nodularity in the parotid tails (arrowheads) and profound atrophy in the sublingual salivary glands (arrow).

Figure 7.3C. Parotid tail atrophy, nodularity, and stones (arrowheads) and profound atrophy of the submandibular glands (SMGs) with some residual nodularity and parotid node prominence (arrows).

Figure 7.3D. Atrophy of the lacrimal glands.

RELEVANT ANATOMY A detailed and complete knowledge of the anatomy of the parotid gland and surrounding structures, as well as an understanding of the anatomic variations and primary drainage fields, is required for the evaluation of parotid infections.

DIFFERENTIAL DIAGNOSIS Not applicable—generally autoimmune sialadenitis

DIAGNOSIS Sjögren syndrome

DISCUSSION Parotid noninfectious inflammatory conditions may be caused by trauma, radiation, or systemic diseases such as sarcoidosis and autoimmune diseases. The autoimmune disease prototype that affects the parotid gland is Sjögren disease or syndrome. Sjögren syndrome causes chronic inflammation of the exocrine glands with destruction of their acinar and ductal epithelial cells, eventually leading to glandular dysfunction. It is primarily diagnosed clinically and confirmed by serologic studies or, in some cases, lip biopsy. Imaging may aid medical decision making in seronegative patients with highly suspicious clinical findings, or it may be the first indication that a parotid disease is related to a systemic condition.

Noninfectious inflammatory conditions of the parotid gland present with unilateral or bilateral pain, tenderness, or enlargement of the parotid gland, which may be exacerbated by meals, and can be associated with lymphadenopathy. They are usually not imaged, but when imaging is performed, it is used for similar reasons and with the same general imaging modality approach as in infections. These conditions alter the glandular architecture and cause similar findings to infectious inflammatory conditions that affect the parenchyma and/or ductal system.

The ductal system becomes obstructed by inspissated debris and/or sialoliths those cysts cause a cascade of events leading to acinar pseudocysts that expanding as there is destruction of the parenchyma. Diffuse parenchymal enhancement is seen in the active phase of the disease and is present to some extent and/or degree in all chronic inflammatory diseases. Such chronic inflammatory diseases, including Sjögren syndrome, may also have broad zones of chronic inflammatory cell accumulation that form parenchymal nodules or confluent masslike components that are difficult to differentiate from a complicating lymphoma.

When the chronicity or severity of the process has caused enough destruction, the final pathway of all inflammatory conditions (infectious or not) is fatty atrophy and/or fibrosis of the parotid gland.

Questions for Further Thought

1. What clinical signs point more toward a noninfectious inflammation of the parotid gland than an infectious cause?
2. What imaging signs point more toward a noninfectious inflammation of the parotid gland?

Reporting Responsibilities

Although these are not typically urgent studies, direct contact with the treating physician should be made in the event of a likely drainable pyogenic abscess or a complicating superimposed malignancy such as a secondary lymphoma.

What the Treating Physician Needs to Know

- If not intrinsic parotid inflammation, what is the likely alternative diagnosis based on imaging?
- If the inflammation is intrinsic to the parotid gland, what is the likely cause?
- Nature and extent of ductal pathology—is the system dilated or focally obstructed?
- Are there stones?
- Are there findings that confirm a systemic etiology or are otherwise morphologically suggestive of a particular etiology?
- Is there an important complicating factor such as superimposed infection or a secondary lymphoma?

Answers

1. History and physical findings of bilateral involvement, less intense symptoms, absence of purulent discharge from the parotid duct orifice, or involvement of other organs such as the eyes, joints, lungs, or lymph nodes
2. Involvement of an additional major salivary gland or findings of nonsalivary origin such as the lacrimal glands and/or cervical lymphadenopathy may signal a noninfectious cause of the inflammation.

> ### LEARN MORE
> See Chapters 178 and 20 in *Head and Neck Radiology* by Mancuso and Hanafee.

CLINICAL HISTORY *A 63-year-old female patient with progressive facial weakness and a solid, enlarging left parotid region mass.*

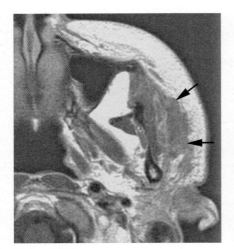

FIGURE **7.4A**

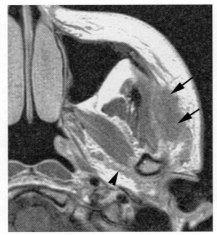

FIGURE **7.4B**

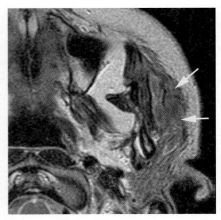

FIGURE **7.4C**

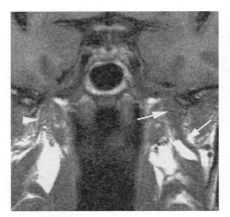

FIGURE **7.4D**

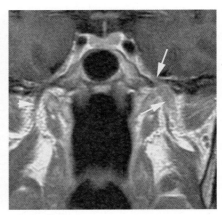

FIGURE **7.4E**

FINDINGS

Figure 7.4A,B. Noncontrast T1W image demonstrates a mass arising from the accessory lobe or the more anterior portion of the parotid gland (arrows). The mass encompasses the expected course of the upper division of the facial nerve.

Figure 7.4C. Contrast-enhanced (CE) T1W image shows soft tissue thickening and enhancement streaming along the auriculotemporal nerve involving the mandibular division of the trigeminal nerve (arrowhead).

Figure 7.4D. Coronal noncontrast T1W image shows thickening and enhancement of the mandibular division of the trigeminal nerve extending proximally to its entrance into the foramen ovale (arrow) compared to the normal nerve on the right (white arrowhead).

Figure 7.4E. Coronal CE T1W image shows the thickened enhancing nerve extending to the junction of the mandibular division of the trigeminal nerve and trigeminal ganglion (arrow).

DIFFERENTIAL DIAGNOSIS Sarcoma of masseter muscle or facial nerve origin, lymphoma

DIAGNOSIS Parotid adenocarcinoma with perineural spread

DISCUSSION Parotid-region masses can be intrinsic or extrinsic, depending on whether they arise from within the parotid gland or the adjacent soft tissues. Intrinsic parotid masses are the most common parotid-region lesions and account for about 80% of all major salivary gland tumors. They are sporadic, and most do not have any associated risk factors, except lymphoepithelial lesions and lymphoma, which are sometimes associated with HIV infection and autoimmune disease. These commonly present as a solitary, palpable, and painless parotid-region mass that may or may not have reduced mobility.

Benign parotid tumors constitute 75% to 80% of the cases in adults and 50% in children. The most common benign parotid neoplasm in adults is a benign mixed tumor or pleomorphic adenoma; in children, it may be a proliferative hemangioma or venolymphatic malformation.

Approximately 25% of parotid tumors and 50% of the remaining major and minor salivary gland tumors are malignant. Malignant salivary neoplasms can be high- or low-grade malignancies. Low-grade neoplasms tend to include mucoepidermoid and acinic cell carcinomas. High-grade neoplasms include adenocarcinomas, mucoepidermoid and poorly differentiated anaplastic, salivary duct, and squamous cell carcinoma. Adenoid cystic carcinoma can have a variable biologic behavior, and almost always there is perineural involvement.

Parotid tumors arise from the many functioning or supporting cells that form the gland as well as from incorporated elements during embryologic development, such as lymphatic and vascular tissue, and components of the branchial apparatus that form part of the face and neck; this leads to a variety of possible histologic and widely variable imaging appearances.

Imaging criteria used to differentiate malignant from benign neoplasms include margins of the lesion (infiltrative vs. well-defined expansion), internal signal characteristics on T2W imaging and diffusion-weighted imaging, and metastatic adenopathy or perineural spread.

The specific diagnosis of a parotid mass requires histologic examination since morphologic features are only suggestive because benign-appearing lesions can eventually prove to be malignant and vice versa. Imaging is most importantly used to define the extent of spread to the surrounding areas, perineural spread, and regional metastatic disease when the parotid-region lesion is shown to be a primary parotid malignancy.

Questions for Further Thought

1. Is FDG-PET uptake a reliable way of differentiating benign from malignant parotid masses?
2. What clinical signs suggest perineural invasion?
3. What imaging signs suggest perineural invasion?

Reporting Responsibilities

Direct communication with the referring physician is mandatory if a tumor is discovered that was not clinically suspected.

What the Treating Physician Needs to Know

- If the mass is intrinsic or extrinsic to the parotid gland
- If not an intrinsic parotid lesion, what is the likely alternative diagnosis based on imaging?
- Full extent of an intrinsic parotid tumor
- Relationship of an intrinsic mass to the facial nerve
- Evidence of perineural spread along the facial and/or auriculotemporal nerves
- If there any regional lymph node involvement? If so, where are the pathologic lymph nodes located? Any evidence for extranodal tumor spread?
- If there is suspicion for tumor recurrence in the posttreatment images

Answers

1. No. FDG uptake is variable in both benign and malignant salivary gland neoplasms, limiting its use in patients with salivary gland tumors.
2. Slowly progressive nerve dysfunction—manifest as worsening pain, paresis, or palsy in a nerve distribution—is frequently associated with an underlying nerve involvement by a malignant neoplasm and warrants a careful evaluation of the entire nerve from its origin to point of most distal distribution.
3. Thickening and enhancement of a nerve and expansion of its corresponding osseous conduits are signs of perineural spread. This can also manifest as obliteration of the fat pad below the stylomastoid foramen when the facial nerve is involved. Spread along the auriculotemporal nerve is strongly suggestive when tumor is seen wrapping around the condylar neck of the mandible, forming a bridge for tumoral extension between the trigeminal and facial nerves. Negative imaging studies do not exclude perineural spread.

LEARN MORE

See Chapters 179 and 22 in *Head and Neck Radiology* by Mancuso and Hanafee.

CLINICAL HISTORY *A 22 year-old male patient with a history of a left mandibular angle mass.*

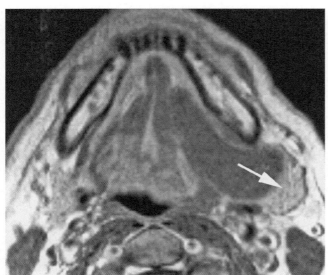

FIGURE 7.5A

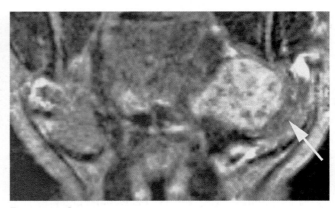

FIGURE 7.5C

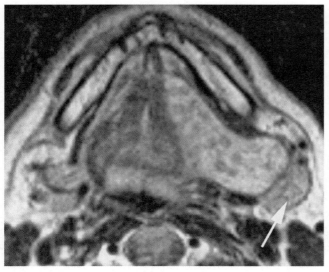

FIGURE 7.5B

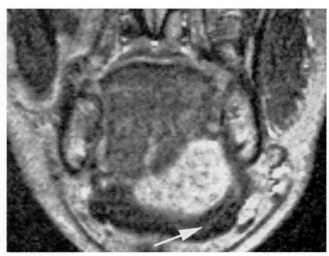

FIGURE 7.5D

FINDINGS

Figure 7.5A. T1W CE image shows a cystic-appearing mass displacing the SMG (arrow).

Figure 7.5B. T2W image shows the cystic mass containing globules displacing the SMG (arrow).

Figure 7.5C. Coronal T2W image shows the cyst displacing the SMG where it extends over the posterior edge of the mylohyoid muscle (arrow).

Figure 7.5D. T2W image shows the cystic mass containing globules displacing the mylohyoid muscle (arrow), identifying a significant component also within the floor of the mouth.

DIFFERENTIAL DIAGNOSIS Ranula, venolymphatic malformation

DIAGNOSIS Dermoid cyst

DISCUSSION Developmental abnormalities involving the submandibular and submental regions are mainly due to venolymphatic malformations and epidermoid and dermoid cysts and, much less commonly, somewhat misplaced branchial apparatus or thyroglossal duct migration anomalies.

Dermoid and epidermoid cysts are typically located in the submandibular and/or submental space, outside of and displacing the SMG. These may tract to the parapharyngeal space, upper deep neck spaces, and floor of the mouth. The floor of the mouth can be potentially accessed through the open back edge or anatomic defects (i.e., areas of passage of a neurovascular bundle and accessory salivary tissue) in the mylohyoid muscle.

These cysts will clinically demonstrate a slow, continuous growth. Intermittent changes in size are more suggestive of a branchial apparatus or thyroglossal duct cyst or a venolymphatic malformation.

Question for Further Thought

1. What is the most common etiology of a submandibular cystic lesion in adults?

Reporting Responsibilities

Direct communication with the referring physician is usually not necessary since these are generally chronic entities, unless there is a potential of airway compromise, when there might be a superimposed infection, or if a tumor is discovered that was not clinically suspected.

What the Treating Physician Needs to Know

- Are the findings due to a developmental cyst or possibly another condition such as a venolymphatic malformation or neoplasm?
- Full extent of the mass, including its relationship to the mandible, floor of the mouth, SMG, and other surrounding spaces

Answer

1. In adults, a submandibular, noninfected, cystic-appearing lesion is far more likely to be a neoplastic lymph node or a ranula, unless there are some characteristic associated developmental findings. If infected, the cystic mass is most like a dental-related abscess.

> ### LEARN MORE
>
> See Chapters 180 and 8 in *Head and Neck Radiology* by Mancuso and Hanafee.

CLINICAL HISTORY *A young adult patient presented with acute submandibular region pain and swelling. It was uncertain whether this was due to dental disease or disease within the SMG.*

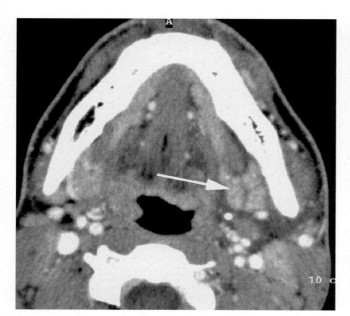

FIGURE 7.6A

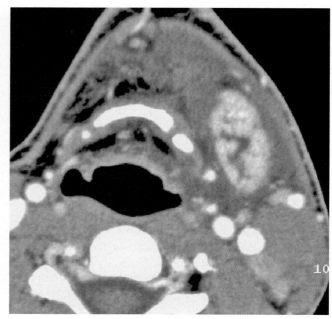

FIGURE 7.6C

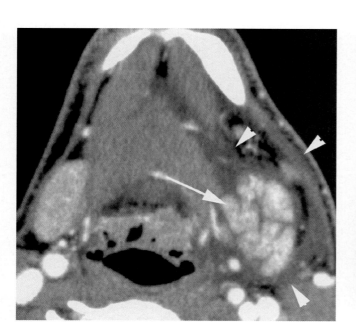

FIGURE 7.6B

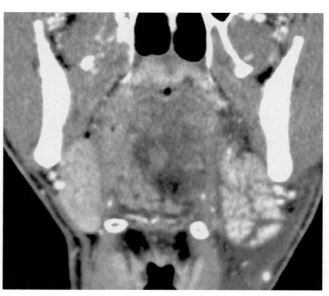

FIGURE 7.6D

FINDINGS CECT in (Fig. 7.6A,B) shows marked enhancement of the SMG (arrows) and very extensive edema around the gland (arrowheads). In the axial section in (Fig. 7.6C) and coronal reformations in (Fig. 7.6D), the glandular parenchymal changes and intense surrounding edema are very evident.

DIFFERENTIAL DIAGNOSIS Dental-related infection, viral sialadenitis

DIAGNOSIS Acute pyogenic sialadenitis without abscess or obstruction of the submandibular duct

DISCUSSION Many SMG and submandibular space (SMS) inflammatory conditions do not come to imaging. Clinical examination of an acutely infected SMG/SMS may be limited by severe pain and toughness of the cervical fascia attachment to the mandible as well as the mandible itself, making imaging a reasonable aid to diagnosis.

Infections of the SMG/SMS that come to imaging are often acute or subacute pyogenic bacterial infections, with studies mainly being done to look for a complicating abscess or underlying cause or if the SMG origin is not certain. The most common infections in the SMS are due to dental disease. Chronic persistent or recurrent bacterial infections are usually studied to identify a cause or complicating factor such as duct obstruction or stones. Occasionally, a chronic inflammatory process will present as a "mass." Fungal infection is rare. SMG tuberculosis and unusual infections such as actinomycosis and parasites are rare and difficult to anticipate prior to tissue sampling and culture.

Pyogenic bacterial infections occur sporadically and more commonly in the pediatric and young adult populations. In older age group diabetes, dehydration or not eating for prolonged periods is a predisposing factor. The latter may be a contributing factor to SMG infections in patients who are critically ill and develop submandibular sialadenitis and/or parotitis in the intensive care unit, especially following surgery. This also occurs in critically ill children. Poor dental hygiene, smoking, and radiation can be contributing risk factors.

Glandular parenchymal changes seen on imaging are variable. Diffuse enhancement may be seen in viral or bacterial disease, as in this case. An abscess may appear only as a zone of fluid density within a diffusely enhancing gland rather than a classic fluid area with some degrees of rim enhancement. A bulging contour of the fluid zone is a clue to a drainable collection even when no discreet enhancing rim is visible. Fluid zones in the gland with or without rim enhancement may be sialoceles representing trapped areas of saliva with the gland similar to the pathophysiology of pancreatic pseudocysts. Sialoceles may become infected, mimicking an abscess or even a mass. Extensive periglandular edema suggests pyogenic cellulitis associated with the glandular infection.

Ductal obstructive patterns, not present in this case, may be manifest in the entire main submandibular duct or more focally when strictures and/or stones are present. The wall of a dilated ductal system may enhance. The more proximal ductal system draining the gland parenchyma may also be dilated. Terminal acinar destruction may produce parenchymal cysts that communicate with the main ductal system.

Questions for Further Thought

1. What predisposing factors are associated with the development of submandibular infections?
2. What information is suggestive of a process other than a bacterial etiology?

Reporting Responsibilities

Although these are not typically urgent studies, direct contact with the treating physician should be made in the event of a likely drainable pyogenic abscess, infections arising in a diabetic or immunocompromised patient, or infections that may pose a risk to the airway.

What the Treating Physician Needs to Know

- If the infection is intrinsic or extrinsic to the SMG
- If not an intrinsic SMG infection, what is the likely alternative diagnosis based on imaging?
- If extrinsic, what is the likely source?
- Is there a related abscess?
- Nature and extent of ductal pathology—is the system dilated or focally obstructed?
- Are there stones?
- Are there findings that suggest a diagnosis other than an infection?

Answers

1. Diabetes mellitus, dehydration, or conditions that cause decreased salivary flow, such as partial/complete obstructions and prolonged periods of no oral ingestion (as with critically ill patients in the intensive care unit), are factors that predispose to the development of salivary gland infections.
2. Bilateral salivary gland inflammatory findings suggest a viral infection, while bilateral chronic changes suggest an autoimmune disease, especially if other major salivary lacrimal glands are affected.

> LEARN MORE
> See Chapters 181 and 13 in *Head and Neck Radiology* by Mancuso and Hanafee.

CLINICAL HISTORY   *A 55-year-old male patient with a solid, enlarging left submandibular region mass.*

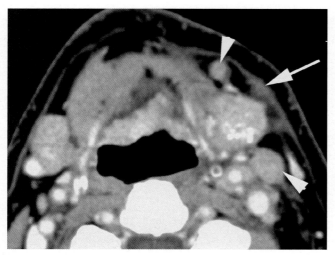

FIGURE **7.7A**

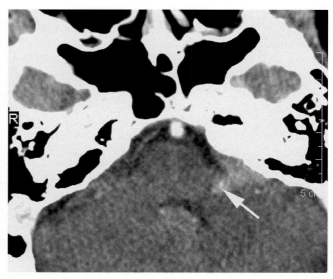

FIGURE **7.7C**

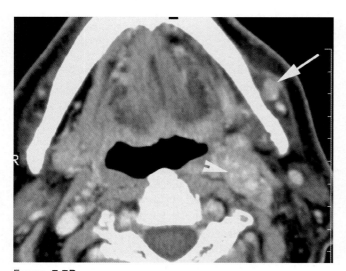

FIGURE **7.7B**

FIGURE **7.7D**

FINDINGS

Figure 7.7A. The mass is centered in the left SMG, spreading to and thickening the superficial musculoaponeurotic system (SMAS) of the face. There are multiple metastatic lymph nodes (arrowheads).

Figure 7.7B. Positive facial lymph node (arrow) and a retrostyloid parapharyngeal space mass (arrowhead) with perineural spread along the carotid sheath.

Figure 7.7C. Cranial spread along the lower cranial nerves associated with the carotid sheath toward the jugular fossa.

Figure 7.7D. Tumor invading the posterior fossa via the jugular fossa, growing transdurally into the posterior fossa and spreading along the lower cranial nerves into their root entry zone at the brainstem (arrow).

DIFFERENTIAL DIAGNOSIS Malignant SMG tumor with perineural spread

DIAGNOSIS Primary adenocarcinoma of the SMG with perineural spread and regional metastatic adenopathy

DISCUSSION Submandibular- and sublingual-region masses—similar to parotid-region masses—can be intrinsic or extrinsic, depending on whether they arise from within the salivary gland or the adjacent soft tissues. Extrinsic masses in these regions are usually due to lymphadenopathy or tumors arising from the structures adjacent to the gland. Intrinsic submandibular or sublingual gland masses have a range of possible histologic diagnosis similar to that of the parotid gland, except for the Warthin tumor, which is unique to the parotid and periparotid region.

Submandibular or sublingual gland neoplasms are malignant in about half of the cases of primary glandular neoplasms. Malignant tumors eventually grow through the gland toward the adjacent tissues, especially the mandible in submandibular masses and the floor of the mouth in sublingual masses. These masses may also grow to communicate with the sublingual and submandibular spaces through the back edge or through anatomic defects of the mylohyoid muscle or by directly invading the muscle.

Imaging criteria used to differentiate malignant from benign neoplasms are similar to those used in parotid intrinsic masses and include aggressive margins, relatively low signal intensity relative to fat on T2W images, evidence of perineural spread, and regional metastatic adenopathy.

Specific diagnosis of a salivary gland mass requires histologic examination since morphologic features are only suggestive, and benign-appearing lesions can eventually prove to be malignant and vice versa. Imaging is most importantly used to define the extent of spread to the surrounding areas, perineural spread, and regional metastatic disease when the lesion is shown to be a primary salivary gland malignancy.

Questions for Further Thought

1. What is a sign that indicates the marginal mandibular branch of the facial nerve may have been invaded? What may have been the neural pathway of spread to the retropharyngeal space and eventually the posterior fossa in this case?
2. What is the significance of new neurologic symptoms in a patient with a history of a malignant salivary gland neoplasm?
3. What is the next best step following a negative needle biopsy of a suspicious SMS lesion?

Reporting Responsibilities

Direct communication with the referring physician is mandatory if a tumor is discovered that was not clinically suspected.

What the Treating Physician Needs to Know

- If not an intrinsic SMG lesion, what is the likely alternative diagnosis based on imaging?

- Full extent of an intrinsic SMG tumor
- Relationship of the intrinsic mass to the surrounding structures
- *Neck lymph nodes:* Are they involved? Where are the pathologic lymph nodes located?
- Is there any evidence of extranodal tumor spread?
- Is there perineural spread?
- *Posttreatment imaging:* Suspicion for tumor recurrence

Answers

1. Invasion of the adjacent SMAS at the level of the mandibular body and slightly below the body may indicate invasion of the marginal mandibular branch of the facial nerve. In the patient under discussion, the sympathetics associated with the SMG where the likely conduit to the carotid sheath since those nerves will travel in the adventitia surrounding the cervical portion of the internal carotid artery.
2. Neurologic symptoms in a patient with a history of a salivary gland malignancy may herald perineural recurrence. Imaging should always be done in light of any new neurologic deficit or symptom; such deficits or symptoms are most commonly those of the trigeminal and facial nerves, but sometimes, as in this case, the sympathetic nerves or lower cranial nerves might be the conduit.
3. If there is a suspicious submandibular mass and no primary site has been found, the next best step is a dissection of the SMS, including removal of the gland. Incisional biopsy or excisional shelling out of a lesion increases the risk of tumor recurrence of even benign lesions. This subsequently increases the surgical morbidity since a wide excision of the biopsy site would then be needed, placing the adjacent structures such as the marginal mandibular branch of the facial nerve at greater risk for injury.

> ### LEARN MORE
> See Chapters 182 and 22 in *Head and Neck Radiology* by Mancuso and Hanafee.

CLINICAL HISTORY *An adult male patient with a solid, enlarging, somewhat tender left floor of the mouth mass.*

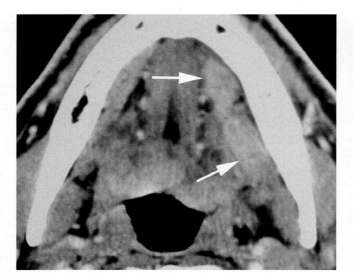

FIGURE **7.8A**

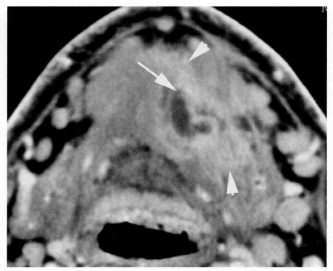

FIGURE **7.8C**

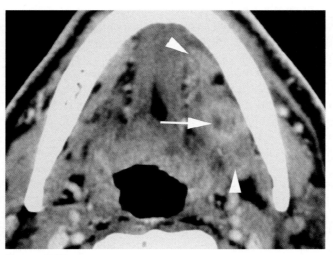

FIGURE **7.8B**

FINDINGS CECT in (Fig. 7.8A) shows diffuse enhancement of the enlarged sublingual gland (arrows) with little or no surrounding edema. In (Fig. 7.8B), there is a focal area of low density within the enlarged sublingual gland (arrowheads) or a lingual lymph node (arrow) with a suggestion of surrounding edema. In (Fig. 7.8C), a low-density, peripherally enhancing (arrow) and necrotic mass (arrowheads) is present deep in the sublingual space and floor of the mouth. There are enlarged level 1 lymph nodes that are also diffusely enhancing.

DIFFERENTIAL DIAGNOSIS Malignant sublingual gland or floor of the mouth tumor with regional lymph node metastases, inflammatory complications arising in a venolymphatic malformation with reactive adenopathy, infected ranula

DIAGNOSIS Sublingual gland pyogenic sialadenitis and reactive adenopathy that completely resolved on antibiotics without surgical intervention.

DISCUSSION Mass lesions in the sublingual gland region may be intrinsic or extrinsic to the sublingual gland. Infiltrating systemic disease such as sarcoidosis, manifestations of autoimmune sialadenitis, and rarely lymphoma can mimic a sublingual gland epithelial-origin tumor if those conditions are not otherwise known to be present. Diagnostic imaging may have a significant impact on sorting out these possibilities and thereby alter medical decision making. The contributions are equally important in some cases of intrinsic glandular epithelial-origin neoplasms.

If the margins or nature of a mass, as in this case, are not clear after physical examination, CT or MR may be done. This case illustrates a primary function of imaging in a mass lesion of this region, namely to define the origin and extent of a sublingual gland/sublingual space mass.

Imaging will first help to determine whether the mass point of origin is intrinsic or extrinsic to the sublingual gland. This factor alone may markedly alter the course of management since submucosal floor of the mouth masses are frequently of nonglandular origin. MR or CT is almost always capable of differentiating an intrinsic sublingual gland neoplasm from an extrinsic mass. Other submucosal masses, such as a ranula, dermoid cyst, venolymphatic malformations, or rare lesions of neural or mesenchymal origin, are fully capable of mimicking an intrinsic sublingual gland lesion. Inflammatory disease will usually manifest some degree of intrinsic surrounding inflammatory appearing change; those findings, however, not being dominant as a clue in this case.

Imaging can also characterize the type of intrinsic or extrinsic lesion and the degree of invasiveness both within and beyond the sublingual gland by determining the full extent of the lesion and whether it has morphology or associated findings suggestive of an invasive and/or malignant process. This includes the margins of the lesion, internal signal characteristics on T2W images, and perhaps behavior on diffusion-weighted imaging. Metastatic adenopathy and perineural spread are almost sure signs of a malignant tumor.

If disease is extrinsic to either or both glands, imaging can determine whether it is a unilateral or bilateral process and whether it is multifocal on one side and/or both. This determination helps to identify whether the process is likely to be due to a systemic process such as autoimmune sialadenitis.

In this case, the abrupt onset, fever (information not provided initially), and tenderness help move the treatment in the right direction.

Questions for Further Thought

1. What are the conduits of spread for a plunging or diving ranula?

2. What is likely the most common developmental mass that arises in the floor of the mouth/sublingual space that comes to imaging?

Reporting Responsibilities

Direct communication with the referring physician is mandatory if a tumor is discovered that was not clinically suspected. An acute infection or potential threat to the airway should also prompt direct, verbal communication, as was done in this case. If a biopsy might lead to excessive bleeding and possible airway encroachment or aspiration of blood, then direct communication is wise. However, in general, determining the origin and extent of a sublingual space mass is the goal of the study at the time of initial imaging, and most of the time these circumstances do not arise, so no special communication is required.

What the Treating Physician Needs to Know

- If the mass/disease process is intrinsic or extrinsic to the sublingual gland or space
- If the findings are multifocal and unilateral or bilateral
- If the mass is likely benign or malignant or poses a risk of airway obstruction or excessive bleeding if biopsied
- If the findings suggest a diagnosis other than a benign or malignant neoplasm—either localized or systemic disease

Answers

1. Over the back edge of the mylohyoid muscle and through a commonly occurring gap in the anterior third of the mylohyoid muscle that serves as a neurovascular conduit and frequently contains normal salivary tissue
2. Venolymphatic malformation

> LEARN MORE
>
> See Chapters 183 and 13 in *Head and Neck Radiology* by Mancuso and Hanafee.

CHAPTER 8

Nasopharynx

CLINICAL HISTORY *A young child presented with upper respiratory obstructive symptoms. A mucosa-covered mass was seen clinically, and fortunately this magnetic resonance (MR) study was obtained before surgery.*

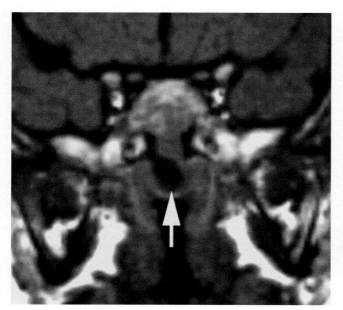

FIGURE 8.1A

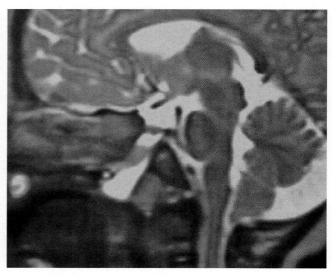

FIGURE 8.1C

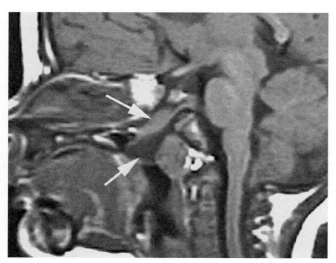

FIGURE 8.1B

FINDINGS

Figure 8.1A. T1W coronal MR image shows a centrally hypointense mass extending inferiorly from the roof of the central skull base (arrow).

Figure 8.1B,C. The sagittal T1W MR image (Fig. 8.1B) shows herniation of the both dysmorphic brain tissue and a meningocele (arrows) into the nasopharynx. This is subsequently confirmed on the sagittal T2W MR image in (Fig. 8.1C).

DIFFERENTIAL DIAGNOSIS None

DIAGNOSIS Meningoencephalocele

DISCUSSION The origin of a nasopharyngeal-level lesion may not be not well understood from the physical examination and may be considered threatening to one or more important and sometimes vital functions until its benign and possible congenital nature origin is established. Imaging typically will facilitate a precise diagnosis in these anomalies.

The primary presentation such as in this case may be that of a mass of uncertain etiology. Airway obstruction to a point of functional limitation is probably the most common chief complaint. Associated pain and swallowing or feeding difficulties are less common. The eustachian tube may be obstructed and cause a secondary middle ear effusion or infection.

In general, tenderness and fever and associated generalized swelling may be present and is much more likely in inflammatory conditions or thrombosed or inflamed venolymphatic malformations.

Developmental abnormalities generally will present during childhood, although presentation may be delayed even into middle age.

The differential diagnosis clinically is based in part on the position in the airway. Encephaloceles and ectopic pituitary tissue are typically in the midline, while branchial apparatus and dermoid or epidermoid cysts will be more likely paramedian or more lateral. The exception to this is the very common acquired Thornwaldt's cyst that arises within the embryologic residual pharyngeal pouch.

The primary imaging observation will most often be that of a mass and whether the origin of the mass can be localized to the nasopharynx. This is followed by an analysis of possible transcompartmental extension. The morphology is often distinctive enough to allow a specific diagnosis.

The imaging appearance of the mass in question will vary with its specific etiology—for example, congenital and acquired cysts may contain air and/or fluid and may appear infected.

Most of these masses have well-defined margins. Irregular or infiltrative margins suggest an alternative malignant or inflammatory etiology or some sort of peripheral reactive change in a congenital mass.

The origin of nasopharyngeal masses may be thought of in terms of frequency of occurrence, precise anatomic site of origin, and/or etiologic categorization—the last option being preferred when suspecting a developmental abnormality. The following is a list of considerations for possible origins:

- Pituitary migratory pathway problems resulting mainly in ectopic glandular tissue (rare). These will present as a submucosal nasopharyngeal mass in or near the midline.
- A central encephalocele
- Branchial apparatus–origin anomalies of the first pouch may produce a cyst that lies along the course of the eustachian tube.
- Dermoid and epidermoid cysts, teratomas, and hamartomas most often present as a paramedian nasopharyngeal submucosal mass.
- Venolymphatic and other vascular malformations
- Some other considerations that are sometimes classified as developmental, such as nerve sheath tumors associated with neurofibromatosis

In this case, the imaging findings leave no room for alternative interpretation. The obvious midline mass filled partly with fluid/cerebrospinal fluid is in connection with the intracranial compartment through a widened craniopharyngeal canal. The soft tissue within the mass has identical signal characteristics as compared to white matter, suggesting dysmorphic brain tissue. All of this together suggests the diagnosis of a meningoencephalocele. Remember that the discovery of one central nervous system (CNS) developmental abnormality requires a diligent search for other craniofacial or CNS abnormalities.

Questions for Further Thought

1. Is biopsy of a submucosal mass ever wise before imaging?
2. Give the differential diagnosis for a submucosal cystic mass occurring in the nasopharynx.

Reporting Responsibilities

In general, developmental abnormalities in the nasopharynx are typically not of high acuity with regard to management decisions and are in the clinical differential diagnosis; thus, routine reporting is sufficient unless there is a potential airway compromise. If an alternative threatening diagnosis such as a malignancy is suspected from the imaging, or biopsy is planned and the mass is connected to brain or potentially vascular, then direct verbal communication would be very wise.

The report should contain precise detail about the full extent of the mass and relationship to critical surrounding anatomic structures that might be the origin of the lesion and/or affected by surgical or other treatment. In general, the most critical of these relationships are how the mass relates to the airway, skull base, and brain.

It is especially important to communicate effectively and promptly if there is a secondary infection, especially if there might be a CNS connection from the anomaly.

Other developmental abnormalities and the possibility of syndromic associations should be considered in all developmental conditions, although most of these rare anomalies are isolated events.

If a vascular malformation is the etiology, the likely nature of flow dynamics should be included. There should also be a determination of whether catheter angiography might be necessary for further clarification of flow dynamics and the possibility of an endovascular treatment option.

If the anterior pituitary migratory pathway is involved, the ectopic tissue can be the source of an ectopic adenoma.

What the Treating Physician Needs to Know

- Precise diagnosis and the degree of confidence in that diagnosis
- Extent of the developmental anomaly and any potential involvement of surrounding critical anatomy
- Any airway compromise
- Any complicating features of the anomaly that might alter medical decision making
- Whether there are associated or other anomalies
- Whether there is a reasonable likelihood of this being syndromic
- If there is any need for further imaging to answer any of these issues

Answers

1. No! Always perform imaging before biopsying a submucosal lesion in order to avoid a dramatic outcome. Rule out high-flow vascular lesions or malformations and lesions such as in this case before considering a biopsy.
2. Retention cyst/postinflammatory, Thornwaldt's cyst, Rathke's cleft cyst, branchial cleft cyst

> **LEARN MORE**
> See Chapters 185 and 8 in *Head and Neck Radiology* by Mancuso and Hanafee.

CLINICAL HISTORY *A 63-year-old male patient presenting with complaint of chronic right-sided headaches.*

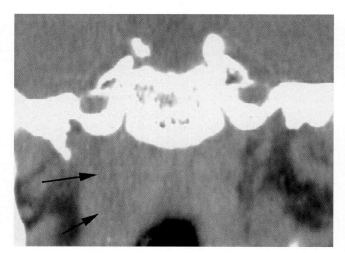

FIGURE 8.2A

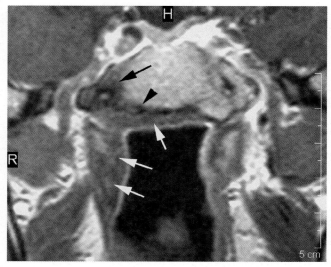

FIGURE 8.2C

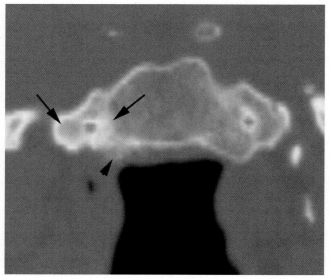

FIGURE 8.2B

FINDINGS

Figure 8.2A. Coronal noncontrast computed tomography (CT) study shows a deeply infiltrating process (arrows).

Figure 8.2B. Coronal noncontrast CT study in bone window shows adjacent skull base reactive changes within the marrow space (arrows) and along the cortical surface of the clivus (arrowheads). The reactive bone has a somewhat fluffy appearance consistent with subacute reactive bony changes.

Figure 8.2C. T1W contrast-enhanced (CE) image shows the infiltrating nasopharyngeal process that does not show extensive enhancement along the lateral wall and roof of the nasopharynx (white arrows). The reactive changes within the cortical bone (black arrowhead) and within the marrow space (arrow) are manifest by diminished signal.

DIFFERENTIAL DIAGNOSIS Carcinoma, lymphoma, or plasmacytoma spreading from the nasopharynx to the skull base or vice versa, Wegener's granulomatosis

DIAGNOSIS Skull base osteomyelitis presenting as a nasopharyngeal mass

DISCUSSION Imaging can properly triage nasopharyngeal infection into one of the following groups and by doing so contributes to successful treatment planning and avoidance of unnecessary complications: (1) pharyngitis without abscess, (2) pharyngitis with suppurative retropharyngeal adenopathy, (3) pharyngitis with abscess, (4) spreading necrotizing infection, (5) infection in the parapharyngeal space, (6) manifestations of skull base osteomyelitis, and (7) infected developmental cyst.

In this case, both clinical presentation and imaging findings favor a more indolent course of the disease. The nasopharyngeal mass shows little enhancement, whereas acute infections would enhance more than muscle. The reactive sclerotic and fluffy bone changes in the skull base suggest a subacute or chronic disease process favoring skull base osteomyelitis. Note the absence of osteolytic bony changes. Skull base osteomyelitis is most commonly associated with necrotizing otitis externa; the presentation is obvious and the infectious agent typically the pseudomonas bacterium. At other times, the portal of entry is via the nasopharynx, perhaps the eustachian tube. The organisms in these latter cases often go unconfirmed and may be bacterial, fungal, or due to less common agents such as actinomycosis. Confirmation of infection is finally presumed based on the therapeutic response.

Most acute infections of the pharynx present an obvious clinical picture, and imaging is reserved for establishing the extent rather than cause of the disease such circumstances might include whether pyogenic adenoiditis is associated with oropharyngeal infection such as a very unusual and advanced tonsillar or peritonsillar an abscess. The very important exception to this is suppurative retropharyngeal adenitis, which should not be mistaken for a retropharyngeal abscess since it is almost completely responsive to medical therapy without any need for surgical intervention.

Contrast-enhanced computed tomography (CECT) and contrast-enhanced magnetic resonance (CEMR) will show a pyogenic process to be one that has a typical cellulitis pattern, and it may show an associated contained or spreading abscess. Both modalities should almost always be able to differentiate "drainable" from "nondrainable" infectious processes. There might be associated bone erosion or vascular complications, the most well known being Lemierre syndrome. Therefore, in patients with any pyogenic pharyngeal infection who come to imaging, it is important to search for evidence of internal jugular vein thrombosis.

In less definitive clinical situations, it may be difficult to decide whether an area of nasopharyngeal swelling is inflammatory or infectious as opposed to neoplastic (i.e., in a low-grade inflammatory process such as Wegener's granulomatosis). This distinction might remain unclear even after biopsy, and watchful waiting might become the default strategy, sometimes with imaging surveillance as an aid. Much inflammatory swelling in the nasopharynx will have a nonspecific imaging appearance when considered independent of the clinical setting. Taken with the clinical setting, the findings are often specific enough to confirm the etiology suspected clinically.

The etiology and presentation of nasopharyngeal infections vary depending on age and immune status. Pyogenic bacterial infections tend to occur more in the younger age groups and present with fever, odynophagia or feeding problems, and possibly suppurative retropharyngeal adenitis or abscess formation. In elderly or immunocompromised patients, there may be little if any fever and fewer local symptoms. However, they may be subject to very aggressive pharyngeal infections (e.g., fungal infections). Epstein-Barr virus infection, including posttransplant lymphoproliferative disorder (PTLD), may mimic lymphoma, and the related adenopathy may trigger imaging. HIV infection can manifest in the lymphoid tissue of Waldeyer's ring.

Question for Further Thought

1. Why is it so important to search for evidence of internal jugular vein thrombosis in patients with any pyogenic pharyngeal infection who come to imaging?

Reporting Responsibilities

The diagnostic radiologist, if asked to assist in this clinical problem, must be immediately available and in verbal contact with the treating physicians. This is mainly to ensure proper communication about the airway status the presence of a pyogenic abscess or a life-threatening condition such as rapidly spreading necrotizing infection or a complication such as Lemierre syndrome.

Infections that arise in a diabetic or otherwise immunocompromised patient usually require some direct communication.

If an unusual etiology is suspected based on the imaging findings, the treating clinician should be informed of this prior to endoscopy and biopsy so that the sampling of material will be appropriate and the pathologist can be forewarned as well.

Reports should include the full extent of potentially drainable purulent material with regard to the spaces and viscera involved. A likely source of the infection should be established if possible. Associated findings such as a retained foreign body or complicating arteritis, thrombophlebitis, or osteomyelitis should be searched for; if such findings are not present, exclusionary language should be included in the report.

What the Treating Physician Needs to Know

- Suppurative retropharyngeal adenopathy is a disease that can be managed with antibiotics alone in most patients.
- CT and magnetic resonance imaging (MRI) will normally be definitive in separating cellulitis and reactive edema due to pyogenic infection from abscess and other drainable collections.
- Spreading necrotizing infections, especially in diabetics, may occasionally mimic edema but require drainage.
- Important complications such as the Lemierre syndrome must be recognized and reported promptly.
- Imaging findings in focal inflammatory diseases can mimic the appearance of malignancy.
- The nasopharynx may the source of infection or secondarily involved in skull base osteomyelitis.

Answer

1. Septic thrombosis may lead to metastatic infection, most commonly in the lungs but also in the joints and liver; rarely, the meninges may be involved or other intracranial complications occur. This complication of a primary oropharyngeal infection is known as Lemierre syndrome. These patients have positive blood cultures for *Fusobacterium necrophorum*, the causative bacterium. If not properly treated, the course of this syndrome may be fatal.

> **LEARN MORE**
> See Chapters 186, 14, and 16 in *Head and Neck Radiology* by Mancuso and Hanafee.

CLINICAL HISTORY *A 53-year-old female patient presenting with unilateral chronic right otitis media and facial pain, clinically considered most likely to be due to a nasopharyngeal carcinoma.*

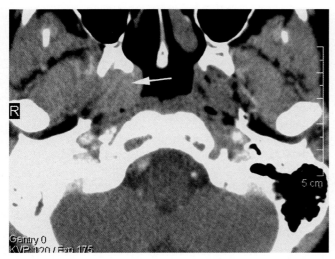

FIGURE **8.3A**

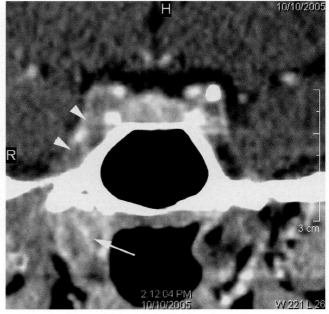

FIGURE **8.3B**

FINDINGS

Figure 8.3A. Axial CECT image showing minimally enhancing soft tissue mass around the eustachian tube (arrow) on the right compared to the normal other side.

Figure 8.3B. Coronal CECT image showing the infiltrating nasopharyngeal process (arrow) spreading to the trigeminal cistern and cavernous sinus (arrowheads).

DIFFERENTIAL DIAGNOSIS Systemic and localized noninfectious inflammatory disease such as Wegener's granulomatosis, skull base osteomyelitis, carcinoma, lymphoma, plasmacytoma

DIAGNOSIS Wegener's granulomatosis

DISCUSSION After physical examination and in less definitive clinical situations, it may be difficult to decide whether an area of nasopharyngeal swelling is inflammatory as opposed to neoplastic. In a low-grade chronic inflammatory process, this distinction might remain unclear even after biopsy; thus watchful waiting might become the default strategy, sometimes with imaging surveillance as an aid.

Wegener's granulomatosis can manifest anywhere in Waldeyer's ring, most typically in the nasopharynx. While, theoretically, sarcoidosis can manifest anywhere in the upper aerodigestive tract mucosa, the nasopharynx will usually be a site of contiguous disease in a patient with sinonasal involvement. Langerhans cell histiocytosis only rarely involves Waldeyer's ring.

Of the autoimmune diseases, none really specifically manifest in the nasopharynx. However, there are a group of patients who will present with self-limited infiltrating processes in the nasopharynx and show a nonspecific rise in "minor immunologic markers." The working diagnosis in these patients is usually Wegener's granulomatosis or cancer, but neither will be confirmed by biopsy that will typically show nonspecific inflammation and a cANCA that remains negative. The inflammations always raise a concern for cancer but turn out to be self-limited and/or responsive to corticosteroid or low-dose cyclophosphamide therapy. It is critical in this situation to be certain that skull base osteomyelitis is excluded and the lesions are followed to clearing so that an early cancer with surrounding inflammation is not missed.

PTLD frequently manifests in Waldeyer's ring, may be considered an inflammatory entity, and may be manifest by an invasive or noninvasive imaging pattern.

Sarcoidosis, Wegener's granulomatosis, and PTLD as seen on CT and MRI will produce nonspecific diffuse or localized infiltrating soft tissue masses in Waldeyer's ring. The nonspecific inflammations that occur do the same. Retropharyngeal and cervical adenopathy of the reactive type may be present. Meningeal involvement may be present as well as manifestations of labyrinthitis. These noninfectious inflammatory conditions will typically mimic cancer if there is not an established diagnosis. Symptoms and signs of eustachian tube dysfunction may dominate the clinical picture. Pain, especially otalgia, is common. Neuropathies related to the cranial nerves of the cavernous sinus and temporal bone or those of the lower cranial nerves are possible.

Because of the nonspecific imaging findings, correlation with the clinical data, laboratory findings, and additional biopsy is mandatory. Biopsy, as mentioned previously, is often not specific, showing only inflammation.

In this case, there was no cervical adenopathy, and when biopsy returned just "inflammatory cells," cANCA was done and Wegener's granulomatosis diagnosed. The patient responded completely to cyclophosphamide.

It is important to remember that atypical clinical and imaging features of nasopharyngeal pathology should raise the possibility of an inflammatory process. These diseases and early nasopharyngeal cancers mimic one another, and both possibilities must be kept in mind when developing a plan of surveillance when the diagnosis is not established definitely.

Question for Further Thought

1. Wegener's granulomatosis can cause nasal septal necrosis. Name three others pathologies that can cause this.

Reporting Responsibilities

Reporting is routine in these cases unless there is some progressive neurologic deficit. If a malignancy is a probable alternative diagnosis, direct communication would be very wise to facilitate planning the next course of action that might include imaging-directed biopsy.

What the Treating Physician Needs to Know

- If the disease process is localized or systemic
- If there is a possible risk of malignancy
- Whether there are any complications affecting adjacent organ systems such as the brain and meninges and orbits/eyes

Answer

1. Sarcoidosis, angiocentric lymphoma, advanced changes due to cocaine abuse

---

LEARN MORE

See Chapters 187 and 17 in *Head and Neck Radiology* by Mancuso and Hanafee.

CLINICAL HISTORY *A 56-year-old male patient presenting with chronic left serous otitis media and eventually developing facial pain.*

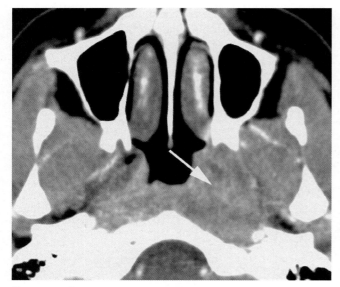

FIGURE **8.4A**

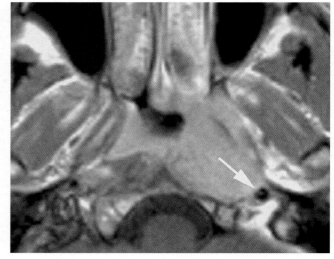

FIGURE **8.4C**

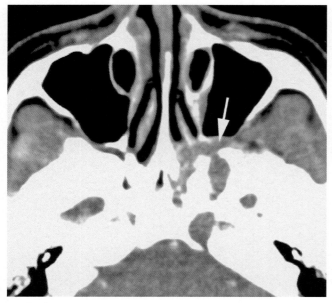

FIGURE **8.4B**

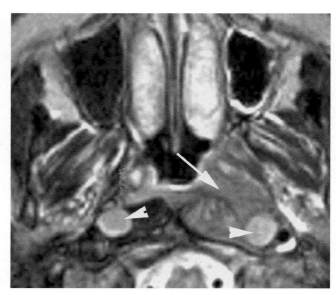

FIGURE **8.4D**

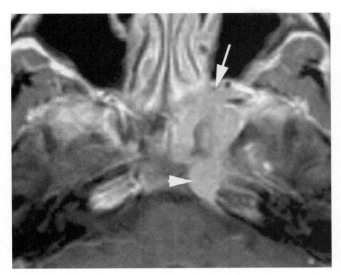

FIGURE 8.4E

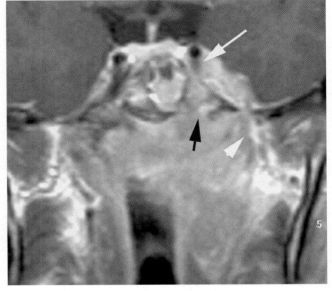

FIGURE 8.4F

FINDINGS

Figure 8.4A. Soft tissue view from a CECT study shows an infiltrating mass with ill-defined margins obliterating the deep soft tissue planes (arrows).

Figure 8.4B. Soft tissue view from a CECT study on a more cranial level than (Fig. 8.4A) shows the tumor spreading into the upper pterygopalatine fossa (arrow) from the sphenopalatine foramen. Note the widening of the pterygopalatine fossa and the obliteration of the fat that is usually visible within the fossa. More posteriorly, there is invasion at the petroclival fissure.

Figure 8.4C. T1W CE image shows the tumor growing into the prevertebral muscles, the retrostyloid parapharyngeal space (RSPS), and toward the carotid artery.

Figure 8.4D. T2W image shows the primary tumor (arrow) and related bilateral retropharyngeal lymph nodes that are obviously positive (arrowheads).

Figure 8.4E. T1W CE image shows the tumor growing into the pterygopalatine fossa (arrow) as well as into the petroclival fissure (arrowhead).

Figure 8.4F. Coronal T1W image with contrast shows the spread into the central skull base at the petroclival fissure (black arrow) and along the carotid artery into the cavernous sinus (white arrow). It also shows a tumor enlarging the third division of the trigeminal nerve (white arrowhead), likely another source of spread into the paracavernous region.

DIFFERENTIAL DIAGNOSIS

- *Nasopharyngeal malignancies:* Carcinoma (85%); lymphoma (10%); others (5%), including adenoid cystic carcinoma, adenocarcinoma, sarcoma (primarily rhabdomyosarcoma in children), plasmocytoma, melanoma
- *Inflammatory lesions:* Wegener's granulomatosis, sarcoidosis, histiocytosis, actinomycosis, pseudotumor, adenitis (all unusual or rare, compared with carcinoma)
- Skull base osteomyelitis

DIAGNOSIS Squamous cell carcinoma of the nasopharynx with skull base invasion and intracranial spread to the cavernous sinus

DISCUSSION Any adult, as in this case, with unilateral serous otitis media unresponsive to medical treatment for 3 to 6 months must have a high-resolution CT or MRI study to exclude a lesion obstructing the eustachian tube.

Facial pain may be due to neuropathy of any or all of the three divisions of the trigeminal nerve due to invasion of the trigeminal ganglion and/or individual divisions. In general, a painless, palpable cervical metastatic node is a common presenting complaint in patients with nasopharyngeal carcinoma. Other possible symptoms include sore throat, headache, neck pain, and neuropathies.

Nasopharyngeal carcinoma may spread submucosally, obviously mucosally, or some combination of the two regardless of histology. No submucosal lesion should ever be biopsied before imaging.

Nasopharyngeal carcinoma can spread in all directions, the most common or first affected regions being as follows:

- Inferior spread, either mucosal or submucosal, along the lateral pharyngeal walls to the tonsil level is common. Tumors invade the retropharyngeal space directly to spread inferiorly.

- Anterior spread through the posterior choana into the posterior nasal cavity occurs in larger lesions.

- Superior spread is primarily to the central and posterior skull base. Invasion of the central skull base, including the sphenoid sinus, is common by the time of presentation. The base of the sphenoid is a particularly common site of early involvement. Another favored site of early central skull base invasion is the region of the foramen lacerum and petroclival fissure since the mucosa of the nasopharyngeal roof and the fossa of Rosenmüller lie essentially on this bone. Advanced tumors erode through the foramen ovale and/or can invade the cavernous sinus with resulting neuropathies.

- Lateral spread can occur when tumor extends through the sinus of Morgagni to the parapharyngeal space and skull base. Direct lateral spread from the prestyloid parapharyngeal space (PSPS) to the infratemporal fossa usually occurs in advanced tumors with destruction of the pterygoid with tumor passing through the plates to the muscles in the space. Lateral spread to the pterygoid plates may direct tumor to the pterygopalatine fossa. Obliteration of the fat pad in the pterygopalatine fossa should prompt a search for subtle spread to the cavernous sinus along the second division of the trigeminal nerve. This route also leads to spread to the orbital apex, inferior orbital fissure, and perhaps nasal cavity. More posterior lateral growth will invade the RSPS. Apparent growth in the RSPS is often due to involvement of the lateral retropharyngeal lymph node. Less well differentiated tumors may follow the carotid artery into its foramen and canal and eventually the cavernous sinus, destroying or sparing adjacent bone of the carotid canal along the way.

Bone involvement and perineural spread may be very subtle. Marrow space invasion is best detected on noncontrast T1W images, whereas subtle cortical bone invasion can best be seen as cortical irregularities on thin-slice CT images in bone window. Perineural spread may manifest as relatively subtle enlargement and enhancement of the nerve or loss of the surrounding fat planes. This can best be appreciated on MR images.

The nasopharyngeal submucosal capillary lymphatic plexus is very extensive, explaining the high incidence of neck metastases in nasopharyngeal carcinoma. The tumor spreads first to the retropharyngeal nodes in almost all cases and then to levels 2 through and including level 5.

Distant metastasis at the time of original presentation is unusual. The most common sites of involvement include the lung, bone, and liver.

The diagnosis is usually obvious at endoscopy, especially for mucosal lesions, but can become ambiguous when the tumor resembles hypertrophic lymphoid tissue (as in lymphoma, PTLD, adenoiditis, and rare diseases such as Wegener's granulomatosis) or when the lesion is entirely submucosal. CT (with or without CT-guided biopsy) and MRI are the main supportive techniques in the evaluation of nasopharyngeal mucosal and submucosal masses. They are used for the differential diagnosis and especially to define the extent of the disease.

A general approach would include the following steps:

- Define where the mass is centered (arises).
- Is the mass well circumscribed, or does it have infiltrating margins?
- Is the morphology more likely inflammatory or neoplastic?
- Is there spread to the skull base, cavernous sinus, or other intracranial areas?
- Is there perineural spread?
- Are there abnormal retropharyngeal or other neck nodes?
- Define the precise margins in all directions.

In this case, as it is often so, the diagnosis of nasopharyngeal carcinoma was already known when the patient presented for imaging, and the question was to define the precise extent of the tumor. The facial pain was suggestive of neural involvement, and that was confirmed with tumor growing into pterygopalatine fossa from the sphenopalatine foramen but also growth into the cavernous sinus along the carotid artery. Furthermore, there was clear invasion of the prevertebral muscles, petroclival fissure, and skull base. This is not an unusual intracranial pattern of spread in less well differentiated nasopharyngeal carcinomas and lymphoma.

Questions for Further Thought

1. What laboratory tests and patient history may influence your differential diagnosis?
2. What are differential diagnostic possibilities for a nasopharyngeal mass with clear evidence of deep infiltration of parapharyngeal fat and muscle bundles?

Reporting Responsibilities

In general, nasopharyngeal carcinoma is known or suspected at the time of imaging, so no special communications is required. When a tumor is discovered or is reasonably likely to be present that was not clinically suspected, immediate direct communication with the referring treatment provider is wise.

It is very important that the report contains a complete assessment of the disease extent and all information that is relevant to treatment planning, reflective of the issues presented in the foregoing Discussion section.

What the Treating Physician Needs to Know

- All submucosal nasopharyngeal masses must be imaged before biopsy.

- Adult patients with nonresolving serous otitis media must have a focused high-resolution MR or CT study of the entire course of the auditory tube interpreted by an observer experienced in ENT imaging issues.
- Whether or not a nasopharyngeal malignancy is likely present with a clearly stated degree of confidence
- If not amenable to endoscopic biopsy, whether imaging-guided percutaneous biopsy is a reasonable alternative
- If cancer is present, the full extent of local and regional disease
- If an alternative diagnosis is more likely, what is the next best course of action?

Answers

1. The differential diagnosis is usually not altered by laboratory findings except in plasmacytoma (abnormal uri-nary and serum proteins), lymphoma/chronic leukemia (white cell differential), and Wegener's granulomatosis (cANCA). A history of transplant and related immunosuppressive therapy would make PTLD a more probable diagnosis.

2. Infiltrating processes may be caused by cancer (most common in adults), adenoiditis, Wegener's granulomatosis, and other noninfectious inflammatory diseases.

LEARN MORE

See Chapters 188 and 21 in *Head and Neck Radiology* by Mancuso and Hanafee.

CASE 8.5

CLINICAL HISTORY   *A 17-year-old male patient presenting with nosebleeds and a polypoid mass in the posterior choana region.*

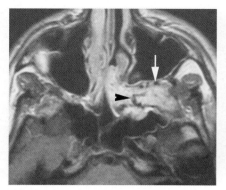

FIGURE 8.5A

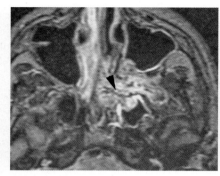

FIGURE 8.5B

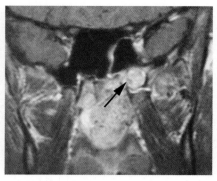

FIGURE 8.5C

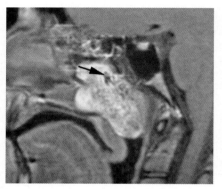

FIGURE 8.5D

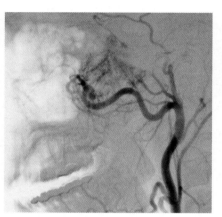

FIGURE 8.5E

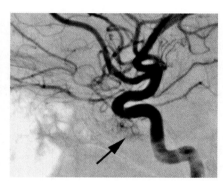

FIGURE 8.5F

FINDINGS

Figure 8.5A. A T1W CE image shows an enhancing mass entering the sphenopalatine foramen to occupy the pterygopalatine fossa and spread to the infratemporal fossa. An enlarged maxillary artery is present (white arrow) as well as flow voids within the lesion (arrowhead).

Figure 8.5B. T2W image shows the flow voids within a mass of mixed signal intensity.

Figure 8.5C. T1W CE mass shows the tumor entering the pterygopalatine fossa, as seen in a coronal plane.

Figure 8.5D. The sagittal T1W image with contrast shows the branching flow void of vascular pattern within the polypoid nasopharyngeal mass. A particularly large vascular pedicle is shown by the arrow.

Figure 8.5E. Angiogram in this patient shows the typical major feeding vessel to be the maxillary artery.

Figure 8.5F. Angiogram shows that the supply from the cavernous segment of the carotid artery is present.

DIFFERENTIAL DIAGNOSIS Differential diagnosis in this age group includes nasal polyps, nasal cavity and nasopha-

ryngeal carcinomas, lymphoma, sarcoma, benign vascular tumors and malformations, large adenoids, and parapharyngeal tumors. An intranasal hemangiopericytoma may occur rarely in this age group.

DIAGNOSIS   Juvenile angiofibroma (JAF)

DISCUSSION JAF is a benign vascular tumor that occurs almost exclusively in adolescent males. This diagnosis is in doubt after the age of 25 years. The tumors will stop growing and may recede once patients are in their early twenties. The point of origin is the mucosa of the high posterior nasal cavity near the sphenopalatine foramen.

The young male patient will present with unilateral nasal obstruction and/or epistaxis. Physical examination shows a polypoid mass that is indistinguishable from other polypoid nasal cavity masses, especially inflammatory fibroangiomatous polyps. This clinical setting should prompt CT and/or MR imaging. Any attempt to biopsy the lesion should be avoided because of the serious risk of hemorrhage. Cheek swelling and proptosis are unusual presenting complaints. Eustachian tube dysfunction may result in a middle ear presentation.

Grossly, the tumor is nonencapsulated, locally invasive with a "pushing" margin, and highly vascular. Growth is always along anatomic paths of least resistance, so continued early extension is directed toward the nasal cavity, the nasopharynx, and into the pterygopalatine fossa from the sphenopalatine foramen. Eventually, the tumor will fill the nasopharynx. Further extension may occur into the infratemporal and buccal space, into the orbit through the inferior orbital fissure, and intracranially through the superior and inferior orbital fissures. Other possible routes of extension include superiorly into the basisphenoid and commonly inferiorly into the pterygoid base and between the pterygoid processes in the pterygoid fossa.

Regressive remodeling and erosion of bone—for example, of the posterior maxillary antral wall—are common features, whereas a permeative or moth-eaten pattern of bone destruction is highly unusual and suggests alternative etiologies.

The predominant blood supply is from the maxillary and ascending pharyngeal arteries. Spread along the cavernous sinus and to the central skull base will appropriate internal carotid supply, greatly complicating a surgical approach following endovascular devascularization. JAF as a rule does not metastasize and has rarely been seen to involve retropharyngeal lymph nodes.

CT and MR typically show intense enhancement and typical spread pattern. An arterialized lesion is suggested indirectly by enlargement of the maxillary and ascending pharyngeal arteries and their distal branches. Noncontrast T1W MR images show a mass, isointense or slightly hyperintense to muscle, containing serpiginous vascular channels usually converging on a vascular pedicle located near the upper pterygopalatine fossa. The vascular pedicle is seen as an area of signal loss due to the flow void phenomenon in this relatively "arterialized" lesion. T2W images will show variable signal intensity throughout the lesion. Bright areas are likely related to slow flow in vascular spaces or myxoid stroma. Darker zones are due to more fibrous stroma. In larger tumors, there may be zones of necrosis and old hemorrhage, although these are the exception in most untreated lesions.

Lack of a typical internal morphology, enhancement, and spread pattern on CT strongly suggests that the mass is not a JAF.

Overall, the diagnosis of JAF is normally very straightforward. The patient's age, gender, and growth pattern and morphology on CECT and/or CEMR and arteriography, if necessary, is definitive. JAF is a benign tumor, but it can lead to death if left untreated. The extent of a JAF determines the therapeutic approach. MR, CT, and catheter angiography help to establish whether there is intracranial extension with a risk of internal carotid, including vidian artery, supply. The geographic limits of the tumor as seen on CT and/or MR will influence the chosen surgical approach or the planning of the radiotherapy. Endovascular devascularization will always precede surgery to minimize blood loss.

The key for the diagnostic images is to make it clear what structures and spaces are involved. Due to the high recurrence rate, preoperative planning is crucial for achieving good outcomes.

Question for Further Thought

1. What is the relevance of the findings in Figure 8.5F?

Reporting Responsibilities

In general, the diagnosis of JAF is suspected at the time of imaging, but some special communication and documentation is well advised if the study shows a likely JAF or an alternative diagnosis likely to be malignant.

If a JAF is diagnosed, it is very important that the report contains a complete assessment of the disease extent and all information that is relevant to treatment planning. The nature of this information should be apparent from the previous Discussion section.

What the Treating Physician Needs to Know

- Most likely alternative diagnosis if not a JAF
- If the diagnosis remains in question, what additional studies or other means of confirmation are appropriate as a next step
- If a JAF, its full extent since it has the potential to alter the approach to treatment: intracranial spread and likelihood of internal carotid supply. This must include detailed comments with regard to the following issues: (1) exactly which parts of the skull base are involved; (2) whether there is orbital or intracranial spread; if so, its precise extent; (3) whether the anatomic spread pattern suggests likely supply from the internal carotid artery on one or both sides, typically from the vidian artery but possibly from the cavernous segment; and (4) whether diagnostic angiography is likely necessary for medical decision making.

Answer

1. Such supply from the internal carotid artery makes complete preoperative embolization challenging and can lead to lack of control of these vessels and substantial blood loss at surgery if not appreciated. It is essential to exclude the internal carotid supply if surgery is contemplated.

> LEARN MORE
>
> See Chapter 189 in *Head and Neck Radiology* by Mancuso and Hanafee.

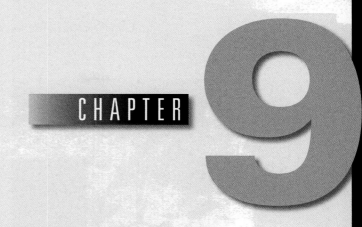

CHAPTER 9

Oropharynx

CLINICAL HISTORY *A teenaged girl with an enlarging submucosal mass in the upper oropharynx involving the soft palate and tonsillar region.*

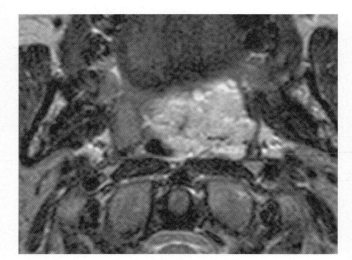

FIGURE **9.1A**

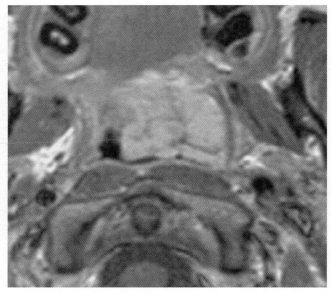

FIGURE **9.1B**

FINDINGS T2W image in (Fig. 9.1A) is consistent with the multiple, static fluid-filled spaces within the mass demonstrated by its fluid signal intensity. In (Fig. 9.1B), the contrast-enhanced (CE) T1W image shows that these spaces enhance and are blood pools.

DIFFERENTIAL DIAGNOSIS Perhaps a neurofibroma

DIAGNOSIS Venolymphatic malformation

DISCUSSION In general, developmental abnormalities present during childhood. Some manifest in infancy; however, the presentation is often delayed beyond infancy, sometimes well into the early adult years, as in this case, and even into middle age. Enlargement due to growth is variable. True growth may be at the same rate of normal structures, but masses may enter a rapid growth phase at times of accelerated growth of the individual—for instance, in adolescence, as in this case. Some, such as high-flow vascular malformations, have internal physiologic dynamics that will allow them to enlarge more rapidly than normal tissues rather than truly proliferate. Enlargement may also be due to infection, bleeding, and vascular thrombosis, especially in the case of venolymphatic malformations. Truly neoplastic developmental conditions such as teratomas or proliferative hemangioma may show relatively rapid true neoplastic growth.

Genetic markers can now separate venous malformations more specifically. There are three types of venolymphatic malformations (VM) based on clinical, epidemiologic, histologic, and imaging features. Some of these disorders of vascular development are now grouped as part of a cere-

brofacial venous metameric syndrome (CVMS). This case is an example of the most common, sporadic type of VM that has no familial associations and is compressible. All of the nonproliferative vascular malformations, as in this case, fit relatively well into a pathologic morphologic classification that includes capillary, venous, cavernous, lymphatic, arterial, and combined categories. These differences are usually suggested by morphologic features as seen on imaging studies. These are further usefully classified into low-flow and high-flow categories; this distinction is usually clear on diagnostic imaging exams. Venous malformations are slow-flow malformations made up of essentially dilated venous space in a fibrous and muscular stroma. Cavernous malformations are simply slow-flow malformations in which the endothelial-lined vascular spaces are nonspecific, and they may have smooth muscle in their walls. Some are well encapsulated, especially those arising in the orbit. Others have a less restrictive margin that allows for a more insinuating pattern of enlargement.

Questions for Further Thought

1. What is the Kasabach-Merritt syndrome?
2. Name some syndromic associations of vascular malformations.

Reporting Responsibilities

VMs are typically not of high acuity with regard to management decisions and are often in the clinical differential diagnosis; thus, routine reporting is sufficient unless there is a potential airway compromise or if a malignancy is suspected as the cause of the submucosal mass. Also, if a vascular mass is discovered, that should likely be reported directly so that the possible untoward effects of an uninformed biopsy of a vascular mass are avoided; these mainly include possible rapid airway encroachment due to any expanding hematoma and extensive aspiration of blood. It is also especially important to communicate effectively and promptly if there is a secondary infection.

The report should contain precise detail about the full extent of the mass and relationship to critical surrounding anatomic structures that might be the origin of the mass and/or affected by surgical or other treatment. In general, the most critical of these relationships are how the mass relates to the airway and surrounding deep neck space, including important nerves and vessels such as the carotid sheath and the lingual and hypoglossal nerves. The relationship to osseous structures, particularly the mandible and maxilla, including any evidence of bony erosion or remodeling may impact treatment planning.

Other developmental abnormalities and the possibility of syndromic associations should be considered in all developmental conditions, although most of these anomalies are isolated events.

If a vascular malformation is the etiology, the likely nature of flow dynamics should be included. There should also be a determination of whether catheter angiography might be necessary for further clarification of flow dynamics and the possibility of an endovascular treatment option.

If the thyroglossal duct migratory pathway is involved it should be noted that if a thyroglossal duct cyst contains functioning thyroid tissue and/or a complicating outgrowth of such tissue and whether other functioning thyroid tissue in its usual and/or ectopic location.

What the Treating Physician Needs to Know

- Precise diagnosis and the degree of confidence in that diagnosis

- Extent of the developmental anomaly and any potential danger to surrounding critical anatomy
- Any airway compromise
- Any complicating features of the anomaly that might alter medical decision making
- Whether there are associated or other anomalies
- Whether there is a reasonable likelihood of this being syndromic
- Is there any need for further imaging to answer any of these issues?

Answers

1. The Kasabach-Merritt syndrome is a secondary disorder associated with large hemangiomas and malformations that cause a thrombocytopenia and a consumptive coagulopathy.

2. Syndromic associations of venolymphatic malformations include Turner, Klinefelter, and Noonan syndromes.

   Most of these disorders of vascular development are now grouped as part of a craniofacial arteriovenous metameric syndrome (CAMS) or CVMS (discussed previously). The current understanding of abnormal migration of neural crest cells relative to the growth directing metameres of craniofacial development now logically explains many of the associations in these conditions that have been largely just described over the history of medicine.

> **LEARN MORE**
> See Chapters 191 and 9 in *Head and Neck Radiology* by Mancuso and Hanafee.

CLINICAL HISTORY *A 32-year-old male patient with a history of a fever, odynophagia, and severe throat pain.*

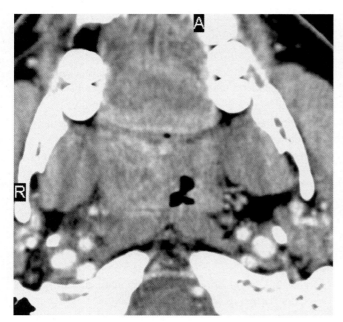

FIGURE 9.2A

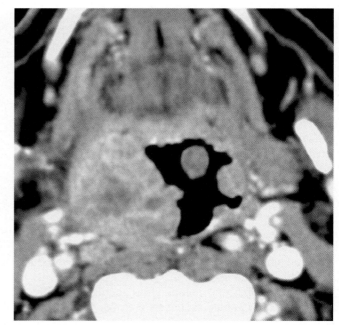

FIGURE 9.2C

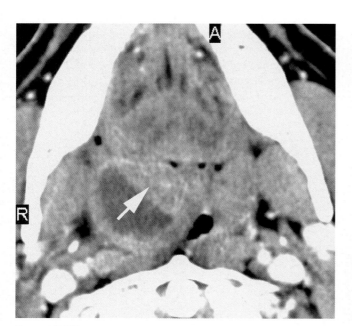

FIGURE 9.2B

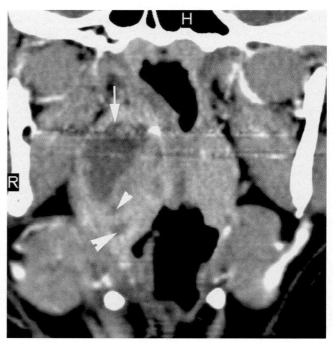

FIGURE 9.2D

FINDINGS

Figure 9.2A. Contrast-enhanced computed tomography (CECT) shows cellulitis and abscess formation along the upper pole of the palatine tonsil.

Figure 9.2B. Accumulation of purulent material spreads mainly in the peritonsillar space, displacing the inflamed tonsillar tissue medially (arrow).

Figure 9.2C. Intense cellulitis in the tonsil and a peritonsillar collection as well as other small abscesses within the tonsillar tissue are present.

Figure 9.2D. Coronal reformations shows a peritonsillar collection (arrow) extending over the superior pole of the tonsil into the supratonsillar recess and smaller abscesses within tonsillar tissue (arrowheads) displacing the main portion of the palatine tonsil inferiorly and medially.

DIFFERENTIAL DIAGNOSIS Tonsillar abscesses

DIAGNOSIS Peritonsillar and tonsillar abscesses

DISCUSSION Inflammatory conditions involving the oral cavity and oropharynx can be noninfectious or infectious. Infections present sporadically in children and young adults, causing fever, intense pain, poor feeding, and lymphadenopathy. In the immunocompromised (i.e., patients with diabetes and HIV infection), they can relatively indolent and/or be unusually aggressive.

Oropharyngeal infections usually have an obvious clinical picture, but when the extent of the disease and complications must be established, their evaluation may be augmented with imaging. Imaged infections are most likely due to an acute or subacute pyogenic bacterial infection, most commonly from a pharyngeal or dental infection complicated by abscess. Viral infections are imaged when they are severe enough to mimic a pyogenic infection or a neoplasm such as lymphoma. Fungal infections occur predominantly in the immunocompromised population.

Imaging findings of infectious processes include the following:

- A cellulitic pattern with infiltration/obliteration of the fat planes. Most infections enhance more than muscle and spread along paths of least resistance, which includes traveling along the adjacent musculature (i.e., styloid muscles) or through penetrating vessels.
- An associated contained or spreading abscess. This should always be identified as "drainable" (usually with a bulging contour) or "nondrainable."
- Signs of osteomyelitis (i.e., cortical bone erosion) or a subperiosteal abscess
- Septic arteritis or thrombophlebitis

Questions for Further Thought

1. When do infections of the oropharynx require drainage?
2. What is the characteristic imaging appearance of inflamed but not necessarily pyogenic tonsillitis?
3. What is the difference between a tonsillar and a peritonsillar abscess?
4. What is Lemierre syndrome?

Reporting Responsibilities

There should always be proper communication with the referring clinician about the airway status and whether there is likely a drainable pyogenic abscess, a life-threatening condition such as rapidly spreading necrotizing infection, or a potentially life-threatening complication such as Lemierre syndrome. Infections that arise in a diabetic or otherwise immunocompromised patient usually require some form of direct communication.

If an unusual etiology is suspected based on the imaging findings, the treating clinician should be informed of this prior to endoscopy and biopsy so that the sampled material will be appropriate and the pathologist can be forewarned as well.

What the Treating Physician Needs to Know

- If the airway appears threatened, recall that the imaging appearance may exaggerate the real risk of airway compromise.
- Computed tomography (CT) and magnetic resonance imaging (MRI) will normally be definitive in separating cellulitis and reactive edema due to pyogenic infection from abscess and other drainable collections.
- Spreading necrotizing infections, especially in diabetics, may occasionally mimic edema but require drainage.
- Imaging findings in focal inflammatory diseases can mimic the appearance of malignancy.
- The oropharynx may be a site of manifestation of systemic inflammatory disease, but this is very uncommonly the only affected site or a significant manifestation of those diseases.

Answers

1. Drainage is needed when abscesses are located in the subperiosteal space or those that show transspatial spread beyond the oropharynx to the parapharyngeal space, submandibular space, or to in the floor of the mouth. Peritonsillar abscess is typically drained by tonsillectomy.
2. Tonsillar tissue that is inflamed with a layered or striated pattern of enhancement is characteristic of inflammation but is nonspecific and not indicative of abscess.
3. Tonsillar abscesses develop within the tonsillar crypts and tonsillar pseudocapsule. When pus spreads outside these confines and into the potential space between the tonsillar tissue and the surrounding pharyngeal constrictor muscles, it becomes a peritonsillar abscess.
4. This is a complication of a pyogenic oropharyngeal infection with a secondary septic thrombophlebitis of the internal jugular vein. This may subsequently lead to septic emboli, most commonly to the lung but also the joints, the liver, and rarely the central nervous system. These patients have positive blood cultures for *Fusobacterium necrophorum*, the causative bacterium. When severe, this can lead to multiorgan failure and death.

> **LEARN MORE**
> See Chapters 192 and 13 in *Head and Neck Radiology* by Mancuso and Hanafee.

CLINICAL HISTORY *A 2-year-old girl presenting with throat pain and tenderness after poking the right tonsil with a sharp pencil.*

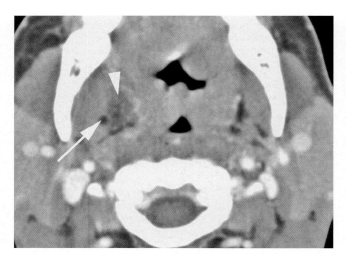

FIGURE **9.3A**

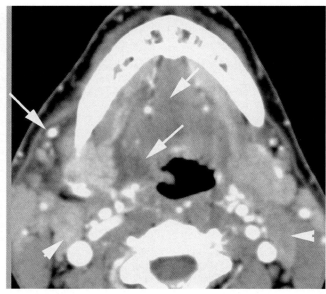

FIGURE **9.3C**

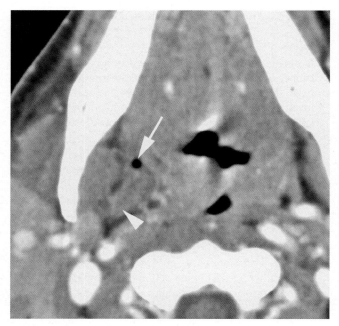

FIGURE **9.3B**

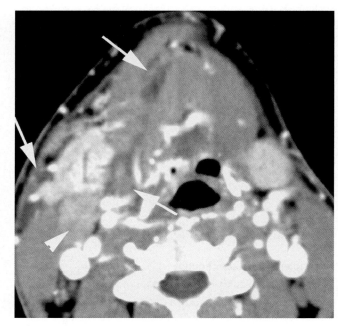

FIGURE **9.3D**

FINDINGS

Figure 9.3A. CECT shows edema and a small amount of gas in the parapharyngeal space deep to the palatine tonsil (arrowhead).

Figure 9.3B. Closer view of the edema (arrowhead) and gas (arrow), with little evidence of surrounding inflammatory change.

Figure 9.3C. Very extensive edema involving the tongue base and adjacent parapharyngeal space as well as the soft tissues of the upper neck (arrows) and very obvious acute reactive adenopathy (arrowheads).

Figure 9.3D. Spreading of the inflammatory changes due to spreading cellulitis and possibly early abscess formation (arrows) in addition to the reactive level 2 adenopathy.

DIFFERENTIAL DIAGNOSIS Posttraumatic cellulitis

DIAGNOSIS Posttraumatic cellulitis and early abscess formation

DISCUSSION The oropharynx and oral cavity can be injured iatrogenically or accidentally. Accidental blunt injuries are mainly due to motor vehicle accidents, assaults, and fights. Penetrating injuries are relatively uncommon and are due to gunshot wounds and swallowed foreign bodies or when children stick sharp objects in the mouth and oropharynx.

Accidental blunt and penetrating injuries often accompany injuries to the face and lower jaw. The identification of these injuries is usually incidental and may be overlooked when there are other extensive injuries in the absence of a life-threatening airway obstruction.

Trauma results in blood and edema that spreads through the deep planes within and surrounding the oropharynx and oral cavity, manifesting as localized swelling and obliteration of the fat planes. Mucosal tears cause air leakage, as seen in the patient under consideration. When there is extensive neck emphysema there may also be more severe injuries also causing bleeding and edema that may compress the airway as well as false passages, fistulas, or denudation of cartilage/bone.

Imaging findings include diffuse or focal mucosal and pharyngeal muscular wall enhancement, either reactive or due to phlegmon; reactive enhancement in the walls of false passages and abscesses. It may also suggest rupture of a major salivary gland with leakage of glandular secretions into surrounding soft tissues. There may also be an associated vascular injury.

Questions for Further Thought

1. When should traumatic injuries to the oral cavity and oropharynx be treated?

2. What are the consequences of a delayed recognition of a traumatic injury to the oral cavity and oropharynx?

Reporting Responsibilities

For acute injuries, immediate verbal communication with the treating trauma team and otolaryngologist and/or oral and maxillofacial surgeon is most important if there is any evidence of severe airway compromise, if an associated significant injury was not expected, or if there is a secondary infection or vascular injury.

What the Treating Physician Needs to Know

- Status of the airway
- Status of the facial skeleton
- Any evidence of false passage or fistula
- Any retained foreign bodies
- Any associated injuries or complications

Answers

1. Once the airway and other potentially life-threatening injuries are stabilized, the diagnostic workup of an injured oral cavity, oropharynx, larynx and/or hypopharynx, and trachea should proceed without delay.

2. Delayed diagnosis can lead to a subacute complication such as an abscess, a salivary gland leak, or a delayed vascular complication.

> LEARN MORE
> See Chapters 193 and 13 in *Head and Neck Radiology* by Mancuso and Hanafee.

CLINICAL HISTORY *An adult patient presenting with a firm, submucosal tongue base mass and swallowing discomfort.*

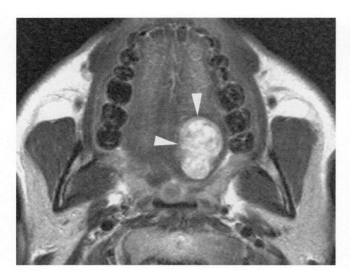

FIGURE **9.4A**

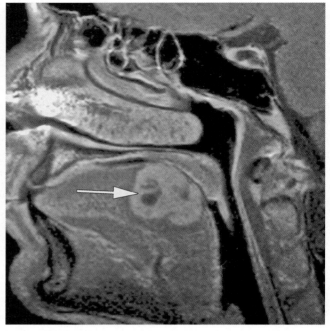

FIGURE **9.4B**

FINDINGS

Figure 9.4A. Axial T2W spin echo image shows a well-circumscribed mass that is hyperintense to muscle and fat in the tongue base on the left side (arrowheads).

Figure 9.4B. Sagittal T1W image, after administration of gadolinium, shows enhancement of the lesion and some areas that lack enhancement perhaps due to a zone of necrosis.

DIFFERENTIAL DIAGNOSIS Minor salivary gland benign or malignant epithelial tumor, squamous cell carcinoma (SCCa), granular cell tumor, sarcoma

DIAGNOSIS Schwannoma

DISCUSSION After physical examination, it is often difficult to decide whether an area of oropharyngeal swelling is neoplastic, inflammatory, traumatic, or degenerative. Even after biopsy, the etiology of a mass may remain obscure since these lesions may be deep seated and the biopsy attempt fails to sample the actual site of interest. As in this case, some patients have processes predominantly occurring beneath intact oropharyngeal mucosa that cause dysphagia and/or odynophagia with no visible mass. Imaging is particularly valuable to the head and neck surgeon to detect or exclude a submucosal lesion that may spread underneath intact and normal-appearing mucosa, causing such symptoms that mimic the initial presentation of the far more common mucosally obvious oropharyngeal squamous cell cancer. Any mass or such symptoms, regardless of etiology, suspicious for a deeply located mass (cancer or otherwise) should be studied primarily with CT or MRI.

Most benign tumors or focal areas of swelling in the oropharynx will have a nonspecific imaging appearance. On occasion, imaging findings will be specific enough to allow an etiologic or sometimes a very likely specific tissue diagnosis. The most fitting and usual use of CT and MRI is to show the extent of the lesion and identify the likely etiology of a submucosal mass. Some of these benign masses will be developmental, and all of them are very uncommon.

Imaging may provide clues but only infrequently suggests a specific diagnosis in these rare tumors. A well-circumscribed mass that appears as if it might be submucosal and enhances considerably suggests a vascular malformation, which may be a true benign neoplasm if it is a proliferative hemangioma. Other tumors, such as muscle-origin tumor and neurogenic tumor including a granular cell tumor, may show more moderate enhancement. A similar mass with cystic or necrotic zones suggests a salivary or neural tissue origin; these features along with the very well demarcated periphery narrow the likelihood to mainly these two possibilities in this case. A more solid mass might suggest a rhabdomyoma or fibrous-origin lesion. Mature fat would indicate a lipoma.

Questions for Further Thought

1. Name three common locations of dense accumulations of minor salivary gland in the oropharynx. What are the most common benign and two most common malignant tumors that arise from these rests?

2. Why do benign salivary gland tumors appear very bright on T2W images?

Reporting Responsibilities

Any time the mass places the airway at risk due to obstruction or if biopsy is planned and the lesion morphology suggests there might be excessive bleeding, immediate direct communication with the referring treatment provider and documentation of that communication is necessary.

If oropharyngeal cancer is suspected clinically but not proven, the study may be used to exclude a deeply infiltrating mass and/or find an alternative explanation for a visible submucosal mass or a symptom such as dysphagia, odynophagia, oropharyngeal region pain, or referred otalgia. Exclusionary language for such possibilities should be part of the report.

It is very important that the report contains a complete assessment of the disease extent and all information that is relevant to treatment planning. This must include precise comments regarding the following issues:

- Full soft tissue extent of the mass including that to the oropharynx, nasopharynx, and suprahyoid deep neck spaces
- Whether the mass might be excessively vascular or of vascular origin, such as a vascular malformation
- Determination of the most likely diagnosis based on imaging and raising the possibility of cancer rather than a benign tumor, if more likely based on the observed spread pattern
- Mandible and maxilla involvement
- Spread along nerves and vessels that in this region may suggest origin from or involvement of the lingual, ascending pharyngeal and maxillary neurovascular bundles as a sign of a neurogenic lesion or as a sign of hypervascularity

What the Treating Physician Needs to Know

- If not SCCa, what is the likely alternative diagnosis based on imaging?
- Exact extent of the mass within the oropharyngeal and related deep soft tissue spaces
- Evidence for bone involvement and its precise extent
- If biopsy might be more hazardous than usual
- If the airway is at risk

Answers

1. Soft palate, tonsillar pillars and retromolar trigone region, tongue base; benign mixed tumor—mucoepidermoid carcinoma and adenoid cystic carcinoma

2. Benign minor salivary gland tumors have microcystic morphology those small cystic spaces filled with relatively watery material.

LEARN MORE

See Chapters 194 and 29 in *Head and Neck Radiology* by Mancuso and Hanafee.

CLINICAL HISTORY *A 54-year-old male patient with a chronic history of smoking and alcohol use presenting with a right-sided throat pain and right-sided otalgia.*

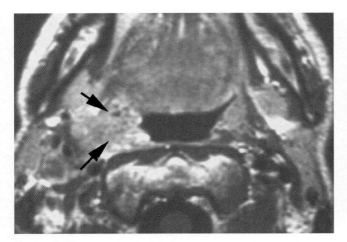

FIGURE **9.5A**

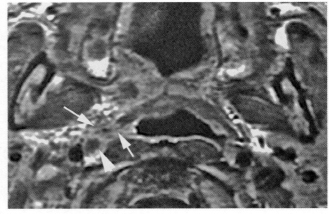

FIGURE **9.5C**

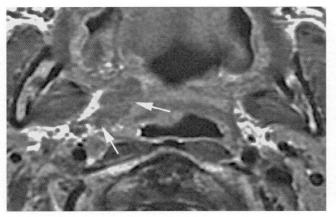

FIGURE **9.5B**

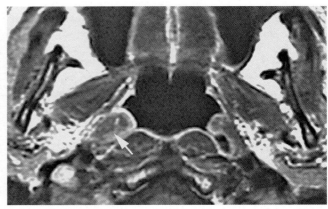

FIGURE **9.5D**

FINDINGS

Figure 9.5A. CE T1W image demonstrates an enhancing tonsillar and glossotonsillar mass infiltrating into the parapharyngeal space along the styloid and constrictor musculature (arrow).

Figure 9.5B. Noncontrast T1W image demonstrates infiltration within the parapharyngeal space (black arrows), invading the palatal musculature (white arrows) and spreading to the retrostyloid parapharyngeal space.

Figure 9.5C. CE T1W image shows continuity of spread between the levator muscle of the palate (arrows) back to a metastatic medial retropharyngeal lymph node (arrowhead).

Figure 9.5D. CE T1W image shows continued spread along the levator muscle of the palate to involve the region of the torus tubarius of the nasopharynx.

DIFFERENTIAL DIAGNOSIS Oropharyngeal lymphoma

DIAGNOSIS Tonsillar SCCa with occult spread to the nasopharynx

DISCUSSION Oropharyngeal and oral cavity malignant neoplasms are SCCa in 95% of cases. The remaining 5% comprise include lymphoma, minor salivary gland epithelial carcinomas, and sarcomas (excluding sinonasal or osseous/dental tumors of the maxilla or mandible). Metastatic lesions rarely mimic primary tumors.

Oropharyngeal and oral cavity SCCa has tobacco use as the main etiologic factor, with alcohol use being both a synergistic factor to tobacco and an independent risk in itself as a carcinogen. Other risk factors include HIV infection and a very important link to papillomavirus infection, the latter being an association that clearly affects treatment strategy and prognosis.

These carcinomas are typically a disease of those over 50 years of age and present with a mass, ulceration, pain, referred otalgia, loose teeth, or trismus or a functional complaint such as alteration of speech, chewing, or swallowing. Cervical adenopathy of uncertain etiology is a common presentation of oropharyngeal SCCa but is virtually never a mode of presentation in oral cavity SCCa.

The tonsillar region includes the anterior and posterior tonsillar pillars and the tonsillar fossa, each with a different spread pattern, clinical findings, prognosis, and treatment when involved by cancer. Tonsillar fossa cancers commonly spread to the posterior tonsillar pillar, oropharynx, glossotonsillar sulcus, and tongue base. Spread to the hypopharynx or invasion of the mandible is seen in advanced lesions. Perineural spread is generally not seen unless the tonsillar pillars are involved. These lesions are among the highest risk of palpable adenopathy at presentation.

Tonsillar fossa carcinomas may be primarily exophytic or endophytic. Endophytic growth penetrates the pharyngeal constrictor to invade the parapharyngeal space. Parapharyngeal space growth or across the supratonsillar recess and soft palate can uncommonly extend to the upper nasopharynx, as in this case, and rarely to the skull base.

Question for Further Thought

1. When is recurrence of a treated malignancy most common, and how does it present?

Reporting Responsibilities

Direct, verbal communication with the referring treatment provider is wise if the tumor places the airway at risk, if there might be a superimposed infection, or if a tumor is discovered that was not clinically suspected.

Routine reporting should include items in the following section.

What the Treating Physician Needs to Know

- If not SCCa, what is the likely alternative diagnosis based on imaging?
- Full soft tissue extent of the tumor, including unexpected spread outside the region of origin
- Bone involvement—presence and extent or exclusion with a very high degree of confidence
- If there is evidence of spread along vessels or nerves
- Evaluation of the presence and extent of cervical and retropharyngeal node metastases
- If the study is done for posttreatment surveillance, the likelihood of control and suggestions for additional follow-up if necessary from an imaging perspective

Answer

1. Recurrence almost always occurs within 2 years of treatment. Recurrences after 5 years are rare and may be difficult to differentiate from a new primary tumor. Recurrence after radiation therapy often presents a return of the original symptoms or new symptoms with persistence and especially worsening of lymphedema beyond 1 or 2 months post radiation therapy. Early recurrence after surgery occurs in a background of an already deformed anatomy following resection or deep within the reconstructed mucosa, making identification of these lesions somewhat challenging.

LEARN MORE
See Chapters 195, 21, and 23 in *Head and Neck Radiology* by Mancuso and Hanafee.

CHAPTER 10

Oral Cavity and Floor of the Mouth

CLINICAL HISTORY *A pediatric patient with a history of poor feeding.*

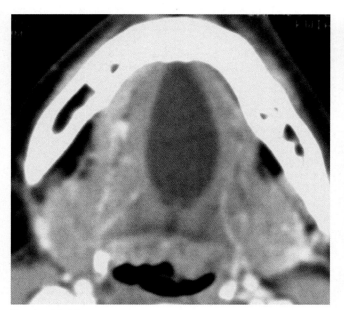

FIGURE **10.1A**

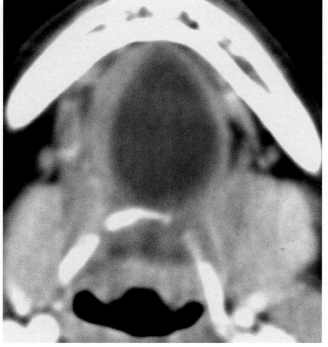

FIGURE **10.1B**

FINDINGS

Figure 10.1A,B. Contrast-enhanced computed tomography (CECT) study demonstrating the midline mass without any fat content.

DIFFERENTIAL DIAGNOSIS Thyroglossal duct cyst (atypical), foregut duplication cyst (rare), epidermoid cyst, venolymphatic malformation (unlikely)

DIAGNOSIS Dermoid cyst

DISCUSSION In general, developmental abnormalities of the oral cavity and oropharynx generally present during childhood; however, this can be delayed well beyond infancy sometimes well into early adulthood and even into middle age. These abnormalities may be discovered incidentally while imaging for other purposes. They more commonly come to medical attention when they become visible; cause pain or interfere with function (i.e., chewing, speech, breathing, or swallowing); or are complicated by infection, bleeding, thrombosis, or a rare case of malignant degeneration.

Developmental cystic abnormalities affecting the oral cavity, floor of the mouth, and oropharynx include dermoids, epidermoids, branchial apparatus cysts, thyroglossal duct cysts, and foregut duplication cysts. Dermoid cysts grow from remnants left behind in developmental migratory pathways.

Question for Further Thought

1. What is the role of ultrasound in the evaluation of developmental abnormalities of the oral cavity and floor of the mouth?

Reporting Responsibilities

Developmental abnormalities of the oral cavity typically are not of high acuity with regard to management decisions and are in the clinical differential diagnosis; thus, routine reporting is sufficient unless there is a potential airway compromise, a compacting infection, or an alternative consideration of a malignancy is likely.

The report should contain precise detail about the full extent of the lesion and relationship to critical surrounding anatomic structures that might be the origin of the lesion and/or affected by surgical or other treatment. In general, the most critical of these relationships is how the mass relates to the airway and surrounding deep neck space, including important nerves and vessels.

The relationship to osseous structures, particularly the mandible and maxilla, including any evidence of bony erosion or remodeling may impact treatment planning.

It is especially important to communicate effectively and promptly if there is a secondary infection.

Other developmental abnormalities and the possibility of syndromic associations should be considered in all developmental conditions, although most of these anomalies are isolated events.

If a vascular malformation is the etiology, the likely nature of flow dynamics should be included as well as the relationship to osseous structures, particularly the mandible and maxilla, with regard to potential for excessive bleeding that might pose a risk during even routine dental procedures. There should also be a determination of whether catheter angiography might be necessary (this is only occasionally the case) for further clarification of flow dynamics and the possibility of an endovascular treatment option.

If the thyroglossal duct migratory pathway is involved it should be determined whether the thyroglossal duct cyst contains functioning thyroid tissue and/or a complicating outgrowth of such tissue and whether other functioning thyroid tissue in its usual and/or ectopic location.

What the Treating Physician Needs to Know

- Precise diagnosis and the degree of confidence in that diagnosis
- Extent of the developmental anomaly and any potential danger to surrounding critical anatomy
- Any airway compromise
- Any complicating features of the anomaly that might alter medical decision making
- Whether there are associated or other anomalies

- Whether there is a reasonable likelihood of this being syndromic
- Is there any need for further imaging to answer any of these issues?

Answer

1. Ultrasound may be sufficient in the evaluation of small, well-defined lesions in the oral cavity and floor of the mouth, but it is often insufficient in defining the anatomic extent of larger lesions; it may provide useful information on the degree of vascularity of a lesion. Ultrasound is frequently not definitive and is cost additive, so its use in general seems unjustified. If it can obviate other more risky studies and provide all information necessary for medical decision making, then it would be of obvious benefit, but this is not the usual circumstance. There is little or no use for ultrasound when the lesions primarily affect the oropharynx.

LEARN MORE
See Chapters 197 and 8 in *Head and Neck Radiology* by Mancuso and Hanafee.

CLINICAL HISTORY *A known intravenous drug abuser presenting with tenderness in the floor of the mouth that was leading to rapid airway compromise.*

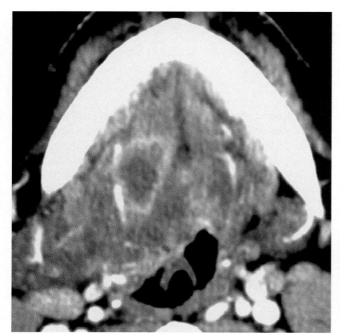

FIGURE **10.2A**

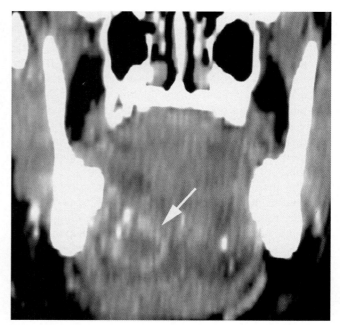

FIGURE **10.2C**

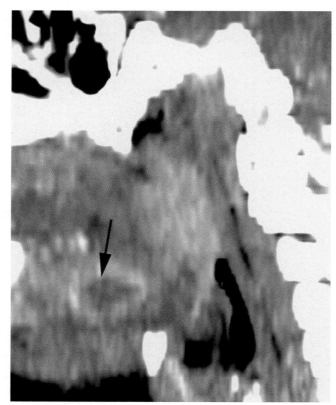

FIGURE **10.2B**

FINDINGS

Figure 10.2A–C. Multiplanar reformatted, contrast-enhanced computed tomography (CECT) shows a ring-enhancing fluid collection in the floor of the mouth with an extraordinary amount of edema. The process is clearly separate from the mandible and teeth. There are no radiodense foreign bodies.

DIFFERENTIAL DIAGNOSIS Infected cancer, purulent sublingual gland sialadenitis, infected ranula or infected developmental cyst

DIAGNOSIS Sublingual space abscess and cellulitis. This infection was not of dental origin but was due to sublingual injections (specific history of sublingual injections withheld).

DISCUSSION The anaerobic abscess due to the sublingual injection route of drug abuse was drained. Note how in this case imaging not only differentiates between a drainable and nondrainable collection but also provides a map for appropriate approach to drainage and some approximation of airway risk as well as possible virulence of the infection.

After physical examination, it may be difficult to decide whether an area of oral cavity swelling is inflammatory or infectious as opposed to neoplastic; however, the clinical presentation will often be very clear, especially in the case of acute pyogenic infections. In low-grade inflammatory processes, this distinction might remain unclear even after biopsy, and watchful waiting might become the default strategy, sometimes with imaging surveillance as an aid.

Much inflammatory swelling in the oral cavity will have a nonspecific imaging appearance when considered independent of the clinical setting. Taken with the clinical setting, the findings are often specific enough to confirm the etiology suspected clinically. Computed tomography (CT) and occasionally magnetic resonance imaging (MRI) are then used for their primary function of mapping the extent of, most commonly pyogenic, infectious inflammatory process.

Most infections of the oral cavity that come to imaging are acute or subacute pyogenic bacterial infections, these being mainly due to dental infections complicated by abscess formation and a few due to extension of pharyngeal infections. The patient under consideration is an example of an unusual source of infection another being a complication of purulent sublingual gland sialadenitis. Actinomycosis infection will most commonly be an extension of a periapical tooth infection. Fungal infection may come from the mandible as well. Syphilis may cause an atrophic glossitis, and a mucosal gumma can mimic tumor until it is biopsied.

Viral infections are usually not so severe that they clinically mimic pyogenic infection enough to trigger imaging

with CT or MRI. Epstein-Barr virus infection, including posttransplant lymphoproliferative disease, may mimic lymphoma, and the related adenopathy may trigger imaging.

Questions for Further Thought

1. What is Ludwig's angina, and what is its most major risk factor that threatens mortality?
2. In what circumstance might an actual abscess mimic only cellulitis?

Reporting Responsibilities

The diagnostic radiologist, if asked to assist in this clinical problem, must be immediately available and in verbal contact with the treating physicians, mainly to ensure proper communication about the airway status as well as if there is a drainable pyogenic abscess present or a life-threatening condition such as rapidly spreading necrotizing infection present. Airway compromise that could prove significant should be verbally communicated immediately.

Infections that arise in a diabetic or otherwise immunocompromised patient usually require some direct communication.

What the Treating Physician Needs to Know

- In occasional cases that appear to threaten the airway, prompt communication is necessary, but the imaging appearance may exaggerate the real risk of airway compromise.
- CT and MRI will normally be definitive in separating cellulitis and reactive edema due to pyogenic infection from abscess and other drainable collections.
- Spreading necrotizing infections, especially in diabetics, may occasionally mimic edema but require drainage.
- Imaging findings in focal inflammatory diseases can mimic the appearance of malignancy.

Answers

1. This cellulitis or abscess of the floor of the mouth was described in the 1800s; its main etiology at that time was pyogenic infection of dental origin. Then and now, although much less frequently nowadays, it can lead to death by rapid airway compromise.
2. Spreading, necrotizing infections that occur in a diabetic or otherwise immunocompromised patient, especially in diabetics, may occasionally mimic edema on CT and MRI but require drainage.

> **LEARN MORE**
> See Chapters 198 and 13 in *Head and Neck Radiology* by Mancuso and Hanafee.

CLINICAL HISTORY *A young adult presenting with a mass medial to the retromolar trigone.*

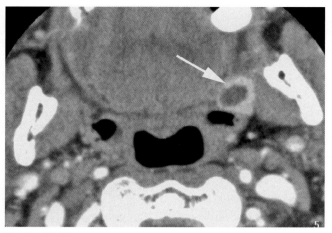

FIGURE **10.3**

FINDINGS

Figure 10.3. CECT image shows a mass medial to the retromolar trigone and along the region of the anterior tonsillar pillar (arrow). It has a thick and focally nodular enhancing periphery and a homogenously low density internal structure. There is no surrounding soft tissue swelling.

DIFFERENTIAL DIAGNOSIS Malignant minor salivary gland epithelial tumor. The rest that follow are very uncommon, if at all likely: atypical granular cell tumor or other benign neurogenic mass, mesenchymal-origin benign tumor or sarcoma, localized venolymphatic malformation, low-grade abscess, thrombosed vessel if a parent vessel could be identified, or history of instrumentation (such as post tonsillectomy).

DIAGNOSIS Benign mixed tumor of minor salivary gland origin

DISCUSSION This mass medial to the retromolar trigone and along the region of the anterior tonsillar pillar lies at the important border zone between the oral cavity and oropharynx. Minor salivary gland tumors are particularly common in the oral cavity in the vicinity of the retromolar trigone. This area, as well as the hard palate, soft palate, and tonsillar pillars, is fairly rich in minor salivary gland tissue.

A benign oral cavity mass may produce problems with speech, chewing, and swallowing as the initial symptom. Sore throat, referred ear pain, and/or pain localized to the oral cavity region would suggest a malignant rather than benign tumor. The more common presentation, as occurred in this patient, is the observation of a submucosal bulge noted by the patient or health care provider, often a dentist.

Physical examination is mainly done by direct inspection and palpation. The physical examination should establish whether there is a visible mucosal lesion. A bluish or reddish hue or abnormal vascularity may be noticed in hypervascular tumors.

Benign masses limited to the oral cavity often mimic the initial presentation of oral cavity cancer. Any mass, regardless of etiology, that is suspicious for deep infiltration or cancer should be studied primarily with CT if imaging is desired as part of the evaluation since a bone origin or involvement will be in question. MRI can be used initially if preferred, especially in young patients. Supplemental MRI, in the situations where it might add meaningful incremental data, is best directed by CT findings to a localized area of interest where its strengths related to better soft tissue contrast resolution may be exploited.

Questions for Further Thought

1. What is the typical morphologic growth pattern of a benign tumor and its affect on bone?
2. What is the typical annual rate of enlargement of the maximum dimension of a benign neoplasm?

Reporting Responsibilities

In general, benign oral cavity masses are in the differential diagnosis at the time of imaging, so no special communication is required. More often, cancer is a concern; if cancer remains a consideration after the study, then direct communication is wise.

Any time the tumor places the airway at risk due to obstruction or if biopsy is planned and the lesion morphology suggests that excessive bleeding might occur, immediate direct communication with the referring treatment provider is necessary.

If oral cavity cancer is clinically suspected but not proven, the study may be used to exclude a deeply infiltrating submucosal mass and/or find an alternative explanation for a visible submucosal mass. Exclusionary language for such possibilities should be part of the report.

It is very important that the report contains a complete assessment of the disease extent and all information that is relevant to treatment planning. This must include precise comments regarding the following issues:

- Full soft tissue extent of the mass, including possible spread to the adjacent oropharynx and sometimes nasopharynx and to the suprahyoid deep neck spaces (mainly the submandibular and parapharyngeal spaces)
- Determination as to whether the mass might be excessively vascular or of vascular origin, such as a vascular malformation
- Determination of the most likely diagnosis based on imaging and raising the possibility of cancer rather than a benign tumor if likely based on spread pattern
- Mandibular and maxillary involvement
- Spread along or origin from regional nerves and vessels

What the Treating Physician Needs to Know

- If not squamous cell carcinoma (SCCa), what is the likely alternative diagnosis based on imaging?
- Exact extent of the mass within the oral cavity and related deep soft tissue spaces

- Evidence for bone involvement and its precise localization and extent
- If biopsy might be more hazardous than usual because of hypervascularity
- If the airway is at risk

Answers

1. These benign masses tend to grow as well-circumscribed spheroids displacing surrounding anatomic structures. They may cause remodeling of adjacent bone but should not appear frankly invasive of surrounding soft tissues or bone.
2. 1 to 3 mm per year—more rapid enlargement in a benign tumor can be related to intratumoral bleeding and/or necrosis.

LEARN MORE
See Chapters 199 and 22 in *Head and Neck Radiology* by Mancuso and Hanafee.

CLINICAL HISTORY *A 54-year-old male patient with a chronic history of smoking and alcohol abuse presenting with progressive difficulty chewing and swallowing food.*

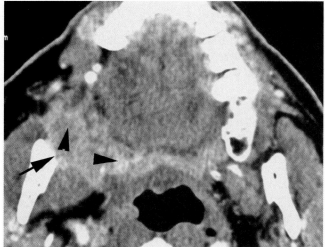

FIGURE **10.4A**

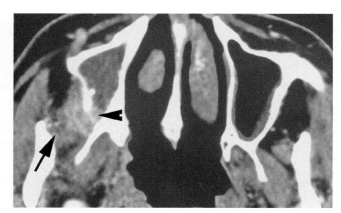

FIGURE **10.4C**

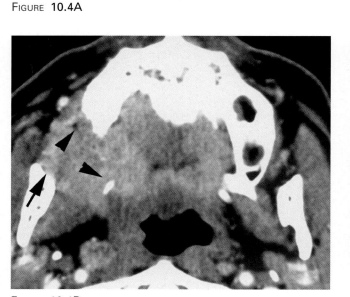

FIGURE **10.4B**

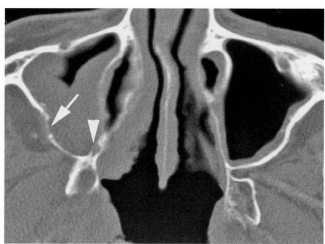

FIGURE **10.4D**

FINDINGS

Figure 10.4A. CECT shows a tumor spreading along the anterior tonsillar pillar to the retromolar trigone region (arrowheads) and involving the pterygomandibular raphe (arrow).

Figure 10.4B. Continued cephalad spread of malignancy along the pterygomandibular raphe (arrow) involving the alveolar ridge, hard palate, and soft palate at the level of the maxillary tuberosity and hook of the hamulus.

Figure 10.4C. Cephalad extension of the tumor involving the mandible along the attachment of the temporalis tendon, an upward extension from the pterygomandibular raphe, and invasion along the posterior wall of the maxillary sinus (arrowhead).

Figure 10.4D. Cephalad extension with perineural spread along the greater palatine canal (arrowhead) and perivascular spread along the posterior superior alveolar vessels (arrow) eroding the adjacent bone.

DIFFERENTIAL DIAGNOSIS Not applicable

DIAGNOSIS "Hybrid" anterior tonsillar pillar and retromolar trigone SCCa

DISCUSSION Retromolar trigone cancers are typically SCCa. Minor salivary gland tumors can also occur here since this is an area where these glands are found in a high concentration. Such cancers tend to occur in a younger patient population (<30 years of age). Retromolar trigone cancers, due to their location at the crossroads of the floor of the mouth, buccal space, oropharynx, and deep spaces of the neck, can spread extensively early on to the adjacent soft tissues, which include the buccal mucosa; the anterior tonsillar pillar, mandibular ridge, and maxilla; the buccinator muscle and fat pad; the pterygomandibular space (which can spread along the inferior alveolar and lingual nerves); and medial pterygoid muscle as well as the mandibular periosteum (mandibular destruction is a sign of advanced lesions).

Retromolar trigone cancers can have extensive distal spread directed by the underlying pterygomandibular raphe. Cephalad extension can be toward the maxillary tuberosity, into the retroantral fat pad, and finally up to its junction with the pterygoid hamulus, which is the highest-most aspect of the pterygomandibular raphe attachment. Once the retroantral fat pad or the posterior wall of the maxillary sinus is invaded, the tumor may involve the posterior superior alveolar neurovascular bundles (permeating the back wall of the maxillary antrum) or continue cephalad to invade the pterygopalatine fossa, skull base, and cavernous sinus. Hard palate invasion may promote perineural growth along the greater and lesser palatine foramina. Caudal spread along the lower margin of the pterygomandibular raphe will cause invasion of the posterior floor of the mouth and the posterior edge of the mylohyoid muscle and finally extend posteriorly, invading the upper neck.

Questions for Further Thought

1. What are signs of perivascular/perineural invasion of the posterior superior alveolar neurovascular bundle?
2. Can CT or MRI distinguish tumor from related inflammatory changes?
3. What is the imaging appearance of oral cavity invasion of the mandible and maxilla?

Reporting Responsibilities

Immediate, direct communication with the referring treatment provider is not necessary in most patients since the tumor is visible and diagnosis is strongly suspected or already biopsy confirmed. Verbal communication might be necessary if the tumor places the airway at risk, if there might be a superimposed infection, or if a tumor is discovered that was not clinically suspected.

Routine reporting should include factors outlined in the following section.

What the Treating Physician Needs to Know

- Full soft tissue extent of the tumor in keeping with spread patterns at particular primary sites
- If there is an unexpected spread outside the region of origin
- If there is an oral tongue and floor of the mouth cancer, what is the proximity to the lingual neurovascular bundle (especially when the tumor breaches the midline to threaten both lingual neurovascular bundles)?

- Is there is bone involvement or not? If so, what is the extent of involvement?
- If there is perineural spread along the inferior alveolar nerve, mandibular division of the trigeminal nerve, greater and lesser palatine nerves, and posterior superior alveolar nerves
- Status of the cervical, retropharyngeal, and facial nodes, including positive nodes, extranodal spread, and possible involvement of critical anatomic structures
- If there are other possible head and neck primaries
- If oral cavity cancer is suspected but not proven, is there a deeply infiltrating mass or an alternative cause that would explain a visible mass or the patient's symptoms?
- If the study is done for posttreatment surveillance, the likelihood of control and suggestions for additional follow-up, if necessary, from an imaging perspective

Answers

1. Obliteration of the retroantral fat pad; subtle plaquelike thickening along the posterior wall of the maxillary sinus with irregularity of the bony wall or thickening around the neurovascular bundle; or distal maxillary artery branches descending from the pterygopalatine fossa that are enlarged with indistinct margins. In the absence of direct imaging findings, perineural/perivascular spread should always be suspected based on the infiltrative appearance of the tumor margins and when tumor tracks along the known anatomic position of the neurovascular bundle at risk. Also, perineural spread occurs more frequently in recurrent and advanced primary SCCa. If this is seen at the time of initial presentation, an unusual histology should be suspected (i.e., sarcoma, melanoma, adenoid cystic carcinoma).
2. No. CT and MRI cannot distinguish tumor from related inflammatory changes. It is best to assume that cancer cells are present wherever the anatomy is deranged by the pathologic changes.
3. When an oral cavity cancer invades the mandible and maxilla, it typically produces a geographic area of bone destruction. The tumor involvement of the marrow space is normally confined to the discrete area of invasion and typically not observed more than 5 mm beyond the invading mucosal lesion. Remodeling of a cortical bone surface or sclerosis adjacent to a juxtacortical tumor mass suggests possible periosteal/early bone invasion.

> LEARN MORE
> See Chapters 200, 21, and 23 in *Head and Neck Radiology* by Mancuso and Hanafee.

CHAPTER 11

Larynx

CLINICAL HISTORY *A young adult patient presenting with hoarseness and a submucosal supraglottic mass.*

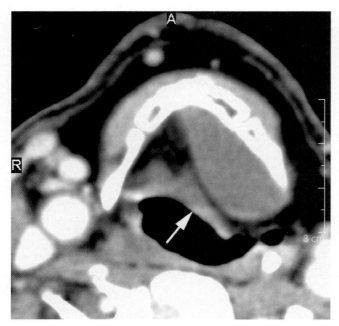

FIGURE 11.1A

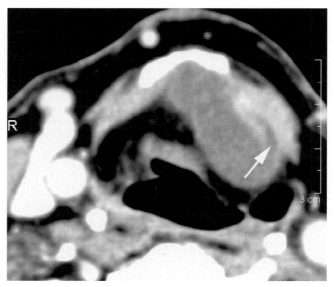

FIGURE 11.1C

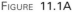

FIGURE 11.1B

FINDINGS Computed tomography (CT) in (Fig. 11.1A) shows deformity of the epiglottis and airway at the hyoid bone level (arrows). Note that the cyst relates to the hyoid bone. In (Fig. 11.1B), the arrow shows the relationship of the mass to the infrahyoid strap muscles and in (Fig. 11.1C) its growth through the thyroid notch. The relationship to the hyoid bone, strap muscles, and thyroid notch are features of particular help in the differential diagnosis.

DIFFERENTIAL DIAGNOSIS Laryngocele or a rare dermoid or epidermoid or duplication cyst

DIAGNOSIS Thyroglossal duct cyst (TGDC)

DISCUSSION Developmental cystic anomalies are spontaneous abnormalities that only infrequently truly affect the larynx. Third branchial arch anomalies secondarily affect the larynx by way of a sinus tract internally that pierces the thyrohyoid membrane. This will connect to the pyriform sinus and may become inflamed and cause laryngeal dysfunction. Infected cysts can also cause recurrent laryngeal nerve dysfunction, thus affecting the larynx secondarily. Duplication cysts of the larynx are rare, likely appearing similar to bronchogenic cysts; it is very difficult to anticipate this diagnosis or that of an epidermoid cyst precisely prior to removal.

The thyroglossal duct migrational abnormalities secondarily involve the larynx at the hyoid bone and occasionally by bulging into the supraglottic larynx. In this case, it is primarily within the supraglottis; however, the relationship of the cyst to the hyoid bone, strap muscles, and thyroid notch are features typical of the thyroglossal duct anomalies. The mainly intralaryngeal position is somewhat atypical and could mimic a laryngocele or a rare developmental cyst of some other etiology.

Questions for Further Thought

1. Is a TGDC frequently associated with a deficiency or absence of normal thyroid tissue?
2. What is the significance of observing functioning thyroid tissue in a TGDC?

Reporting Responsibilities

In general, a TGDC is in the differential diagnosis at the time of imaging, so no special communication is required unless the mass places the airway at risk due to obstruction or is infected.

What the Treating Physician Needs to Know

It is very important that the report contains a complete assessment of the nature and extent of the anomaly, including all information that is relevant to surgical planning. This should include precise comments regarding the following issues:

- Diagnosis and degree of confidence in the diagnosis
- If significant diagnostic uncertainty exists, the odds that the condition may be a benign or malignant neoplasm as an alternative diagnosis
- For a TGDC, if there is significant nodularity, morphology, or adenopathy that suggest a malignancy is complicating the ectopic or otherwise anomalous thyroid tissue
- Site of origin and all anatomic compartments or spaces of the larynx, hypopharynx, and neck involved
- Relationship to critical nerves and vessels
- Other developmental abnormalities and the possibility of any syndromic associations

Answers

1. No. There is typically a normal-appearing gland, of normal volume in its normal anatomic location, when a TGDC is discovered.
2. Ectopic or otherwise anomalous thyroid tissue associated with a TGDC raises the risk of an adenoma or malignancy developing in that tissue

---

LEARN MORE
See Chapters 202 and 8 in *Head and Neck Radiology* by Mancuso and Hanafee.

CLINICAL HISTORY *An older adult with hoarseness and a submucosal laryngeal mass.*

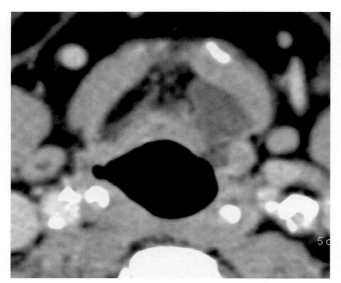

FIGURE **11.2A**

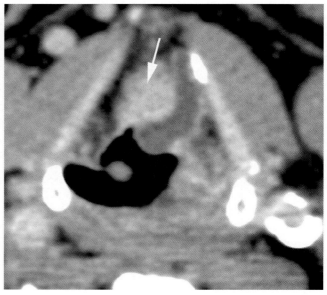

FIGURE **11.2C**

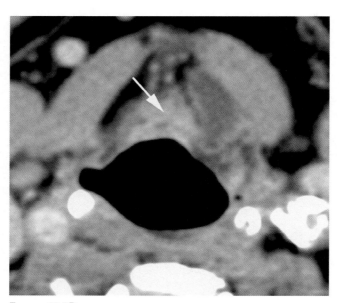

FIGURE **11.2B**

FINDINGS In (Fig. 11.2A,B), contrast-enhanced computed tomography (CECT) shows the internal laryngocele tracking in the paraglottic space. In (Fig. 11.2C), there is enhancing tissue in the paraglottic and low pre-epiglottic space (arrows in Fig. 11.2B,C).

DIFFERENTIAL DIAGNOSIS Internal laryngocele—uncomplicated

DIAGNOSIS Internal laryngocele shown to be due to an obstructing tumor

DISCUSSION Laryngoceles arise spontaneously or due to obstruction of the saccule (appendix) of the laryngeal ventricle. A laryngocele presupposes a saccule, which is not present in all patients.

The clinical classification of laryngocele is based on its location. If the mass is entirely contained within the endolarynx, primarily in the false vocal fold and aryepiglottic fold, it is classified as *internal*. An *external* laryngocele extends laterally superior to the superior border of the thyroid cartilage. Laryngoceles with components of both types are considered to be *combined*.

The presence of a laryngocele requires a search for tumor obstructing the outlet of the saccule. In this case an obstructing mass was found by imaging and confirmed as an entirely submucosal squamous cell carcinoma (SCCa) in this patient.

Questions for Further Thought

1. Given all entirely submucosal lesions that present in the larynx, what percent are likely to be due to a laryngocele? To other lesions? What type?
2. What are the two most likely complications of a laryngocele aside from a causative obstructing mass?

Reporting Responsibilities

In general, laryngocele is known or suspected at the time of imaging, so no special communication is required. The one exception is in significant airway encroachment wherein the matter should be handled as an emergency and the referring provider immediately contacted.

If there is a causative mass lesion or, more rarely, some other type of infiltrating pathology, verbal communication of that finding or suspicion is wise.

What the Treating Physician Needs to Know

- If a laryngocele is the correct diagnosis
- Extent of the laryngocele
- Whether there are any complications such as infection or severe airway narrowing
- Whether there is imaging evidence of an obstructing mass
- Imaging cannot completely exclude a small, mucosally based obstructing mass—that requires endoscopy by a very skilled observer.

Answers

1. About 50% are due to a laryngocele—the other 50% split between submucosal SCCa and more rare benign and malignant tumors and venolymphatic vascular malformations.
2. Infection (laryngopyocele) and airway obstruction

LEARN MORE

See Chapters 203 and 8 in *Head and Neck Radiology* by Mancuso and Hanafee.

CLINICAL HISTORY *A febrile and toxic-appearing young adult patient with progressive throat pain, dysphagia, and dyspnea.*

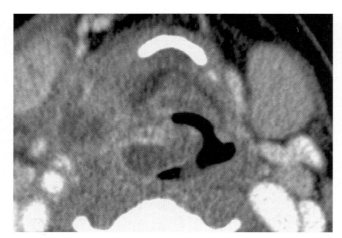

FIGURE **11.3A**

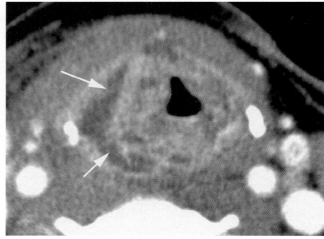

FIGURE **11.3C**

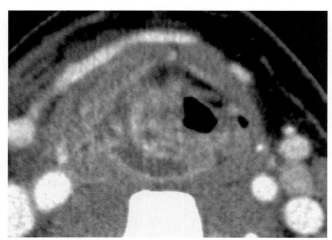

FIGURE **11.3B**

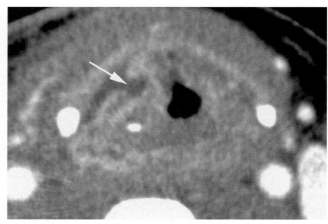

FIGURE **11.3D**

FINDINGS CECT in (Fig. 11.3A) shows extensive edema along the pharyngeal wall and within the supraglottic larynx on the right but no definitely drainable fluid collection. This was considered to be consistent with severe supraglottitis. In (Fig. 11.3B–D), the pharyngeal and laryngeal infection had likely matured to a drainable collection of purulent material (arrows) extending along the paraglottic space. In (Fig. 11.3D), communication with the saccule is likely present (arrow).

DIFFERENTIAL DIAGNOSIS Given the proper clinical situation, imaging will always be able to sort out epiglottitis/supraglottitis from croup and other infections, including laryngopyocele, spread of an acute suppurative deep neck or pharyngeal infection to the larynx, or pyogenic infection related to penetrating or blunt trauma or retained foreign bodies.

Laryngeal tuberculosis and other rare granulomatous infectious might have this appearance but are differentiated on the basis of chronicity, age, and perhaps other clinical circumstances.

DIAGNOSIS Acute bacterial supraglottitis complicated by abscess formation

DISCUSSION Acute bacterial epiglottitis is also known as supraglottitis since it involves not only the epiglottis but may also involve the entire supraglottis, including the aryepiglottic fold. The disease may critically narrow the airway at the level of the laryngeal vestibule. It is caused by *Haemophilus influenzae* type B in 90% of cases.

Epiglottitis/supraglottitis is predominantly a disease of 3 to 5 year olds; in adults, is more commonly referred to as adult supraglottitis and tends to be less immediately life threatening, perhaps because the airway is larger or perhaps related to the ability to mount an immunologic response.

Epiglottitis/supraglottitis causes severe mucosal disease in the supraglottis with secondary edema that spreads freely within the loose spaces of the supraglottis. Those deep spaces are relatively tight at the true cord level, so the vocal cords are relatively less affected. Rarely, an epiglottic/supraglottic abscess develops in adult patients; formation of an epiglottic abscess is much rarer in children.

Question for Further Thought

1. What is a major clinical imaging consideration when this disease is suspected?

Reporting Responsibilities

The diagnostic radiologist, if asked to assist in this clinical problem, must be immediately available and in verbal contact with the treating physicians.

What the Treating Physician Needs to Know

- No imaging study should be performed in a patient at risk for acute loss of the airway due to bacterial epiglottitis/

supraglottitis until an expert at managing the airway is closely supervising the case.
- CT imaging can provide an excellent assessment of the airway, especially if there is some reason to avoid direct laryngoscopy.
- Imaging findings in focal inflammatory diseases can mimic the appearance of malignancy.
- The larynx can be a site of manifestation of systemic inflammatory diseases, causing significant anatomic and functional airway problems.

Answer

1. No imaging study should be performed until an expert at managing the airway is supervising the patient and directing care.

LEARN MORE
See Chapters 204 and 13 in *Head and Neck Radiology* by Mancuso and Hanafee.

CLINICAL HISTORY *An adult presenting with a submucosal supraglottic mass and hoarseness.*

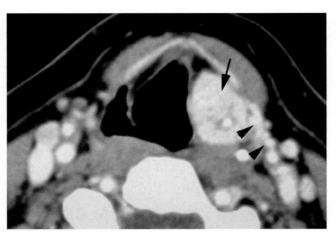

FIGURE **11.4**

FINDINGS

Figure 11.4. CECT shows an excessively enhancing mass centered within the aryepiglottic fold (arrow). There is also a very prominent superior laryngeal neurovascular bundle (arrowheads) that identifies this as a potentially arterialized lesion.

DIFFERENTIAL DIAGNOSIS
A well-circumscribed mass that appears as if it might be submucosal and that enhances considerably aside from a vascular SCCa suggests a mesenchymal-origin tumor (benign or malignant) such as a leiomyoma or sarcoma. Other possibilities include paraganglioma, hemangiopericytoma, neurogenic tumor, minor salivary gland tumor, granular cell tumor, or vascular malformation.

DIAGNOSIS Paraganglioma

DISCUSSION
Submucosal laryngeal lesions raise the differential of an entirely submucosal SCCa or laryngocele as the most common diagnostic considerations. Otherwise, a rare malignant tumor of some other etiology, laryngeal deformity due to trauma or developmental variation, or an atypical TGDC might be considered though would be very unusual. A low-grade inflammatory lesion of the laryngeal skeleton or mucosal or submucosal tissues might mimic these benign tumors.

Most benign tumors or focal areas of swelling in the larynx will have a nonspecific imaging appearance. On occasion, imaging findings will be specific enough to allow an etiologic or, rarely, a very likely specific tissue diagnosis. The most fitting and usual use of CT and magnetic resonance imaging (MRI) is to show the extent of the lesion and iden-tify the likely etiology of a submucosal mass and to identify any potential and otherwise unforeseen potential danger of tissue sampling.

A paraganglioma of the larynx arises from those cells known to populate aryepiglottic folds of the supraglottic larynx. These tumors are rare.

Question for Further Thought

1. What is the single most important information to transmit to the treating provider in this case?

Reporting Responsibilities

Any time the tumor places the airway at risk due to obstruction or if biopsy is planned and the lesion morphology suggests there might be excessive bleeding, immediate direct communication with the referring treatment provider is necessary. If the mass is suspicious for cancer, verbal communication is wise at the time of initial diagnosis.

What the Treating Physician Needs to Know

- If not SCCa, what is the likely alternative diagnosis based on imaging?
- Exact extent of the mass within the laryngeal soft tissues
- Evidence for involvement of the laryngeal framework and its precise extent
- Evidence for extralaryngeal tumor extension and its extent when present
- If biopsy might be more hazardous than usual
- If the airway is at risk

Answer

1. Excessive bleeding, which might lead to very significant blood aspiration or rapid airway compromise, is a clear risk of biopsy in this patient. An angiogram and prebiopsy devascularization might be a wise next course of action.

LEARN MORE
See Chapters 205 and 33 in *Head and Neck Radiology* by Mancuso and Hanafee.

CLINICAL HISTORY *An adult presenting with what was believed to be true vocal cord (TVC) paralysis. CT images are shown below:*

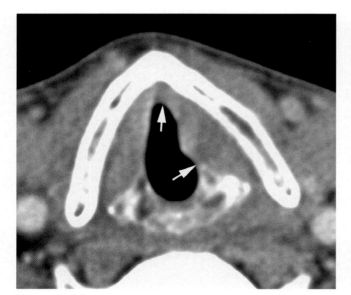

FIGURE **11.5A**

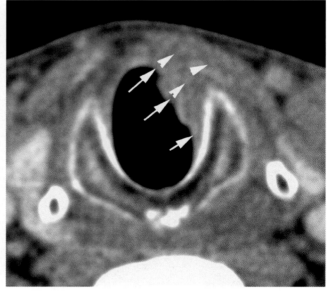

FIGURE **11.5C**

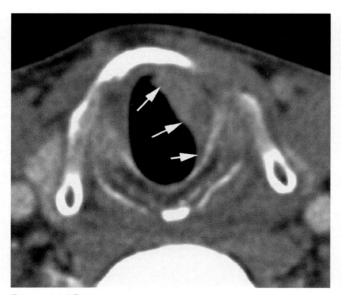

FIGURE **11.5B**

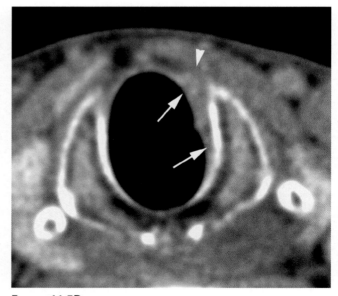

FIGURE **11.5D**

FINDINGS

Figure 11.5A. An infiltrating process that involves the entire true cord up to the anterior commissure (arrows).

Figure 11.5B. Subglottic spread is present (arrows).

Figure 11.5C. The subglottic spread (arrows) extends through the cricothyroid membrane into the soft tissues beneath the infrahyoid strap muscles (arrowheads).

Figure 11.5D. There is continued subglottic spread almost to the bottom of the cricoid cartilage (arrows).

DIFFERENTIAL DIAGNOSIS Vagal or recurrent laryngeal nerve neuropathy—possibly infiltrative or compressive, other endolaryngeal pathology causative of vocal cord dysfunction (see following discussion)

DIAGNOSIS Squamous cell cancer growing entirely beneath intact mucosa

DISCUSSION TVC dysfunction believed clinically to be due to recurrent laryngeal or vagal neuropathy will on occasion be caused by an entirely submucosal laryngeal pathology; the most frequent cause is cancer. CT is the preferred modality since it not only provides a good evaluation of the larynx but also can easily be extended to include the upper thoracic cavity or intracranial structures when the cause is not endolaryngeal. Adjunctive MRI may be used selectively to evaluate the cisternal course of the vagus nerve and its brainstem nuclei.

CT study from the posterior fossa to the aortopulmonary window in this patient showed no abnormality along the vagus or recurrent laryngeal nerves. It did, however, show an infiltrating tumor of the larynx that was entirely submucosal.

Some patients have squamous cell cancers growing entirely beneath intact mucosa, as in this case. These malignancies may begin on the mucosa within the laryngeal ventricle and the false vocal cord (FVC) and grow in the paraglottic space. This illustrates that any evaluation of vocal cord dysfunction must include detailed images of the larynx since a submucosal cancer or other endolaryngeal problems might mimic vocal cord weakness due to a vagal or recurrent nerve neuropathy.

A partial list of other submucosal processes that might cause vocal cord dysfunction includes an enchondroma or chondrosarcoma, more specifically diagnosed by CT than MRI. Other submucosal cancers from minor salivary and benign mesenchymal tumors are rare but often cannot be distinguished from squamous cell cancers until biopsied. Deformity of the laryngeal skeleton due to old trauma may also cause laryngeal dysfunction.

Questions for Further Thought

1. Is CT or MRI better for detecting cartilage invasion in larynx cancer?
2. Is FDG-PET essential in the evaluation of most laryngeal cancers?

Reporting Responsibilities

In general, laryngeal carcinoma is known or suspected at the time of imaging, so no special communication is required unless the diagnosis is unsuspected, as in this case, where it would be wise to verbally communicate this initial suspicion of submucosal cancer.

Some other special circumstances arise that require direct and possibly urgent communication with the referring treatment provider in already suspected or known laryngeal cancers include the following:

- Any time the tumor places the airway at risk
- When there might be superimposed infection
- A circumstance where it may be anticipated from imaging that a tracheostomy might cross tumor

- In a post radiation therapy patient where the larynx has become necrotic and may collapse and the patient has not had a tracheostomy

What the Treating Physician Needs to Know

- Extent of invasion along mucosal structures within larynx as well as the tongue base, hypopharynx, trachea, and esophagus
- Subglottic extent
- Spread to deep tissues spaces within the larynx including the preepiglottic space and paraglottic space.
- Spread to the laryngeal skeleton and cartilage invasion
- Extralaryngeal spread to the deep neck
- *Perineurovascular spread:*
  - Involvement of the recurrent laryngeal or superior laryngeal neurovascular bundle
  - Evaluation of regional lymph nodes, emphasizing levels 2 through 6

Answers

1. CT and MRI vastly improve the clinical detection of subtle cartilage invasion. A less than 3 mm slice thickness (SLT; preferably 0.5 to 1 mm) is required for this task, so CT is the better choice as the primary examination. There have been suggestions that MRI is better than CT for detection of early cartilage invasion. CT and MRI are both imperfect in detecting early macroinvasion and, of course by definition, cannot directly show microinvasion. Variation in ossification of the cartilages and the related marrow spaces makes interpretation difficult. Volume averaging aggravates the effects of these anatomic variations. Foci of cartilage/bone invasion larger than 3 to 5 mm should be visible or strongly suggestive of early macroinvasion if imaging techniques are adequate. CT sections of 1- to 2-mm SLT and reformations facilitate the search for small defects and early marrow space invasion. Enhanced MRI might also facilitate the diagnosis in highly selected cases.

2. In most laryngeal neoplasms, FDG-PET has a modest, if any, primary role since this technique does not allow one to reliably assess the anatomic extent of the lesion and the possible invasion of the tumor into adjacent structures. Its value in determining or planning gross tumor volume for radiation therapy planning is controversial, especially in smaller laryngeal cancers. While it might improve neck staging, this will only have a significant treatment decision impact in highly selected cases.

LEARN MORE

See Chapters 20b and 21 in *Head and Neck Radiology* by Mancuso and Hanafee.

CLINICAL HISTORY *A patient suffered injury to the neck in a car accident. Extensive swelling in the neck impeded physical examination of the larynx.*

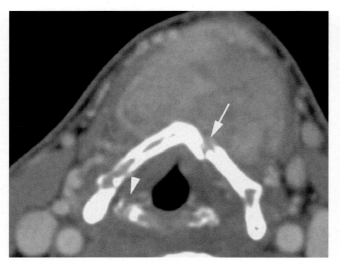

FIGURE **11.6A**

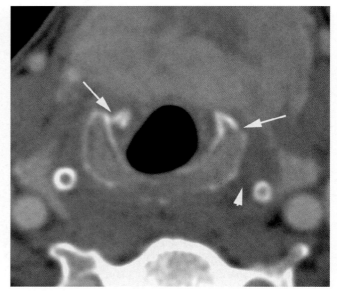

FIGURE **11.6C**

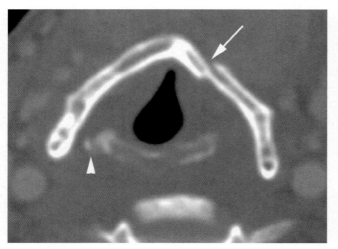

FIGURE **11.6B**

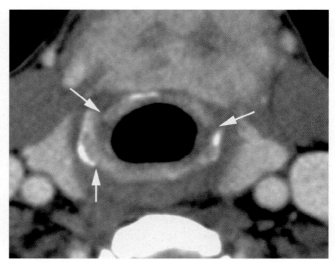

FIGURE **11.6D**

FINDINGS

Figure 11.6A–D. CECT study. In (Fig. 11.6A), the large neck hematoma due to a ruptured thyroid overlies the larynx. There is a left paramedian thyroid lamina fracture (arrow) and a likely dislocated and possibly fractured arytenoid cartilage on the right (arrowhead). In (Fig. 11.6B), a close-up view for bone detail shows the minimally displaced thyroid lamina fracture (arrow) and the posteriorly dislocated arytenoid (arrowhead). In (Fig. 11.6C), there are somewhat displaced fractures of the cricoid arches (arrows) that continue inferiorly in (Fig. 11.6D).

DIFFERENTIAL DIAGNOSIS Not applicable

DIAGNOSIS Neck trauma with displaced fracture of the larynx and a ruptured thyroid gland and related hematoma

DISCUSSION This case illustrates how extensive soft tissue swelling might interfere with the clinical evaluation of the larynx and the type of information useful in determining what the approach to laryngeal skeleton repair might entail. In this case, the laryngeal skeletal injury to the cricoid is relatively minor and that to the thyroid lamina likely not significant. The arytenoid dislocation would need to be repaired. The overall prognosis for restoration of glottic function is good.

The larynx is most commonly injured by blunt trauma or iatrogenically, with the latter causing mainly endolaryngeal findings. The treatment principles for the injured larynx have been in place for decades and well before the advent of CT and MRI. Treatment has varied little since this earlier experience except that triage, planning, and prognosis are executed in a more informed context because of diagnostic imaging input. Imaging, almost entirely nowadays with CT, shows the extent of injury to the laryngeal skeleton and related tissues. CT as a study that can provide such information and occasionally other studies takes, their place alongside endoscopy on the critical path for triage of laryngeal injuries to proper management plans.

In summary, an adequate imaging evaluation of an injured larynx should proceed with an orderly consideration of the following factors:

- *Soft tissue injury:* The extent of swelling or possible tears along mucosal structures within larynx as well as involving the tongue base, hypopharynx, trachea, and esophagus and/or related false passage or fistula should be reported whether the examination is by CT, MRI, or swallowing study.

  Hematoma, fluid collections, or abscess within the deep tissues spaces of the larynx, including the pre-epiglottic and paraglottic spaces, should be described and a contrast study suggested if indicated.

  Extralaryngeal gas, soft tissue swelling, or fluid collections to the deep neck should be noted and contrast studies done if vascular injury or abscess is a reasonable consideration.

- *Laryngeal skeleton evaluation:* The status of the cricoid cartilage in particular and a precise accounting of any fracture, dislocation, or deformity of the laryngeal cartilages and their connecting membranes must be part of the report.

- *Neurologic or vascular injury:* The likelihood of injury of the recurrent laryngeal nerve should be described. If contrast is given, any evidence of major arterial injury should be noted.

- *Complications of treatment:* For example, is tube placement and status appropriate?

Question for Further Thought

1. The status of what part of the laryngeal skeleton is most important for predicting the likelihood of restoration of adequate laryngeal function?

Reporting Responsibilities

For acute injuries, immediate verbal communication with the treating trauma team and laryngologist is most important if there is any evidence of severe airway compromise or the laryngeal injury was not expected. It is very important that the report contains a complete assessment of the extent of injury and all information that is relevant to treatment planning.

What the Treating Physician Needs to Know

- Status of the airway
- Status of all parts of the laryngeal skeleton
- Any evidence of false passage or fistula
- Any associated injuries or complications

Answer

1. That of the cricoid cartilage

LEARN MORE
See Chapter 207 in *Head and Neck Radiology* by Mancuso and Hanafee.

CLINICAL HISTORY *A patient suffering dyspnea on exertion and increased dysphonia and a history of left vocal cord paralysis. A noncontrast CT study was done.*

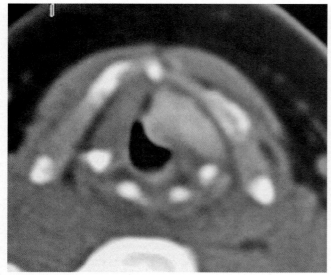

FIGURE 11.7A

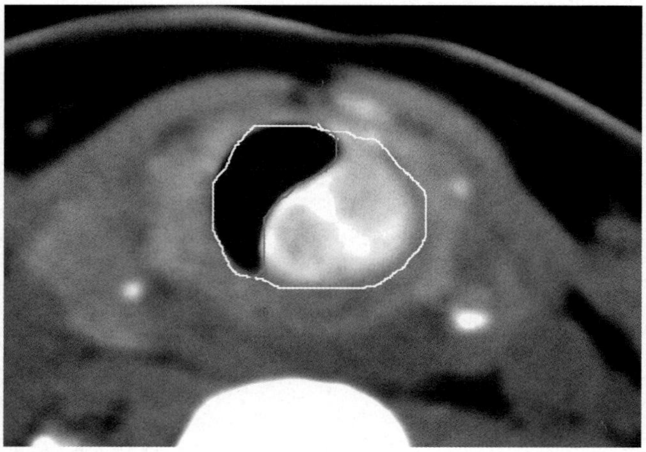

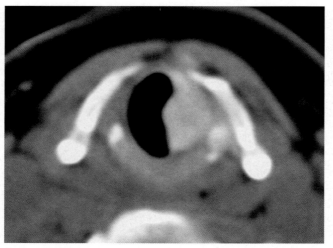

FIGURE 11.7B

FIGURE 11.7C

FINDINGS In (Fig. 11.7A), the left true cord was medialized by a high-density "mass," the constituents of which spread deep to the conus elasticus to occlude more than 50% of the subglottic airway (Fig. 11.7B,C).

DIFFERENTIAL DIAGNOSIS Not applicable

DIAGNOSIS Injection of the left TVC with Teflon to treat an idiopathic left vocal cord paralysis. The volume of injected material was excessive and caused "subglottic stenosis."

DISCUSSION Subglottic stenosis is a common complication of intubation or tracheostomy placement. It is by far the most commonly encountered iatrogenic injury to the larynx.

Other, less common, iatrogenic causes of laryngeal stenosis are surgery related to restoration of laryngeal function in a patient with TVC paralysis, as in this case, and operations to improve laryngeal and tracheal stenosis following complications of intubation or trauma.

Patients may have complaints of persistent pain, hoarseness, those related to aspiration and airway encroachment (dyspnea and stridor) following intubation, tracheostomy (emergent or routine) and surgery for vocal cord dysfunction, trauma, and subglottic stenosis. Throat pain is a less usual symptom.

One common procedure to restore glottic competency is TVC injection of Teflon or other foreign substance into the paretic or paralyzed, abducted, or sagging cord. This is done so that the poorly functioning cord will be medialized and the contralateral vocal cord will then create a competent glottis during speech and swallowing without airway compromise. Since Teflon is of higher density than soft tissues and does not create artifacts noncontrast CT can precisely localize the injection sites, as seen in this case. Misplaced injection, inadequate injection, and overinjection can be recognized and may account for otherwise inexplicable postoperative symptoms. Fat can also be injected for the same purpose and is easy to recognize similar to those seen with Teflon injection complications on CT images unless the fat is replaced by fibrosis.

Question for Further Thought

1. What is the meaning of the graphics applied in Figure 11.7C, and what is their significance clinically?

Reporting Responsibilities

For chronic subglottic stenosis, immediate verbal communication with the treating physician and laryngologist is usually only important if there is any evidence of severe laryngeal airway compromise that was not expected. This might include observations in a patient without a tracheostomy suggesting that the larynx is inflamed and/or just structurally weakened in such a way that airway collapse is possible. This latter circumstance is most commonly encountered in osteoradionecrosis following radiation therapy.

In general, the diagnosis of subglottic stenosis or other airway or TVC function compromise is known or suspected at the time of imaging, so no special communication is required. It is very important that the report contains a complete assessment of the extent of structural abnormality and all information that is relevant to treatment planning. In summary, the report must include precise comments and might be organized in the following manner:

- *Soft tissue injury:* The extent of endoluminal swelling or possible false passage or fistula should be reported if material has been injected into the endolaryngeal space and soft tissue (TVC/FVC); the location of the injected material should be described relative to the TVC, FVC, paraglottic space, and extralaryngeal soft tissues.

The cross-sectional area of the subglottis should be measured and reported as a percentage of reduction from normal. This is usually reasonably accomplished by outlining the contour of the cricoid cartilage inner margin and the estimated inner margin of the cricothyroid membrane as an estimate of the normal area (and the denominator) and then outlining the inner margin of the airway column (as the numerator) and computing the percentage reduction.

Extralaryngeal gas, soft tissue swelling, or fluid collections in the deep neck around the larynx, in particular, as possible signs of chondritis or other complication should be noted

and contrast studies done if the patient complains of pain, is febrile, and/or is tender around the laryngeal skeleton.

- *Laryngeal skeleton evaluation:* The status of the cricoid cartilage in particular and a precise accounting of any dislocation or deformity of the laryngeal cartilages and their connecting membranes must be part of the report. Cartilage sclerosis, erosion, or fragmentation may be signs of chondritis. Any unusual placement, displacement, or erosion of graft or other material used to construct the laryngeal skeleton should be reported.
- *Neurologic or vascular injury:* The likelihood of injury of the recurrent laryngeal nerve should be described. In acute settings, vascular leaks may be an issue.

What the Treating Physician Needs to Know

- Status of the airway, including the vertical extent of any stenosis and subglottic cross-sectional area.
- Status of all parts of the laryngeal skeleton, but mainly the cricoid cartilage
- Any evidence of false passage or fistula
- Any associated injuries or complications

Answer

1. In Figure 11.7C, the method of calculation of the degree of encroachment on this subglottic airway is demonstrated. The white line circles the expected dimension of the low subglottic airway as the denominator for the calculation. The red line outlines the residual lumen, which would be the numerator for the calculation of residual airway lumen area, and subtracting that from 100% would give the degree of airway area reduction. Such a calculation is possible in almost all patients.

This measured area is the best correlate for airway functional studies. This area is a key factor in medical decision making. Those treating subglottic and tracheal stenosis understand that reduction of airway luminal area leads to proportionate decrease in airflow and worsening functional capacity of the patient. In adults, less than 25% reduction of airway cross-sectional area usually causes few symptoms. A 25% to 50% reduction causes dyspnea with fairly extreme exertion, while 50% to 75% reduction might produce dyspnea with mild exertion. Greater than 75% reduction may cause symptoms at rest and audible stridor. The time course of any airway obstruction is also critical. Acute airway obstruction is much more poorly tolerated than a more chronic, progressive process.

> **LEARN MORE**
> See Chapters 208 and 12 in *Head and Neck Radiology* by Mancuso and Hanafee.

CHAPTER 12

Trachea

CLINICAL HISTORY *A 3-year-old boy with a history of sleep apnea, noisy respirations, and frequent cough spells while eating.*

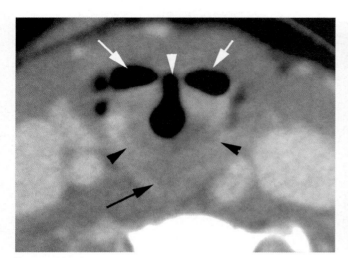

FIGURE **12.1A**

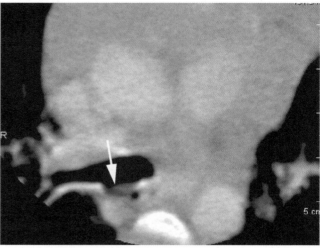

FIGURE **12.1C**

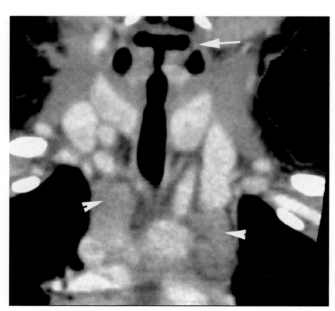

FIGURE **12.1B**

FINDINGS

Figure 12.1A. Laryngeal cleft with an abnormal relationship between the pharynx (arrows) and laryngeal vestibule (white arrowheads) and an abnormal cricoid (black arrowheads) and the postcricoid hypopharynx.

Figure 12.1B. Dysmorphic larynx and migrational variation of the thymus that presents as two different migratory cords rather than a single midline mediastinal organ.

Figure 12.1C. Tracheoesophageal fistula.

DIFFERENTIAL DIAGNOSIS Congenital laryngotracheoesophageal cleft, congenital tracheoesophageal fistula, acquired tracheoesophageal fistula

DIAGNOSIS Congenital tracheoesophageal fistula and laryngeal cleft

DISCUSSION Most congenital abnormalities of the trachea present as airway or feeding problems or as neck masses that are usually evaluated clinically with direct endoscopy and rarely with imaging. They are less frequently discovered incidentally on imaging studies done for other purposes.

Developmental abnormalities that primarily involve the trachea are mostly caused by an abnormal structural development (but could also be acquired) such as tracheal esophageal clefts and fistulas, tracheal stenosis, or tracheomalacia. These are largely sporadic, although sometimes syndromic, disorders of embryogenesis that result from failure of development such as tracheal agenesis; separation such as tracheoesophageal fistula; recanalization such as atresia, stenosis, or webs; or obliteration of the midline elements such as tracheal esophageal clefts.

Laryngeal abnormalities and secondary involvement of the trachea from developmental cysts such as duplication cysts, epidermoids, and dermoids, masses such as cervical teratomas, and vascular malformations can also present with a similar clinical picture to intrinsic tracheal problems.

The only branchial system–related anomalies affecting the trachea are those of thymic-origin abnormal migration and other rare cysts of the third and fourth division of the branchial apparatus.

Questions for Further Thought

1. How do developmental abnormalities affect the trachea?
2. Are congenital tracheal abnormalities frequently imaged?
3. What is the role of imaging in these cases?

Reporting Responsibilities

Direct communication with the referring physician is mandatory if any developmental anomaly places the airway at risk due to obstruction, aspiration, or infection that may be rapidly progressive.

What the Treating Physician Needs to Know

- Precise diagnosis and the degree of confidence in that diagnosis
- Extent of the developmental anomaly
- Any complicating features of the anomaly that might alter medical decision making
- How threatened is the airway, and what is its precise status?
- If there are associated or other anomalies
- If there is a possibility of any syndromic associations
- If there is any need for further imaging to answer any of these issues

Answers

1. Most developmental abnormalities affect the trachea primarily, such as structural anomalies, or secondarily, as developmental cysts, masses, or vascular lesions.
2. No. Most will not come to imaging since they are evaluated clinically with direct endoscopy.
3. Although imaging plays an adjunctive role to endoscopic examination, which is definitive in most cases, it has the potential to affect medical decision making in some conditions.

LEARN MORE
See Chapter 210 in *Head and Neck Radiology* by Mancuso and Hanafee.

12.2

CLINICAL HISTORY *A 59-year-old Central American immigrant female patient with a remote history of a mixed connective tissue disorder. She now presents with progressive dyspnea and hoarseness.*

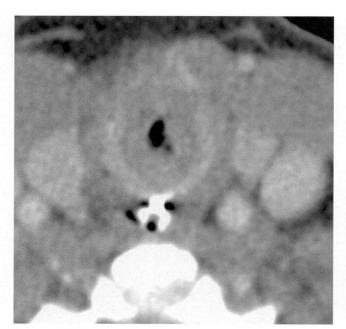

FIGURE **12.2A**

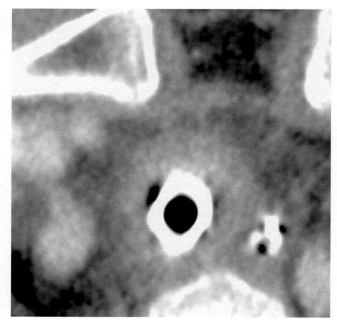

FIGURE **12.2C**

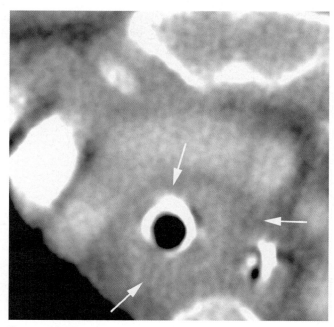

FIGURE **12.2B**

FINDINGS

Figure 12.2A. Endoluminal soft tissue thickening causing near complete obliteration of the subglottic airway.

Figure 12.1B,C. Inferior extension into the distal cervical trachea (arrows) and mediastinal trachea.

DIFFERENTIAL DIAGNOSIS Infectious process involving the trachea, noninfectious inflammation of the trachea related to an underlying systemic disease, primary infiltrative subglottic malignancy extending into the trachea

DIAGNOSIS The etiology was never established. The patient was treated for both infectious etiologies and possible auto-immune-type disease.

DISCUSSION Infectious and noninfectious inflammatory disorders that affect the trachea often involve the adjacent larynx, usually the subglottis, as well. Tracheal manifestations of these disorders may be focal and subepithelial or widespread and infiltrative.

When infectious granulomatous processes involve the trachea, their specific etiology is often not discovered. Rhinoscleroma is an infection that may predominantly involve the trachea. This is caused by a *Klebsiella* infection and is endemic in Central and South America. Other infections typically have dominant laryngeal and pharyngeal findings.

Almost all patients with a systemic inflammatory disease will have a known diagnosis, with the airway being an uncommon site of involvement. Differentiating laboratory and other data aid in the diagnosis in those with an unknown etiology.

Questions for Further Thought

1. How do inflammatory disorders of the trachea present at imaging?
2. How is a definitive diagnosis made?
3. What is the role of imaging in these situations?

Reporting Responsibilities

Direct communication with the referring physician is mandatory if the airway is at risk due to obstruction or infection that may be rapidly progressive.

What the Treating Physician Needs to Know

- Computed tomography (CT) and magnetic resonance (MR) images can provide excellent static and dynamic images of tracheal pathology, especially if there are reasons to avoid direct laryngoscopy.
- Imaging findings of focal inflammatory diseases can mimic the appearance of malignancy.

Answers

1. Inflammatory disorders that affect the trachea typically present with nonspecific soft tissue thickening that may involve the mucosa, tracheal cartilage, membranous walls, and soft tissues outside the trachea.
2. Tissue sampling and culture, as well as clinical and laboratory data, is required for a definitive diagnosis. Imaging is limited in this regard but perhaps useful in differentiating some viral and bacterial laryngeal infections—for instance, croup from epiglottitis/supraglottitis and occasionally suggesting a multifocal systemic disease such as amyloidosis.
3. Imaging in inflammatory laryngotracheal diseases, except in relapsing polychondritis, is generally nonspecific for diagnosis purposes and is usually done to assess the airway status or look for complications. Imaging may be used to assess dynamic tracheal problems as an occasional adjunct to endoscopy.

LEARN MORE

See Chapters 211 and 13 in *Head and Neck Radiology* by Mancuso and Hanafee.

CLINICAL HISTORY *A 47-year-old male patient with a history of tracheolaryngeal papillomatosis and tobacco use. He now presents with progressive exertional dyspnea and chronic cough.*

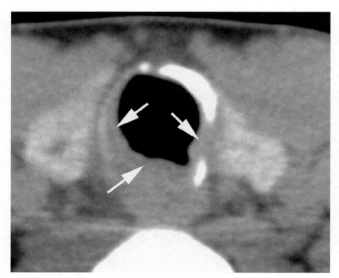

FIGURE **12.3A**

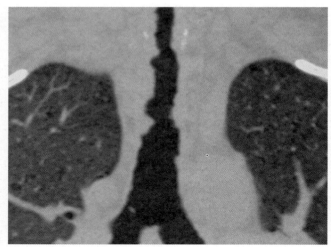

FIGURE **12.3C**

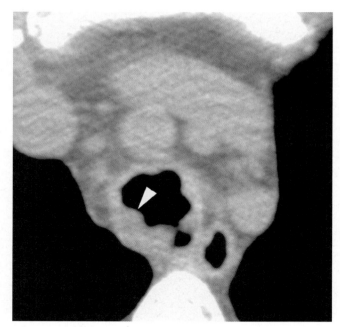

FIGURE **12.3B**

FINDINGS

Figure 12.3A. Endoluminal mass arising from the upper trachea with extension along the common (membranous) wall between the trachea and esophagus (arrows).

Figure 12.3B. Coronal reformatted image of the trachea demonstrating tracheal papillomatosis.

Figure 12.3C. Papillary polyps circumferentially involving the lumen of the trachea (arrowhead).

DIFFERENTIAL DIAGNOSIS Tracheal papillomatosis with malignant degeneration, tracheal papillomatosis with superimposed focal inflammation, diffuse inflammatory process of the trachea

DIAGNOSIS Tracheal papillomatosis with malignant degeneration of the lesion seen in Figure 12.3A

DISCUSSION Approximately 10% of primary tracheal tumors are benign, with the most common being a papilloma.

Other benign tumors include pleomorphic adenoma, granular cell tumor, and those of cartilage origin. Benign masses limited to the trachea and malignant tumors have essentially the same initial presentation. Laryngeal papillomatosis occurs in children and young adults due to human papillomavirus infection, and it predisposes to squamous cell carcinoma. Tracheal squamous cell carcinoma is a disease essentially of older smoking adults. Infectious and noninfectious inflammatory conditions can mimic cancer and can only be differentiated histologically.

Squamous cell carcinoma is the most common primary tracheal malignancy. Other frequent tracheal malignancies, although all are relatively rare, are adenoid cystic and mucoepidermoid carcinoma. Sarcomas are rare and sporadic, with most occurring in children and young adults. Chondrosarcoma is the most common of these lesions. Lymphoma and plasmacytoma usually occur in systemic disease. Tracheal metastases occur rarely but virtually always in the setting of a known primary. Local malignant spread may occur along the mucosa, submucosa (which is invisible endoscopically), or transmurally and into the adjacent structures since there are no real anatomic barriers in the trachea. Lymphatic spread is most commonly to cervical groups 4, 5B, and 6 as well as the mediastinal lymph nodes.

Questions for Further Thought

1. Are primary tracheal malignancies common?
2. What features favor a primary tracheal malignancy over secondary tracheal invasion?
3. What is the role of imaging in tracheal tumors?

Reporting Responsibilities

Direct communication with the referring physician is mandatory if the airway is at risk for progressive obstruction either by the mass or a potential airway complication that might arise as a result of biopsy. Additionally, the report must contain a complete assessment of the disease extent and all information that is relevant to treatment planning.

What the Treating Physician Needs to Know

- If the tumor is more likely benign or malignant
- If the tumor is arising from the trachea or from another source
- What is the degree of airway encroachment, and what is the possibility of worsening to a life-threatening obstruction with tissue sampling and/or treatment?
- Is there evidence of tracheal wall invasion? If so, does it spread beyond the wall, and what adjacent structures are involved?
- What is the status of the cervical and mediastinal lymph nodes?

Answers

1. No. Intrinsic tracheal tumors are uncommon, and benign tumors are rare, except for papillomas. The trachea is far more commonly involved secondarily by spread of tumors from adjacent sites such as the larynx, hypopharynx, and thyroid.
2. Transmural spread of a primary tracheal malignancy tends to present with airway symptoms long before there is extensive spread beyond the trachea. A primary source other than the trachea should be considered when there is more tumor growth outside than within the trachea.
3. Imaging, although histologically nonspecific, is essential since it provides additional information concerning the depth and regional spread of disease. It is used as an adjunct to endoscopy with biopsy for staging and medical decision making. It can also be very useful when the pattern of disease spread suggests a primary site other than the trachea.

LEARN MORE
See Chapters 212 and 21 in *Head and Neck Radiology* by Mancuso and Hanafee.

CLINICAL HISTORY *A patient suffering laryngotracheal trauma was intubated. Contrast-enhanced computed tomography (CECT) images are shown below:*

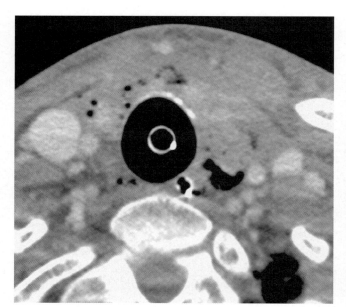

FIGURE **12.4A**

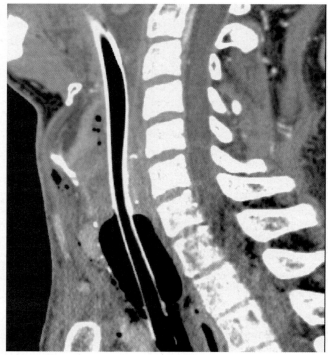

FIGURE **12.4C**

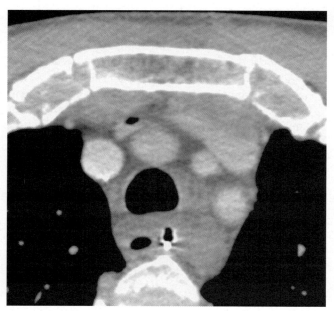

FIGURE **12.4B**

FINDINGS In (Fig. 12.4A), the endotracheal tube is seen centrally and the airway overdistended, as can be judged from the image below the level of the balloon in (Fig. 12.4B), which shows the normal tracheal dimensions. The air in the soft tissues suggests a false passage; tracheal wall necrosis is a second consideration. An overall perspective of the overdistended balloon can be gained from (Fig. 12.4C), which shows the balloon in the upper trachea markedly distending the airway.

DIFFERENTIAL DIAGNOSIS Not applicable

DIAGNOSIS Overdistended endotracheal tube balloon that might lead to pressure necrosis of the mucosa and subsequent tracheal injury. Soft tissue free air due to likely false passage cannot exclude tracheal wall injury.

DISCUSSION The trachea is commonly injured with the larynx accidentally or iatrogenically. Direct injury, pressure necrosis from an endotracheal or tracheostomy tube or chronic irritation can begin as a mucosal injury and progress, causing long-term airway disability. The common pathway of tracheal mucosal injury is that lining becoming denuded due to direct injury, pressure necrosis, or chronic irritation. For instance, pressure necrosis occurs during prolonged intubation when the cuff pressure exceeds capillary perfusion pressure, causing a chain of events starting with mucosal ischemia and necrosis. This eventually leads to exposure of underlying cartilage, chondritis, and granulation tissue formation. This was the risk in this patient. The end stage of this common pathogenesis is a final maturation into firm scar tissue that reduces the lumen of the airway. The tracheal wall may weaken, and a dynamic component due to tracheomalacia may add to the airway compromise. Caustic aspiration and burns can lead to the same chain of events. Extension of the inflammatory process may produce false passages or a fistula to the esophagus or brachiocephalic vessels. Secondary infection can result in infectious chondritis and/or a deep neck abscess. Tracheal stenosis and tracheomalacia are frequent sequela of tracheal injuries or surgical reconstructions.

Imaging takes its place alongside endoscopy for evaluation of these injuries for proper development of management plans. Imaging is used to assess the extent and associated complications, but weakening of the wall is established endoscopically.

Granulation tissue in the subacute phase of an injury (10 to 30 days post trauma) is hypodense to muscle in noncontrast CT, similar in appearance to hemorrhage and edema in the acute phase, but hyperdense in CECT. This will organize and contract over time, forming soft tissue webs and circumferential stenoses. Gas at the margins of the cartilage, as well as cartilage erosions, fragmentation, and/or sclerosis, may be seen as signs of chondritis.

Questions for Further Thought

1. When should tracheal and laryngeal injuries be treated?
2. What structure is a critical prognostic factor for laryngotracheal injury?
3. What CT information about the airway provides the best correlate for airway functional studies and is a key factor in medical decision making?

Reporting Responsibilities

In the circumstances of this case, the referring clinical service should be notified immediately about the overdistension of the balloon to avoid tracheal mucosal injury due to pressure-induced necrosis. More generally, for acute injuries, immediate verbal communication with the treating trauma team and laryngologist is most important if there is any evidence of severe airway compromise or the laryngeal injury was not expected.

It is very important that the report contains a complete assessment of the extent of injury and all information that is relevant to treatment planning. In summary, the report must include precise comments regarding the extent of injury and might be organized in the following manner:

- *Soft tissue injury:* The extent of swelling or possible tears along mucosal structures within trachea, larynx, hypopharynx, and esophagus and/or related false passage or fistula should be reported whether the examination is by CT, MR, or swallowing study. The level and length of the injured segment should be identified and cross-sectional area and measurements of the maximal airway narrowing

computed and recorded. Hematoma, fluid collections, or abscess within the deep tissues spaces of the neck compressing the trachea or within the trachea should be noted. A contrast study should be suggested if indicated.

- *Laryngeal and tracheal skeleton evaluation:* The status of the cricoid cartilage in particular at the cricotracheal junction and a precise accounting of any fracture, dislocation, or deformity of the cartilages and their connecting membranes must be part of the report. Peritracheal soft tissue swelling and/or gas within or immediately external to the tracheal wall can be an indication of early pressure necrosis.

- *Neurologic or vascular injury:* The likelihood of injury of the recurrent laryngeal nerve should be described. If contrast is given, any evidence of major arterial injury should be noted.

- *Complications of treatment:* For example, is tube placement and status appropriate?

What the Treating Physician Needs to Know

- Status of the airway and all parts of the laryngeal and tracheal skeleton, especially the cricoid cartilage at the cricotracheal junction
- Extent of the soft tissue injury, including possible tears along mucosal structures and/or related false passage or fistula
- Cross-sectional area measurements of the maximal airway narrowing and percentage of reduction from normal
- Any associated injury or complications

Answers

1. Acute injuries should be treated within 3 to 7 days to improve the functional outcome since delay in treatment can lead to scarring and chronic stenosis.
2. The status of the cricoid cartilage
3. The percent relative reduction in the cross-sectional area of the maximal airway narrowing is the best correlate for airway functional studies and a key factor in medical decision making since the cross-sectional area of the airway is directly proportional to the amount of airflow and functional airway capacity of the patient.

> LEARN MORE
>
> See Chapter 213 in *Head and Neck Radiology* by Mancuso and Hanafee.

CLINICAL HISTORY *Progressive stridor in an adult patient with a remote history of intubation and surgery. Noncontrast CT images are shown below:*

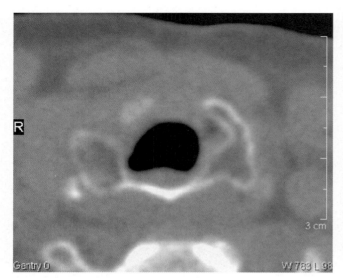

FIGURE **12.5A**

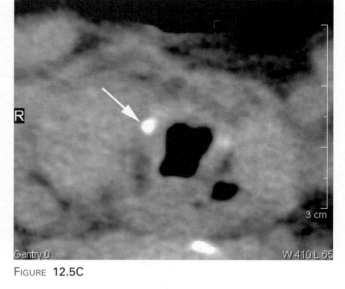

FIGURE **12.5C**

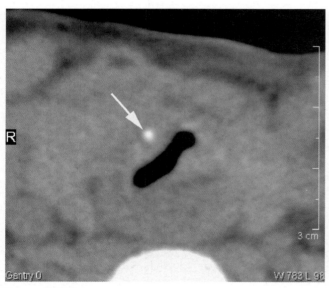

FIGURE **12.5B**

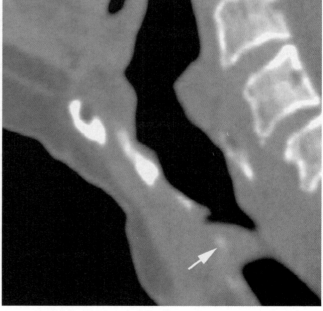

FIGURE **12.5D**

FINDINGS

Figure 12.5A. Extensive distortion of the cricoid cartilage with luminal narrowing due to chronic scar.

Figure 12.5B. Extensive distortion of the upper tracheal cartilage with luminal narrowing due to soft tissue and collapse.

Figure 12.5C,D. Severe short-segment stenosis with a small amount of residual strut (history withheld) between the cricoid and the upper trachea remaining (arrows in Fig. 12.5B,C). The distorted airway and residual strut bone (arrow) can be seen on the sagittal reformation.

DIFFERENTIAL DIAGNOSIS Tracheomalacia

DIAGNOSIS Tracheal stenosis due to intubation where the tube was placed so that the balloon was blown up in the low subglottis and upper trachea. This study shows the results of many years of unsuccessful chronic attempts to repair this problem.

DISCUSSION This is an example of a follow-up study in a patient with chronic recurrent symptoms and unsuccessful treatment (history of prior attempted cricotracheal bony strut placement was withheld) of an endotracheal tube misadventure. Tracheal stenosis and tracheomalacia are common complications of intubation or tracheostomy placement and by far are the most frequently encountered consequences of iatrogenic injury to the trachea seen in an imaging practice. Less common iatrogenic causes of tracheal stenosis are surgical constructs made necessary by other medical conditions, such tumor invasion that requires tracheal resection. Tracheal stenosis and tracheomalacia are also a final common pathway of insults to the trachea due to blunt and penetrating trauma, caustic substance aspiration, burns, inflammatory diseases, tumors, and the effects of a tracheoesophageal fistula. An acute event, endotracheal tube overinflation, that might to lead to such a circumstance was presented in Case 12.4; the pathogenesis of tracheal stenosis and tracheomalacia is presented in the discussion of that case. That pathogenesis is akin to the mechanisms that produce postintubation subglottic stenosis. To summarize that disease progression, the endotracheal tube denudes the mucosa of the trachea, as it might the subglottis, either due to pressure necrosis or chronic irritation This leads to the series of changes described in Case 12.4 that may ultimately lead to a permanent stenosis that matures to firm scar tissue. If the balloon is inadvertently blown up in the subglottis, the effects may be even worse since it is inherently stiff and in children is the narrowest portion of the airway. The act of intubation or other injury can also excoriate the mucosa and produce a localized masslike area of chondritis. This can be rarely mistaken for tumor, but the larger problem is the increased risk of tracheomalacia or the formation of a stenosis that may eventually become very hard or calcific.

CT demonstrates the cross-sectional area of the residual airway in the trachea whether an injury may be due to solely or mainly mucosal injury or injury to both the tracheal mucosa and cartilage. This measured area is the best correlate for airway functional studies and is a key factor in medical decision making along with the level and length of the stenosis and/or segment of tracheomalacia. A reduction of airway luminal area leads to proportionate decrease in airflow and worsening functional capacity of the patient. In adults, less than 25% reduction of airway cross-sectional area usually causes few symptoms. A 25% to 50% reduction causes dyspnea with fairly extreme exertion, while a 50% to 75% reduction might produce dyspnea with mild exertion. Greater than 75% reduction may cause symptoms at rest and audible stridor.

Questions for Further Thought

1. Describe the Myer-Cotton system for classifying upper airway stenosis?
2. What thickness sections should be used to study these problems, and is contrast used routinely for these studies?

Reporting Responsibilities

For these chronic conditions, immediate verbal communication with the treating physician and laryngologist is most important if there is any evidence of severe airway compromise that was not expected. This might include observations in a patient without a tracheostomy, suggesting that the trachea or subglottis is inflamed and/or just structurally weakened in such a way that airway collapse is possible.

In general, the diagnosis of tracheal and/or subglottic stenosis or other airway compromise is known or suspected at the time of imaging, so no special communication is required. It is very important that the report contains a complete assessment of the extent of structural abnormality and all information that is relevant to treatment planning.

In summary, the report must include precise comments regarding the following issues and those issues might be used as a format for producing an adequate report:

- *Soft tissue injury:* The extent of endoluminal swelling or possible false passage or fistula should be reported whether the examination is by CT, MRI, or swallowing study. The cross-sectional area of the trachea should be measured and reported as a percentage of reduction from normal, as demonstrated in Case 11.7. This is usually reasonably accomplished by outlining the contour of a reference normal tracheal ring cartilage inner margin as an estimate of the normal area (and the denominator) and then outlining the inner margin of the airway column (as the numerator) and computing the percentage reduction. The length and level of the stenosis should also be documented.
- *Tracheal and laryngeal skeleton evaluation:* The status of the cricoid cartilage in particular and a precise accounting of any dislocation or deformity of the tracheal and laryngeal cartilages and their connecting membranes must be part of the report. Cartilage sclerosis, erosion, or fragmentation may be signs of chondritis that still could be active. Any unusual placement, displacement, or erosion of graft or other material used to construct the trachea and/or subglottis should be reported.

What the Treating Physician Needs to Know

- Status of the airway, including the vertical extent of any stenosis and luminal cross-sectional area
- Status of all parts of the trachea, including a careful assessment of the subglottis and especially the cricoid cartilage
- Any evidence of false passage or fistula
- Any associated injuries or complications

Answers

1. The Myer-Cotton staging system stages mature, firm, circumferential stenosis confined to the subglottis. It also describes the stenosis based on the percent relative reduction in cross-sectional area of the subglottis, which is determined by differing sizes of endotracheal tubes. Four grades of stenosis are described with this system: Grade I lesions have less than 50% obstruction, grade II lesions have 51% to 70% obstruction, grade III lesions have 71% to 99% obstruction, and grade IV lesions have no detectable lumen or complete stenosis.
2. Sections should be no thicker than 1 mm so that the quality of information on reformatted images is ensured. Contrast is used only in selected cases, mainly to look for infectious complications. Perfusion imaging has some potential to differentiate active scar from end-stage fibrotic scar, but the potential to make such a differentiation and its treatment implications have not been established.

LEARN MORE

See Chapter 214 in *Head and Neck Radiology* by Mancuso and Hanafee.

CHAPTER 13

Hypopharynx

CLINICAL HISTORY *A 7-year-old boy with dysphagia.*

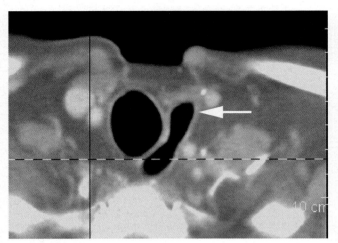

FIGURE **13.1A**

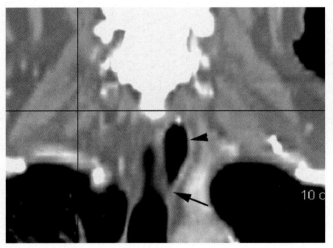

FIGURE **13.1B**

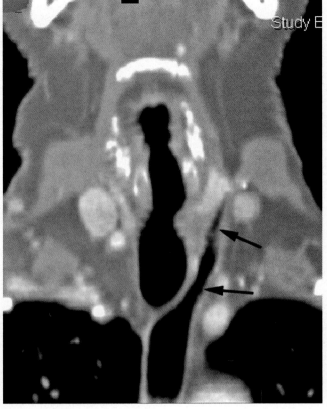

FIGURE **13.1C**

FINDINGS

Figure 13.1A. Axial section shows the fairly wide mouth diverticulum projecting laterally.

Figure 13.1B,C. The diverticulum (arrowhead) projects toward the lumen of the pharynx and esophagus near the thoracic inlet.

DIFFERENTIAL DIAGNOSIS Esophageal or foregut duplication cyst, Zenker's diverticulum

DIAGNOSIS Pharyngeal diverticulum of the Killian-Jamieson type

DISCUSSION Developmental anomalies of the hypopharynx and cervical esophagus generally present during childhood as masses or because they interfere with function, causing dysphagia, odynophagia, or aspiration. They are also frequently discovered incidentally in adults while imaging for other purposes. They are typically painless unless there is a complicating factor such as infection of a developmental cyst that connects to the hypopharynx/cervical esophagus, or infection, bleeding, or thrombosis of a vascular malformation. In the hypopharynx, they can cause referred otalgia.

Hypopharyngeal-cervical esophageal diverticuli arise from developmental deficiencies or at least some predisposition based on the anatomy of the esophageal verge or inlet, where the lower margin of the functional zone of the inferior constrictor of the pharynx (cricopharyngeus muscle) and the proximal esophageal muscles overlap. The more common diverticuli occur at the Killian dehiscence of the lower inferior constrictor muscle above the functional zone (cricopharyngeus muscle) in the midline (Zenker's type) and between the inferior margin of the lower inferior constrictor and the lateral muscular wall of the proximal cervical esophagus (Killian-Jamieson type) below the cricopharyngeus muscle.

Questions for Further Thought

1. When are hypopharyngeal-esophageal diverticuli considered congenital?
2. What is the difference between a Zenker diverticulum and a Killian-Jamieson type of diverticulum?
3. How does Killian-Jamieson type diverticuli present?

Reporting Responsibilities

Direct communication with the referring physician is mandatory if any developmental anomaly places the airway at risk due to obstruction or an infection that may be rapidly progressive or if a tracheoesophageal fistula might be present.

What the Treating Physician Needs to Know

- Precise diagnosis and the degree of confidence in the diagnosis
- Extent of the developmental anomaly
- Any complicating features that may alter medical decision making
- If the airway is at significant risk
- If there are any associated or additional anomalies
- If there is a likelihood of the finding to be syndromic
- If there is any need for further imaging to answer any of these issues

Answers

1. Although most hypopharyngeal-cervical esophageal diverticuli are acquired, congenital diverticuli should be considered any time they are found in children. They are more likely to be lateral than midline posterior on a congenital basis.

2. The more common Zenker diverticulum occurs at the Killian dehiscence of the inferior constrictor muscle, which is a triangular area located *above* the functional zone (cricopharyngeus muscle) in the posterior midline. The Killian-Jamieson type of diverticulum occurs between the inferior margin of the cricopharyngeus muscle and the lateral muscular wall of the proximal cervical esophagus, *below* the cricopharyngeus muscle. A Zenker diverticulum would then be technically considered a *midline posterior* postcricoid portion hypopharyngeal diverticulum and a Killian-Jamieson type diverticulum would be a *lateral* esophageal verge/proximal cervical esophageal diverticulum.

3. The Killian-Jamieson type of diverticuli typically present as a fairly wide mouth diverticulum projecting laterally in the region of the esophageal verge/lateral proximal cervical esophagus.

LEARN MORE

See Chapter 216 in *Head and Neck Radiology* by Mancuso and Hanafee.

CLINICAL HISTORY *A 48-year-old immunocompromised female patient with mild hoarseness and odynophagia.*

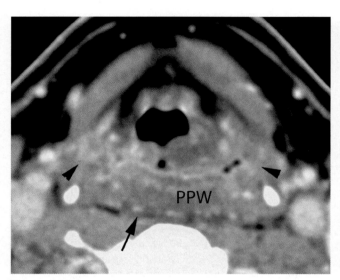

FIGURE 13.2A

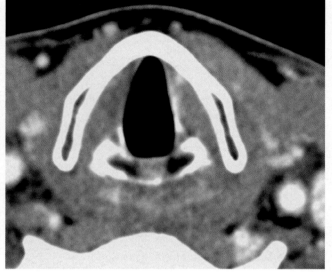

FIGURE 13.2B

FINDINGS

Figure 13.2A,B. Subtle loss of fat planes lateral to the pyriform sinuses (arrowheads) and thickening of the posterior pharyngeal muscular wall *(PPW)*. There is retropharyngeal edema (arrows).

DIFFERENTIAL DIAGNOSIS Postradiation changes, squamous cell carcinoma (SCCa) of the hypopharynx, hypopharyngeal infection

DIAGNOSIS Bacterial hypopharyngeal infection

DISCUSSION Many infectious and noninfectious inflammatory disorders may affect the hypopharynx and esophagus, most of which never come to imaging. Imaging is usually obtained to aid in the diagnostic process when the etiology is uncertain, especially when the disease mimics cancer, or for a noninvasive assessment of the static airway dimensions.

Inflammatory disorders of the hypopharynx usually arise in conjunction with laryngeal diseases or are secondary to diseases arising from the adjacent structures causing reactive changes in the wall. They may also mimic the initial presentation of cancer.

Bacterial infections of the hypopharynx are usually secondary to a laryngeal infection such as epiglottis, acute bacterial laryngopyocele, pyogenic infection related to penetrating or blunt trauma or retained foreign body, or spread from an acute deep neck infection. They may complicate a pharyngeal/esophageal diverticulum or communicating duplication cyst and may also be the cause or effect of a tracheoesophageal fistula or spinal infection.

Chronic hypopharyngeal mycotic infections occur primarily in immunocompromised patients and are rare in immunocompetent individuals. Other than *Candida*, *Cryptococcus*, *Aspergillus*, and *Coccidioides* are the most common agents.

Chronic bacterial hypopharyngeal infections are usually granulomatous agents such as tuberculosis, syphilis, leprosy, and rhinoscleromas.

Hypopharyngeal manifestations of systemic inflammatory diseases can range from focal and subepithelial to widespread and infiltrative.

Questions for Further Thought
1. When should the imaging features of hypopharyngeal pathology raise the possibility of an inflammatory process rather than cancer?
2. What is the role of computed tomography (CT), magnetic resonance (MR), and FDG-PET in the evaluation of inflammatory disorders of the hypopharynx?

Reporting Responsibilities
Direct communication with the referring physician is mandatory if any inflammatory process affecting the hypopharynx places the airway at risk due to obstruction or infection that may be rapidly progressive.

What the Treating Physician Needs to Know
• No imaging study should be performed in a patient at risk for acute loss of the airway due to likely pyogenic laryngeal or pharyngeal infection until an expert at managing the airway is closely supervising the case.

- CT imaging can provide an excellent assessment of the airway, especially if there is some reason to avoid direct laryngoscopy.
- Imaging findings in focal inflammatory diseases can mimic the appearance of malignancy.
- The hypopharynx and esophagus are only rarely a site of manifestation of systemic inflammatory diseases causing significant anatomic manifestations on CT and MR studies. Mucosal disease and motility problems may manifest on swallowing studies, but those are typically visualized in the more distal esophagus.

Answers

1. When the imaging and clinical features of hypopharyngeal pathology are atypical, the possibility of an inflammatory process rather than cancer should be raised.

Low-grade inflammatory lesions of the mucosal or submucosal tissues are suspected clinically, but these are rare and usually mimic neoplasms on imaging.

2. Any condition that is suspicious for a deep infiltration or cancer should be studied primarily by CT. MR should be used as a supplemental problem-solving tool directed by CT to a localized area of interest where its strengths related to better soft tissue contrast resolution can be exploited. FDG-PET is currently limited to cancer evaluation.

> **LEARN MORE**
> See Chapters 217 and 13 in *Head and Neck Radiology* by Mancuso and Hanafee.

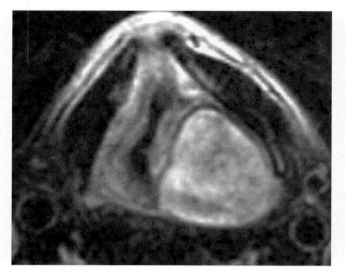

FIGURE **13.3A**

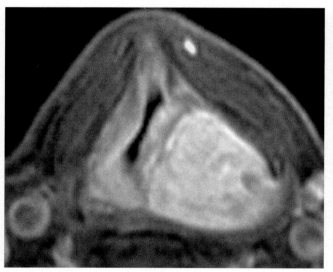

FIGURE **13.3B**

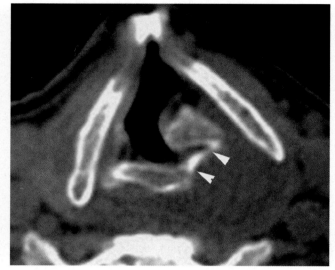

FIGURE **13.3C**

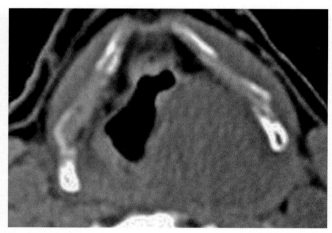

FIGURE **13.3D**

FINDINGS

Figure 13.3A. T2W image showing a mass at the lower pyriform sinus region with homogenous bright internal characteristics.

Figure 13.3B. Contrast-enhanced fat-suppressed T1W image showing homogeneous enhancement of the mass.

Figure 13.3C. Noncontrast CT image to correlate with (Fig. 13.3A) and (Fig. 13.3B).

Figure 13.3D. Noncontrast CT image at the level of the pyriform sinus apex showing remodeling of the cricoid cartilage in the region of the cricoarytenoid joint (arrowheads).

DIFFERENTIAL DIAGNOSIS Benign epithelial (likely minor salivary gland) or mesenchymal tumor of the hypopharynx/larynx, paraganglioma, vascular malformation ("hemangioma"), aneurysm, malignant tumor of the hypopharynx/larynx, sarcoma, plasmacytoma, minor salivary gland tumor, submucosal SCCa

DIAGNOSIS Schwannoma of the larynx arising from the aryepiglottic fold

DISCUSSION Benign tumors of the hypopharynx are rare, typically have no particular etiology, and are usually not in the differential diagnosis at the time of imaging, with submucosal

SCCa cancer being of greater concern. Most of these are adenomas and mesenchymal tumors (except chondromas, which are rare and are usually low-grade chondrosarcomas). They often present with dysphagia and odynophagia and/or aspiration due to the pharyngeal dysfunction caused by the submucosal involvement or secondary compression by abnormal neighboring structures. They may also have dysphonia or a palpable cervical mass. Although they often mimic the initial presentation of cancer, sore throat, referred ear pain, and/or localized pain to the laryngeal skeleton are more suggestive of a malignant tumor rather than a benign tumor.

Most submucosal masses intrinsic to the hypopharynx usually have a nonspecific imaging appearance and in about half the cases are SCCa, which should be included in the differential diagnosis unless the imaging findings are specific enough to allow an etiologic-specific type of tissue diagnosis. The diagnosis is usually a "surprise" following review of the material obtained for pathologic evaluation. Submucosal hypopharyngeal masses should always be imaged before biopsy to exclude an underlying cause that could be disastrous, if sampled, such as a paraganglioma, vascular malformation, or aneurysm.

Benign tumors tend to grow as a well-circumscribed spheroidal mass in the deep planes displacing the surrounding anatomic structures. They frequently involve both the larynx and hypopharynx. They may cause demineralization and remodeling of the laryngeal skeleton but should not frankly invade it. Most of these tumors usually enhance more than muscle. Hypervascular lesions may produce enlargement of the superior and/or inferior neurovascular pedicle. They replace fat and may spread along the neurovascular bundles or other natural areas of weakness.

Questions for Further Thought

1. How are benign hypopharyngeal lesions treated?
2. What are the expected imaging findings in benign lesions treated with radiation therapy?
3. What are the imaging features of neurogenic tumors of the hypopharynx that distinguish those from other benign tumors?

Reporting Responsibilities

Any time a tumor places the airway at risk due to obstruction, or if biopsy is planned and the lesion morphology suggests that there might be excessive bleeding, immediate direct communication with the referring treatment provider is necessary.

What the Treating Physician Needs to Know

- If not SCCa, what is the likely alternative diagnosis based on imaging?
- Exact extent of the mass within the hypopharyngeal and laryngeal soft tissues
- Evidence for involvement of the laryngeal framework and its precise extent
- Evidence for extrapharyngeal tumor extension and its extent when present
- If biopsy might be more hazardous than usual, such as increased risk for excessive bleeding from endoscopic biopsy
- If the airway is at risk

Answers

1. These lesions are generally treated surgically, sparing the larynx, by partial laryngeal resection and reconstruction or even total or near-total laryngectomy if much of the cricoid is involved. Others can be treated by radiotherapy or observation.
2. Benign lesions are treated with doses well under those used for malignancy and should not produce changes other than minimal edema that should completely resolve. Although some lesions may shrink, most stabilize in response to radiation therapy.
3. Neurogenic tumors usually present as submucosal masses with considerable enhancement, with or without cystic or necrotic zones. They can be indistinguishable from paragangliomas, leiomyomas, or a tumor of salivary origin.

> **LEARN MORE**
> See Chapters 218 and 29 in *Head and Neck Radiology* by Mancuso and Hanafee.

CLINICAL HISTORY *Patient 1 (Fig. 13.4A,B) and Patient 2 (Fig. 13.4C,D) are adult patients with a history of right-sided ear pain and odynophagia.*

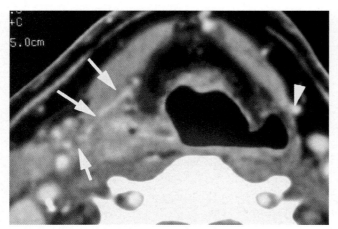

FIGURE 13.4A

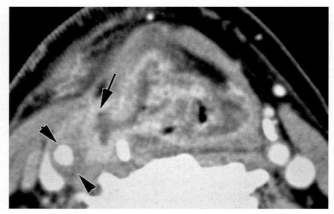

FIGURE 13.4C

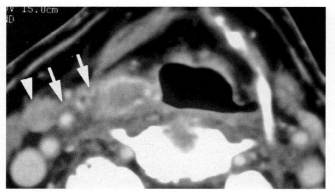

FIGURE 13.4B

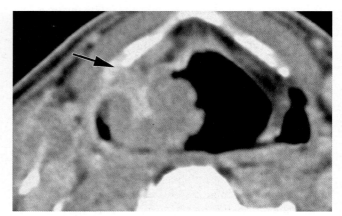

FIGURE 13.4D

FINDINGS

Figure 13.4A. Locally aggressive–appearing pyriform sinus carcinoma invades the right superior laryngeal neurovascular bundle (arrows) and spreads outside the larynx.

Figure 13.4B. The spread pattern along the superior neurovascular bundle can be seen again (arrows), and there is associated metastatic lymph node.

Figure 13.4C. Aggressive cancer can be seen growing through the thyrohyoid membrane along the superior laryngeal neurovascular bundle (arrows). The carotid artery is encased by this tumor growth (arrowheads).

Figure 13.4D. The tumor, which on its surface appears relatively lobulated and exophytic, shows evidence of probable early thyroid lamina invasion (arrow).

DIFFERENTIAL DIAGNOSIS Not applicable

DIAGNOSIS SCCa of the hypopharynx with spread beyond the larynx along the superior laryngeal neurovascular bundle

in both patients 1 and 2 and in Patient 2 also encasing the common carotid artery

DISCUSSION Hypopharyngeal cancer is about four times less common than laryngeal cancer and is also clearly linked to cigarette smoking. Greater than 95% of malignant hypopharyngeal tumors are SCCa. They usually present with sore throat and, in later stages, dysphagia, globus, otalgia, bloody saliva, aspiration, and voice changes. Localized pain or tenderness over the thyroid lamina suggests gross cartilaginous invasion.

Hypopharyngeal tumors may be infiltrative or exert mass effect with well-defined borders. There is no real anatomic barrier that restricts spread, with submucosal spread beyond the visible mucosal margins being a common finding. Infiltrating tumors replace the normal fat separating other anatomic structures, and may spread along neurovascular bundles or natural areas of weakness in the pharyngeal wall and laryngeal skeleton. They may also spread along the adjacent musculature, being distinguished by their increased vascularity and related increased enhancement and high signal on T2W images when compared to normal muscle.

SCCa of the posterior pharyngeal wall tends to include both mucosal and submucosal spreading lesions with extensive cephalic spread, but it tends to not extend caudally beyond the level of the arytenoids.

Pyriform sinus carcinomas are the most common hypopharyngeal carcinomas. They frequently produce significant submucosal spread. Spread into the larynx is common, but extension into the cervical esophagus constitutes an uncommon late event. Lateral wall pyriform sinus cancers show relatively early invasion of the posterior thyroid lamina and posterior superior margin of the cricoid cartilage. Invasion of the upper lobe of the thyroid gland follows the cartilaginous invasion or through the cricothyroid membrane.

Postcricoid carcinomas frequently spread to and beyond the esophageal wall.

Establishing the superior and inferior extent of all hypopharyngeal cancers is an essential factor in planning the treatment approach to these cancers. Imaging therefore serves as a vital adjunct to the physical examination for evaluating specific growth patterns of interest in medical decision making as well as for characterizing metastatic lymphadenopathy. CT is usually the initial examination to evaluate the primary site and regional disease as well as for detection of recurrent tumor. FDG-PET may used for staging and identifying recurrent disease after treatment. MR is reserved for the evaluation of the postcricoid portion, esophageal verge, and proximal cervical esophagus; the data help to plan the lower margin of resection and appropriate pharyngeal reconstruction.

In these cases, the spread along the superior laryngeal neurovascular bundle alters management. In Patient 1, the vessel was taken much nearer its external carotid origin than usual; in Patient 2, gross total resection was not possible, and therapy was switched to chemoradiation.

Questions for Further Thought

1. Name some potential routes of perineural spread or hypopharyngeal carcinomas.
2. Is nodal metastatic disease common with hypopharyngeal carcinomas, and what nodal groups are at risk?

Reporting Responsibilities

In general, hypopharyngeal carcinoma is known or suspected at the time of imaging, so no special communication is required. It is very important that the report contains a complete assessment of the disease extent and all information that is relevant to treatment planning. The nature of this information should be apparent from study of the prior sections on treatment options. This must include precise observations shown in the following section.

Some special circumstances arise that require immediate direct communication with the referring treatment provider. These include the following:

- Any time the tumor places the airway at risk
- A circumstance where it may be anticipated from imaging that a tracheostomy might cross tumor
- In a post radiation therapy patient where the larynx and hypopharynx have become necrotic and may collapse and the patient has not had a tracheostomy
- If a tumor is discovered that was not clinically suspected

What the Treating Physician Needs to Know

Primary site evaluation:

- Extent of invasion along mucosal structures within hypopharynx and adjacent oropharyngeal walls superiorly and inferiorly the trachea and esophagus. Of particular importance is spread to the postcricoid region and esophageal verge and cervical esophagus.
- Spread to deep tissues spaces within the larynx, including the pre-epiglottic and paraglottic spaces
- Spread to the laryngeal skeleton with possible cartilage invasion
- Extrapharyngeal spread to the deep neck, including prevertebral muscles (rare)

Perineurovascular spread:

- Involvement of the recurrent laryngeal or superior laryngeal neurovascular bundle
- Evaluation of regional lymph nodes, emphasizing levels 2 through 6 and the retropharyngeal nodes

Answers

1. Perineural spread can be along the superior laryngeal neurovascular bundle; recurrent laryngeal, glossopharyngeal, and vagus nerves; and the sympathetic chain.
2. The incidence of nodal metastatic disease associated with early-stage hypopharyngeal lesions is higher than that observed in other primary head and neck tumor sites. At presentation, 75% of patients have clinically positive nodes. Hypopharyngeal malignancies tend to metastasize to levels 2, 3, and 4 with a secondary risk to level 5. Retropharyngeal node involvement increases with extensive neck disease as well as lesions in the upper hypopharyngeal wall. Malignancies of the pyriform sinus apex and postcricoid region place level 6 nodes at a significant risk.

LEARN MORE

See Chapters 219 and 21 in *Head and Neck Radiology* by Mancuso and Hanafee.

CLINICAL HISTORY *A 27-year-old male patient with a history of blunt trauma to the neck while in a bar fight.*

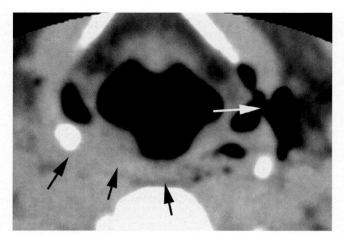

FIGURE **13.5A**

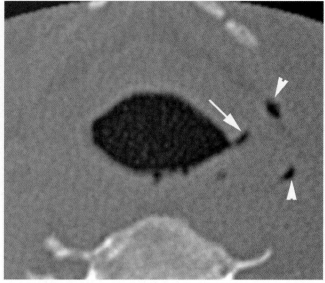

FIGURE **13.5C**

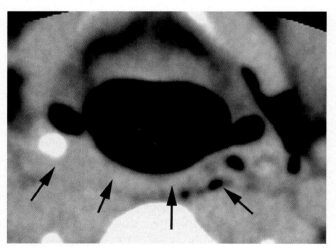

FIGURE **13.5B**

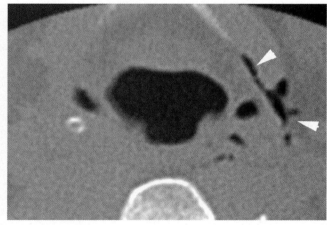

FIGURE **13.5D**

FINDINGS

Figure 13.5A,B. There is a tear in the lateral wall of the pyriform sinus (white arrow in Fig. 13.5A) and a tract of air extending into the neck. There is also soft tissue swelling of the contralateral posterior pharyngeal wall and retropharyngeal edema (black arrows).

Figure 13.5C,D. There is a small mucosal tear (white arrow in Fig. 13.5C) and multiple areas of air distributed peripherally along and outside the thyrohyoid membrane (arrowheads).

DIFFERENTIAL DIAGNOSIS Incidental laryngocele or pharyngocele

DIAGNOSIS Posttraumatic hypopharyngeal tear and false passage to the peripharyngeal soft tissue spaces

DISCUSSION Hypopharyngeal and cervical esophageal injuries most often accompany injuries to the larynx and trachea. These can be accidental or iatrogenic in nature.

Blunt trauma is most commonly due to a force applied from anterior to posterior with compression of the visceral neck between the source of force and the cervical spine, although other factors may influence this pattern of injury. Penetrating injuries are most frequently related to stab or gunshot wounds. Iatrogenic injuries are most commonly due to intubation injuries.

Acute injuries result in blood and edema spreading through the adjacent deep planes, causing edema, and obliteration of the fat planes within the peripharyngeal tissue spaces, resulting in various degrees of mass effect. Mucosal lesions cause additional air leakage and neck emphysema as well as formation of false passages. Penetrating injuries may leave tracts of gas, blood, edema, and foreign bodies along their pathway.

Subacute injuries (10 to 30 days post trauma) may be associated with infection. Granulation tissue in this phase may look the same as hemorrhage and edema in the acute phase; over time, it will organize and contract, resulting in soft tissue webs, adhesions, and stenosis. Contrast-enhanced studies show more enhancement in granulation tissue than muscle.

Chronic injuries may be classified as mucosal or submucosal, deep space and framework distortion, and mixed. Untreated false passages or false diverticuli can become a source of chronic/recurrent infections and fistulous formations. The spaces surrounding the injured regions may become infiltrated by granulation tissue that heals with varying amounts of scarring and retraction.

Failure to acutely establish the extent of hypopharyngeal and laryngeal injuries can lead to swallowing disorders and laryngeal stenosis that can insidiously complicate, becoming more difficult to manage with a less satisfactory outcome.

Questions for Further Thought

1. In what situations are hypopharyngeal and laryngeal injuries most commonly missed?
2. How are hypopharyngeal/laryngeal injuries evaluated for management?
3. What is the possible spectrum of CT findings seen in hypopharyngeal injuries?

Reporting Responsibilities

Direct communication with the referring physician is mandatory if any there is any evidence of severe airway compromise, false passage, or complicating infection or the associated laryngeal injury was not expected.

What the Treating Physician Needs to Know

- Status of the airway
- Any evidence of a foreign body, false passage, or fistula
- Any associated injuries or complications
- Status of all parts of the laryngeal skeleton

Answers

1. Hypopharyngeal or laryngeal injuries are often seen in patients treated for other life-threatening injuries who were intubated and the neck not evaluated with CT at the time of initial imaging evaluation.

2. CT and endoscopy will normally provide all information necessary for management. Water-soluble contrast swallow studies are reserved for identification of an otherwise undetectable false passage.

3. Soft tissue findings on noncontrast CT include edema, blood, extraluminal gas, false passages, fistula formation, mucosal lacerations, injuries to the laryngeal skeleton, avulsed soft tissue structures, and radiodense or radiolucent foreign bodies. Contrast-enhanced CT can additionally demonstrate diffuse or focal mucosal/muscular enhancement that may be reactive or due to a phlegmon, reactive enhancement of the walls of false passages, abscess, or evidence of vascular injuries.

> **LEARN MORE**
> See Chapter 220 in *Head and Neck Radiology* by Mancuso and Hanafee.

CHAPTER 14

Cervical Esophagus

CLINICAL HISTORY *A neonate who had abnormal feeding and an inflamed neck mass.*

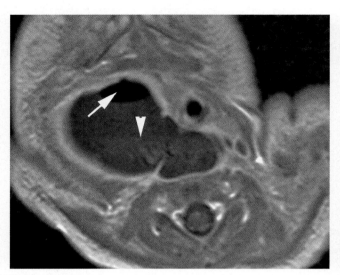

FIGURE **14.1A**

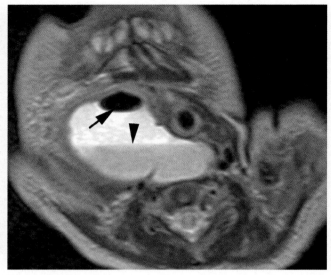

FIGURE **14.1C**

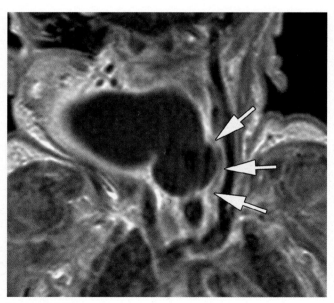

FIGURE **14.1B**

FINDINGS Cystic mass with an enhancing wall seen on contrast-enhanced T1W images (axial in Fig. 14.1A; coronal in Fig. 14.1B) and a T2W axial image (Fig. 14.1C). The mass also had fluid–fluid levels (arrowheads) and gas (arrows).

DIFFERENTIAL DIAGNOSIS Branchial apparatus cyst, bronchogenic cyst, esophageal diverticulum

DIAGNOSIS Infected esophageal duplication cyst

DISCUSSION Some developmental conditions present as masses or because they interfere with function. In the region of the cervical esophagus, an esophageal duplication cyst or other developmental cysts may produce dysphagia or odynophagia, with the latter two symptoms manifesting as poor feeding in an infant, as in this patient, or symptoms of associated anomalies. Such cysts, when they present as a mass, are typically not painful unless there is some complicating factor. Such complicating factors include infection in an esophageal or foregut duplication cyst that connects to the cervical esophagus, as seen in this case, or bleeding, thrombosis, or infection of a vascular malformation. Developmental abnormalities may also be discovered incidentally on imaging studies done for other purposes.

Question for Further Thought

1. What is the anatomic basis for developmental pharyngeal diverticuli that arise at the hypopharyngeal–esophageal junction?

Reporting Responsibilities

In general, dermoid, epidermoid, teratoma, hamartoma, and duplication and branchial apparatus origin cysts are usually in the differential diagnosis at the time of imaging, so no special communication is required.

Any time one of these anomalies places the airway at risk due to obstruction, communication with the referring treatment provider is necessary. If a tumor rather than congenital cyst or complicating acute or subacute infection is suspected, direct communication is wise. Direct communication might also be wise if there is a tracheoesophageal fistula or if the cyst is likely infected since either or both circumstances threaten possibly catastrophic episodes of aspiration. In this case, both the airway risk and likely infection prompted such communication.

It is very important that the report contains a complete assessment of the nature and extent of the mass, including all information that is relevant to surgical planning. This should also include precise comments regarding the factors outlined in the following section.

What the Treating Physician Needs to Know

- Precise diagnosis and the degree of confidence in that diagnosis
- Extent of the developmental anomaly
- Any complicating features of the anomaly that might alter medical decision making
- Is the airway at significant risk?
- Whether there are associated or other anomalies
- Whether there is a reasonable likelihood of this being syndromic
- Is there any need for further imaging to answer any of these issues?

Answer

1. The acquired cervical esophageal-pharyngeal diverticuli have some basis in development, or at least some predisposition with regard to their point of origin, based on the anatomy of the pharyngeal muscular wall as it develops in an individual. The more common diverticuli occur at the Killian dehiscence of the lower inferior constrictor (cricopharyngeus) muscle in the midline and between the inferior margin of the inferior constrictor and the lateral muscular wall of the esophagus.

> **LEARN MORE**
> See Chapters 222, 10, and 13 in *Head and Neck Radiology* by Mancuso and Hanafee.

CLINICAL HISTORY *A 54-year-old male patient presenting with dysphagia and hoarseness.*

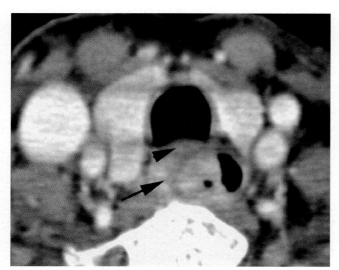

FIGURE **14.2A**

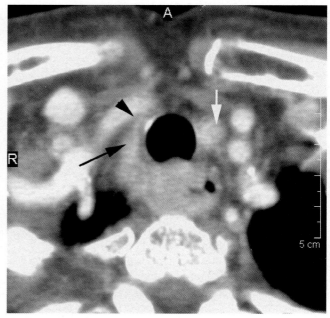

FIGURE **14.2C**

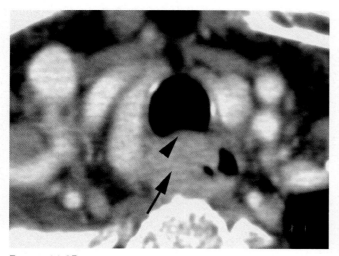

FIGURE **14.2B**

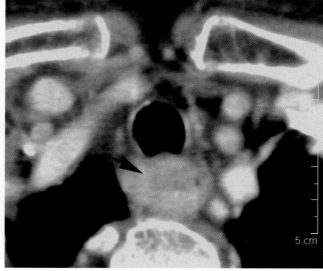

FIGURE **14.2D**

FINDINGS

Figure 14.2A. A mass invades outside the muscular wall of the esophagus (arrow) and likely invades the common membranous wall between the trachea and esophagus (arrowhead).

Figure 14.2B. An entirely submucosal mass invades outside the muscular wall of the esophagus (arrow) and likely the common membranous wall between the trachea and esophagus (arrowhead).

Figure 14.2C. The mass invades along the lateral wall of the trachea (black arrow), coming very near to the brachio-cephalic artery (arrowhead). There is a metastatic left level 6 lymph node (white arrow).

Figure 14.2D. The mass spreads inferiorly both within and outside the muscular wall of the esophagus.

DIFFERENTIAL DIAGNOSIS Malignant tumor of the cervical esophagus

DIAGNOSIS Entirely submucosal squamous cell carcinoma of the cervical esophagus

DISCUSSION Cancer of the cervical esophagus is relatively uncommon, and it is far more likely for this esophageal segment to be secondarily involved by a cancer in the thyroid or hypopharynx. It tends to present in the older age group, with a peak incidence in people in their fifties and sixties. Squamous cell carcinoma is the most common type, with the risk increased in smokers, alcohol use, or a previous head and neck cancer. Other primary malignancies and benign tumors of the cervical esophagus are rare without a consistent etiology.

The most common presentation is dysphagia and/or odynophagia and weight loss. Hoarseness can be secondary to direct extension to the larynx or invasion of the recurrent laryngeal nerve.

Squamous cell carcinoma of the esophagus arises from the surface epithelium and is normally a mucosally spreading disease; however, submucosal spread within its muscular wall and mucosal skip areas are frequent. There are no true anatomic barriers that limit the spread of malignancy beyond the esophageal wall and into the adjacent structures. Lymph node metastasis rates are proportional to the length of the primary lesion. The most common groups involved include levels 2 through 6 as well as the supraclavicular and upper mediastinal nodes.

Infiltrating tumors enhance more than muscle, replace the adjacent fat, and may spread along neurovascular bundles or through the membranous wall of the trachea.

Recurrence of tumor after definitive reconstruction is uncommon in cervical esophageal cancer and most frequently occurs in the primary site and/or regional lymph nodes.

Questions for Further Thought

1. What is involved in a curative surgical procedure for cervical esophageal carcinoma?
2. Why is curative surgery for cervical esophageal cancer such an extensive procedure?
3. When is cervical esophageal carcinoma considered incurable?

Reporting Responsibilities

Direct communication with the referring physician is mandatory if the tumor places the airway at risk for compression or due to a secondary tracheoesophageal fistula, when there might be a superimposed infection, when a tracheostomy might cross tumor, or if a tumor is discovered that was not clinically suspected.

What the Treating Physician Needs to Know

- Nature and full extent of any mass of uncertain etiology that affects the cervical esophagus
- If a lesion cannot be seen at endoscopy, it can be safely and usually successfully biopsied percutaneously under imaging guidance.
- In known primary tumors, the full extent of the cancer, especially within the muscular wall of the esophagus and spread outside the confines of its muscular wall to surrounding adjacent structures
- In known primary cancers, the extent of regional lymphadenopathy
- Imaging can be used for surveillance, but recurrent tumor is very difficult to cure; thus, surveillance for second primaries may have more benefit than detecting a recurrence.

Answers

1. Curative surgery includes a cervical/total esophagectomy, possibly with laryngopharyngectomy, ipsilateral thyroidectomy (total if the thyroid gland is invaded), or unilateral/bilateral neck dissection with or without resection of the anterior superior mediastinal nodes. Reconstruction includes a variety of flaps and grafts with gastric transposition and tubed vascularized soft tissue grafts being most commonly done.
2. The rationale for an extensive surgical procedure is that cancer of the esophagus has a propensity for lymph node metastasis and submucosal skip lesions regardless of the imaging findings.
3. Involvement of the brachiocephalic vessels, spine, or trachea usually makes the tumor unresectable for cure and generally unlikely to be cured at all.

> LEARN MORE
>
> See Chapters 223, 21, and 23 in *Head and Neck Radiology* by Mancuso and Hanafee.